Regist
Acce

SPRINGER PUBLISHING COMPANY
CONNECT™

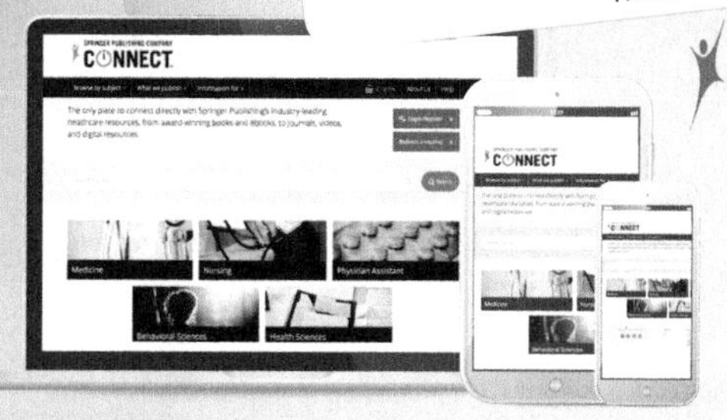

Your print purchase of *Complications of Acute Stroke* **includes online access to the contents of your book—** increasing accessibility, portability, and searchability!

Access today at:

http://connect.springerpub.com/content/book/978-0-8261-2479-1 or scan the QR code at the right with your smartphone and enter the access code below.

Y3CUM2G0

Scan here for quick access.

If you are experiencing problems accessing the digital component of this product, please contact our customer service department at cs@springerpub.com

The online access with your print purchase is available at the publisher's discretion and may be removed at any time without notice.

Publisher's Note: New and used products purchased from third-party sellers are not guaranteed for quality, authenticity, or access to any included digital components.

Complications of Acute Stroke

A Concise Guide to Prevention, Recognition, and Management

Editors

Réza Behrouz, DO
Associate Professor
Division of Cerebrovascular Diseases
Department of Neurology
School of Medicine
University of Texas Health Science Center San Antonio
San Antonio, Texas

Lee A. Birnbaum, MD
Associate Professor
Division of Cerebrovascular Diseases
Department of Neurology
Division of Endovascular Neurosurgery
Department of Neurological Surgery
Department of Radiology
School of Medicine
University of Texas Health Science Center San Antonio
San Antonio, Texas

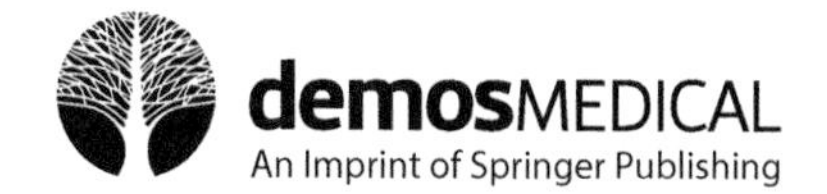

Visit www.springerpub.com and http://connect.springerpub.com

ISBN: 9780826123541
ebook ISBN: 9780826124791
DOI: 10.1891/9780826124791

Acquisitions Editor: Beth Barry
Compositor: Exeter Premedia Services Private Ltd.

Demos Medical Publishing is an imprint of Springer Publishing Company, LLC.

Medicine is an ever-changing science. Research and clinical experience are continually expanding our knowledge, in particular our understanding of proper treatment and drug therapy. The authors, editors, and publisher have made every effort to ensure that all information in this book is in accordance with the state of knowledge at the time of production of the book. Nevertheless, the authors, editors, and publisher are not responsible for errors or omissions or for any consequences from application of the information in this book and make no warranty, expressed or implied, with respect to the contents of the publication. Every reader should examine carefully the package inserts accompanying each drug and should carefully check whether the dosage schedules mentioned therein or the contraindications stated by the manufacturer differ from the statements made in this book. Such examination is particularly important with drugs that are either rarely used or have been newly released on the market.

Library of Congress Cataloging-in-Publication Data

Names: Behrouz, Réza, editor. | Birnbaum, Lee A., editor.
Title: Complications of acute stroke : a concise guide to prevention, recognition, and management / editors, Réza Behrouz, Lee A. Birnbaum.
Description: New York : Springer Publishing Company, [2019] | Includes bibliographical references.
Identifiers: LCCN 2018048991| ISBN 9780826123541 | ISBN 9780826124791 (ebook)
Subjects: | MESH: Stroke--complications | Stroke--therapy
Classification: LCC RC388.5 | NLM WL 356 | DDC 616.8/1--dc23
LC record available at https://lccn.loc.gov/2018048991

Réza Behrouz: https://orcid.org/0000-0002-3684-434X

Publisher's Note: **New and used products purchased from third-party sellers are not guaranteed for quality, authenticity, or access to any included digital components.**

Printed in the United States of America.
19 20 21 22 23 / 5 4 3 2 1

To my wife for her unconditional love, to my mother for giving me life, and to my father for showing me the light.

—Réza Behrouz

To my family for their limitless love and to my mentors for their tough love.

—Lee A. Birnbaum

Contents

Contributors

Kanita Beba Abadal, MD, Clinical Fellow in Vascular Neurology, Department of Neurology, Beth Israel Deaconess Medical Center, Harvard Medical School, Boston, Massachusetts

Mohammed H. Aref, MD, FRCSC, Clinical Fellow in Skull Base Surgery, Department of Neurological Surgery, University of Colorado School of Medicine, Aurora, Colorado

Niraj A. Arora, MD, Clinical Fellow in Neurocritical Care, Department of Neurology, University of Miami Miller School of Medicine, Miami, Florida

Réza Behrouz, DO, Associate Professor, Division of Cerebrovascular Diseases, Department of Neurology, School of Medicine, University of Texas Health Science Center San Antonio, San Antonio, Texas

Lee A. Birnbaum, MD, Associate Professor, Division of Cerebrovascular Diseases, Department of Neurology, Division of Endovascular Neurosurgery, Department of Neurological Surgery, Department of Radiology, School of Medicine, University of Texas Health Science Center San Antonio, San Antonio, Texas

Katharina M. Busl, MD, MS, Associate Professor, Division of Neurocritical Care, Department of Neurology, University of Florida College of Medicine, Gainesville, Florida

Bilal Butt, MD, Assistant Professor, Department of Neurology, Southern Illinois University, Springfield, Illinois

Pablo Coss, MD, Resident in Neurology, Department of Neurology, School of Medicine, University of Texas Health Science Center San Antonio, San Antonio, Texas

Dar Dowlatshahi, MD, PhD, Associate Professor, Division of Neurology, Department of Medicine, University of Ottawa Faculty of Medicine, Ottawa, Ontario, Canada

Lucas Elijovich, MD, Associate Professor, Departments of Neurology and Neurological Surgery, Director, Neurocritical Care, Director, Vascular Anomalies Clinic, Lebonheur Children's Hospital, University of Tennessee Health Sciences Center, Semmes-Murphey Neurologic and Spine Institute, Memphis, Tennessee

Johanna T. Fifi, MD, Associate Professor, Departments of Neurology, Neurological Surgery, and Radiology, Director of Endovascular Ischemic Stroke; Associate Director, Cerebrovascular Center, Icahn School of Medicine at Mount Sinai, New York, New York

Daniel Agustín Godoy, MD, Medical Director, Neurointensive Care Unit, Sanatorio Pasteur; Assistant Professor, Critical Care, Intensive Care Unit, Hospital San Juan Bautista, Catamarca, Argentina

Joshua N. Goldstein, MD, PhD, Associate Professor, Department of Emergency Medicine, Harvard Medical School, Boston, Massachusetts

Juan Jose Goyanes, MD, Staff Physician, Department of Neurology, University of Tennessee Health Sciences Center, Memphis, Tennessee

Shaheryar Hafeez, MD, Assistant Professor, Division of Neurocritical Care, Department of Neurological Surgery, School of Medicine, University of Texas Health Science Center San Antonio, San Antonio, Texas

Christeena Kurian, MD, Clinical Fellow in Vascular Neurology, Department of Neurology, Icahn School of Medicine at Mount Sinai, New York, New York

Christos Lazaridis, MD, EDIC, Associate Professor, Departments of Neurology and Neurological Surgery, Pritzker School of Medicine, University of Chicago, Chicago, Illinois

Jessica D. Lee, MD, Associate Professor, Department of Neurology, University of Kentucky College of Medicine, Lexington, Kentucky

Stefania Maraka, MD, Assistant Professor, Department of Neurology, University of Illinois at Chicago, Chicago, Illinois

Justin Mascitelli, MD, Assistant Professor, Department of Neurological Surgery, School of Medicine, University of Texas Health Science Center San Antonio, San Antonio, Texas

Cameron McDougall, MD, Assistant Professor, Department of Neurological Surgery, School of Medicine, University of Texas Health Science Center San Antonio, San Antonio, Texas

Kristine H. O'Phelan, MD, Associate Professor, Division of Neurocritical Care, Department of Neurology, University of Miami Miller School of Medicine, Miami, Florida

Alejandro A. Rabinstein, MD, Professor, Division of Neurocritical Care, Department of Neurology, Mayo Clinic College of Medicine, Rochester, Minnesota

Eugene L. Scharf, MD, Assistant Professor, Department of Neurology, Mayo Clinic College of Medicine, Rochester, Minnesota

Ali Seifi, MD, Associate Professor, Division of Neurocritical Care, Department of Neurological Surgery, School of Medicine, University of Texas Health Science Center San Antonio, San Antonio, Texas

Hazem Shoirah, MD, Assistant Professor, Departments of Neurology and Neurological Surgery, Icahn School of Medicine at Mount Sinai, New York, New York

Brian Silver, MD, Professor and Interim Chair, Department of Neurology, UMass Memorial Medical Center/University of Massachusetts Medical School, Worcester, Massachusetts

Laura Stein, MD, Assistant Professor, Department of Neurology, Icahn School of Medicine at Mount Sinai, New York, New York

Vignan Yogendrakumar, MD, Resident in Neurology, Division of Neurology, Department of Medicine, University of Ottawa Faculty of Medicine, Ottawa, Ontario, Canada

A. Samy Youssef, MD, PhD, Professor, Department of Neurological Surgery, University of Colorado School of Medicine, Aurora, Colorado

Preface

The practice of stroke medicine has become quite complex over the past two decades. Fortunately, this is for good reasons. The intricacies associated with management of ischemic and hemorrhagic strokes reflect improved understanding of the disease process, advances in neuroimaging, and development of novel treatment options. Appropriate management of acute stroke is multifaceted and does not end with emergent therapy. In the first 24 to 72 hours of hospitalization, stroke patients are susceptible to a whole host of cerebral (neurological) and extracerebral (medical) complications. Being familiar with these complications and having the knowledge to properly identify and manage them can reduce length of hospital stay, adverse functional outcomes, and mortality.

Our goals with this book, *Complications of Acute Stroke: A Concise Guide to Prevention, Recognition, and Management,* are manifold. First, we hope that practitioners will appreciate acute stroke management as a dynamic process and understand the uniqueness of acute stroke as a clinical entity with its potential for complications that may be a direct or indirect consequence of the initial brain injury. Second, by developing an understanding of how and why complications occur in the first place, practitioners will not only recognize but also effectively manage complications and minimize any negative impact. Lastly, an understanding of potential complications enables prevention strategies that reduce the odds or severity of future events.

Based on these goals, we have divided each chapter (except one) into distinct subheadings of prevention, recognition, and management. In addition, each chapter will begin with a brief discussion on the pathophysiology of the condition or topic. Each chapter will touch upon specific complications that may occur in stroke patients during the acute phase. The chapters on extracerebral complications are loosely based on organ systems.

This book is meant to educate and assist any healthcare professional who has the privilege of caring for patients with acute stroke. Although it is particularly helpful for clinicians who are involved with critical decision making, such as those working in the intensive care units, practitioners at all levels of training can use this book as a guide. We hope our work is of benefit to you and gives you additional tools and knowledge necessary to provide the optimal care for patients with acute stroke.

Réza Behrouz, DO
Lee A. Birnbaum, MD

1 Complications of Acute Stroke: An Introduction

Réza Behrouz and Lee A. Birnbaum

KEY POINTS

- One-half of all in-hospital deaths after stroke are attributed to serious complications.
- Complications can:
  - Occur in nearly 50% of patients with acute stroke
  - Have a high impact on short-term and long-term functional outcomes
  - Be cerebral (neurological) or extracerebral (medical)
- Medical complications can result from exacerbation of preexisting conditions, or de novo adverse events.
- Stroke patients should be cared for in settings wherein:
  - Standardized prevention strategies can be implemented
  - Close surveillance allows timely identification of complications
  - Complications can be managed effectively

INTRODUCTION

Any pathological process can have complications, from common cold to cancer. As with any acute illness, patients with acute stroke are at high risk of complications. Every year, 15 million people worldwide suffer a stroke, resulting in 6 million deaths and 5 million left with permanent disability (1). An individual who suffers a stroke is susceptible to a wide range of complications, particularly in the acute phase. These complications often impede neurological recovery and can profoundly impact functional outcomes, in addition to prolonging length of hospital stay and delaying successful rehabilitation (1–3). Occurrence of early complications influences patient outcome not only in the acute phase after stroke, but also in the 3 months after the event (4). Furthermore, up to one-half of all in-hospital deaths after stroke are attributed to serious

© Springer Publishing Company DOI: 10.1891/9780826124791.0001

complications (5,6). Patients with advanced age, high prevalence of comorbidities, previous disability, and more severe stroke tend to have the highest risk for complications (7). In ischemic stroke patients, an increased baseline National Institutes of Health Stroke Scale score is associated with an increased risk of medical and neurological complications (8).

Due to heterogeneity in definition, the precise rate of complications in acute stroke is difficult to decipher. Studies using variable methodologies have reported a range of 13.9% to as high as 95% (9,10). By and large, studies of high quality on complications after stroke are challenging and require a systematic approach, prospective design, close observation, honest reporting, and completeness of recording (11). Accurate delineation of clinically meaningful complication rate also depends upon when the study was conducted. With enhanced knowledge of pathophysiology, improvements in pharmacology and surgical techniques, and advancement of technology, the rate of serious complications has declined over the years (12).

Many of these complications cannot be predicted and by the time they are identified, the patient has already sustained irreparable injury. Still, prevention, identification, and management of acute stroke complications are considered to be essential aspects of modern stroke care, and perhaps just as important as acute reperfusion or resuscitative therapy in improving short-term and long-term prognoses after stroke.

PATHOPHYSIOLOGY

Complications in the setting of acute stroke can be grouped into two broad categories: *cerebral* and *extracerebral*; or neurological and medical, respectively. Both types can place the patient at risk for death and influence functional outcomes after stroke. Cerebral complications are those that are directly related to the initial insult to the brain. They result from continuation or progression of the primary injury, or secondary injurious biochemical processes in the brain that ensue. Some examples of cerebral complications are expansion of brain infarction or intracerebral hemorrhage, cerebral edema, increased intracranial pressure, and cerebral vasospasm after subarachnoid hemorrhage. Iatrogenic complications directly involving the brain also fit into this category.

Extracerebral complications can arise from exacerbation of preexisting disorders or incipient pathological events. This broad category encompasses a whole host of complications including infections, metabolic derangements, and morbidities related to systemic dysfunction or failure. In the acutely ill patient such as one with stroke, virtually every organ system is susceptible to complications, from cardiovascular to integumentary. Table 1.1 provides a list of the most common and important complications in the acute stroke patient. Accounting for all potential medical complications after acute stroke is beyond the scope of this chapter. However, the most common extracerebral complications after acute stroke are fever, chest infections, urinary tract infections, venous thromboembolism, and myocardial infarction (12). Stroke mortality is significantly influenced by in-hospital medical complications all the way into the chronic stage (13). Some preexisting conditions, such as hypertension and diabetes mellitus, are risk factors for medical complications after stroke (14).

Table 1.1 Most Common Complications in Acute Stroke, Categorized According to Organ System

CEREBRAL (NEUROLOGICAL)	
	Central nervous system infection due to instrumentation
	Cerebral edema
	Cerebral procedural complications
	Cerebral vasospasm after subarachnoid hemorrhage
	Delirium and encephalopathy
	Expansion of cerebral infarction
	Expansion of intracerebral hemorrhage
	Hemorrhagic transformation of cerebral infarction
	Increased intracranial pressure
	Seizures
EXTRACEREBRAL (MEDICAL)	
Cardiac	Cardiac arrest
	Cardiac arrhythmia
	Congestive heart failure
	Myocardial ischemia/infarction
	Neurogenic stunned myocardial syndrome
Pulmonary	Aspiration
	Exacerbation of obstructive lung disease
	Mucous plugging of bronchi and bronchioles

(*continued*)

Table 1.1 Most Common Complications in Acute Stroke, Categorized According to Organ System (*continued*)

EXTRACEREBRAL (MEDICAL)	
	Pulmonary edema (neurogenic and non-neurogenic)
	Pulmonary embolism
	Respiratory failure
Infectious	Chest and bronchial infections
	Fever
	Urinary tract infections
Metabolic	Acid–base derangements
	Accumulation of intrinsic toxins (e.g., ammonia, lactate)
	Drug toxicity
	Electrolyte abnormalities
	Kidney failure
Hematological	Deep vein thrombosis
Gastrointestinal	Constipation, pseudo-obstruction, and ileus
	Gastrointestinal hemorrhage

Cerebral complications tend to occur earlier than the ones that are extracerebral (medical) (15). However, cerebral and extracerebral complications may occur in a continuum and mutually influence one another, regardless of timing. These complications can influence future risk of stroke as well. A study of 7,593 stroke patients in China showed that in-hospital medical complications were independent risk factors for stroke recurrence in patients with initial ischemic stroke at 3 months (9). It is conceivable that physical or mental deterioration in acute stroke arises from an interplay of cerebral factors, new extracerebral derangements, and exacerbation of preexisting cerebral or extracerebral diseases (Figure 1.1).

PREVENTION

Complications not only measure the success and quality of care, but also underscore the necessity for proper surveillance and preventive therapy. The setting wherein the stroke patient is cared for is particularly important. Patients who are managed in an organized inpatient stroke unit are more likely to survive, return home, and regain independence than those managed in conventional

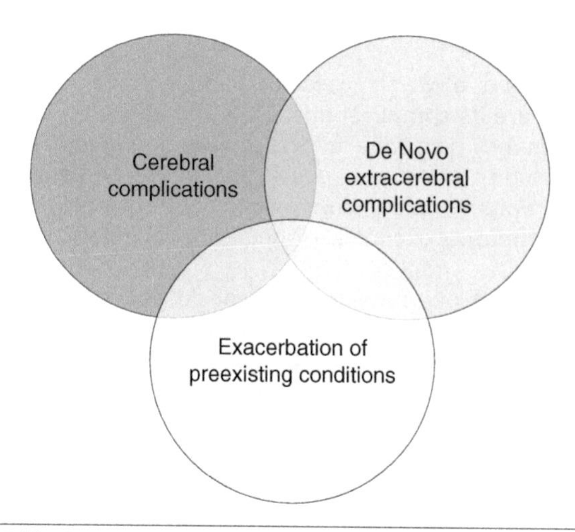

Figure 1.1 The interplay of complicating factors that ultimately lead to death or poor functional outcome after stroke.

care settings (16). Specialized stroke care units reduce the risk of death after stroke primarily through prevention and treatment of complications (17). These units are often equipped with proper surveillance apparatus and staffed by a cadre of specialized nurses who follow standardized guidelines and protocols for prevention of complications and subsequently, result in improved outcomes. Multidisciplinary teams conduct frequent, meticulous inspections to address pitfalls that predict or lead to complications. Examples are implementation of deep vein thrombosis prophylaxis, aspiration precautions, close neurological monitoring, optimizing hemodynamics, glycemic control, and early mobilization. That said, every effort should be made to move the patient from the emergency department to the stroke unit as soon as possible. Delays in transferring from the emergency department may lead to an increase in complications (18).

In essence, best efforts should be made to ensure that in spite of acute stroke, homeostasis is maintained, thereby averting the risk of common complications. As previously mentioned, several factors that have been shown to increase the risk of complications include advanced age, comorbidities, previous disability, and stroke severity on presentation (7). Special attention to those who have one or more of these characteristics is an important aspect of preventive strategy.

IDENTIFICATION

Prevention is not always successful. Just as stroke itself is unpredictable, so are its complications. Early identification of complications—when they do occur—allows strategizing to manage them in a timely fashion and before irreversible damage is sustained. Acute stroke care units are particularly proficient in recognizing and acting upon symptoms of clinical or neurological deterioration due to complications.

In an acute stroke patient, physical deterioration is probably the most early and sensitive sign of disarray. The hallmark of cerebral complications is neurological worsening, which can manifest as decline in the level of consciousness, increase in severity of neurological deficit, or seizures. Close neurological monitoring is central to timely identification of complications. The National Institutes of Health Stroke Scale was designed to be a standardized and repeatable assessment of stroke patients and can be used by all medical specialties and paramedical personnel. It allows quantification of neurological deficit and interval comparison. Full-scale or the modified National Institutes of Health Stroke Scale, or other standardized neuromonitoring exams should be done frequently to capture signs of neurological deterioration as early as possible.

Extracerebral complications may manifest in relatively more subtle signs and symptoms with physical deterioration lagging behind the actual onset of complication. Constitutional signs and symptoms such as fever, tachycardia, and laboratory abnormalities, such as leukocytosis may represent early evidence for a life-threatening complication. Although worsening of neurological deficit can occur in stroke patients with medical complications, identification of subtle clinical signs may be difficult in stroke patients with severe disability.

MANAGEMENT

Even with best prevention strategies, early recognition, and management, patients with stroke inherently remain at high risk of complications. Management of acute stroke complications depends upon the type and the number of coexisting complications. Complication severity and timing are also important, although even minor complications can worsen and transform into severe conditions. Intervention must be tailored to the system or systems involved, with priority being protection of the brain from further injury. Management strategies specific to organ systems are discussed in subsequent chapters.

CONCLUSION

In acute stoke, a variety of complications may result from not only the brain injury itself but also from the unique aspect of immobility. This combination of major organ injury and immobility makes acute stroke patients especially susceptible to complications. Unfortunately, data to guide the management of stroke-related complications is limited. We hope that this book will help the reader prevent, identify, and manage complications in acute stroke.

REFERENCES

1. The global burden of stroke. Word Heart Federation. http://www.world-heart-federation.org/cardiovascular-health/stroke
2. Wang PL, Zhao XQ, Du WL, et al. In-hospital medical complications associated with patient dependency after acute ischemic stroke: data from the China National Stroke Registry. *Chin Med J.* 2013;126:1236–1241.
3. Koennecke HC, Belz W, Berfelde D, et al. Berlin Stroke Register Investigators. Factors influencing in-hospital mortality and morbidity in patients treated on a stroke unit. *Neurology.* 2011;77:965–972. doi:10.1212/WNL.0b013e31822dc795
4. Grube MM, Koennecke HC, Walter G, et al. Berlin Stroke Register (BSR). Influence of acute complications on outcome 3 months after ischemic stroke. *PLoS One.* 2013;8:e75719. doi:10.1371/journal.pone.0075719
5. Heuschmann PU, Kolominsky-Rabas PL, Misselwitz B, et al. Predictors of in-hospital mortality and attributable risks of death after ischemic stroke: the German Stroke Registers Study Group. *Arch Intern Med.* 2004;164:1761–1768. doi:10.1001/archinte.164.16.1761
6. Silver FL, Norris JW, Lewis AJ, et al.. Early mortality following stroke: a prospective review. *Stroke.* 1984;15:492–496. doi:10.1161/01.STR.15.3.492
7. Davenport RJ, Dennis MS, Wellwood I, et al. Complications after acute stroke. *Stroke.* 1996;27:415–420. doi:10.1161/01.STR.27.3.415
8. Boone M, Chillon JM, Garcia PY, et al. NIHSS and acute complications after anterior and posterior circulation strokes. *Ther Clin Risk Manag.* 2012;8:87–93.
9. Wang P, Wang Y, Zhao X, et al. In-hospital medical complications associated with stroke recurrence after initial ischemic stroke: a prospective cohort study from the China National Stroke Registry. *Medicine (Baltimore).* 2016;95:e4929. doi:10.1097/MD.0000000000004929
10. Johnston KC, Li JY, Lyden PD, et al. Medical and neurological complications of ischemic stroke: experience from the RANTTAS trial. RANTTAS Investigators. *Stroke.* 1998;29:447–453. doi:10.1161/01.STR.29.2.447
11. Indredavik B, Rohweder G, Naalsund E, et al. Medical complications in a comprehensive stroke unit and an early supported discharge service. *Stroke.* 2008;39:414–420. doi:10.1161/STROKEAHA.107.489294

12. Bovim MR, Askim T, Lydersen S, et al. Complications in the first week after stroke: a 10-year comparison. *BMC Neurol.* 2016;16:133. doi:10.1186/s12883-016-0654-8
13. Bae HJ, Yoon DS, Lee J, et al. In-hospital medical complications and long-term mortality after ischemic stroke. *Stroke.* 2005;36:2441–2445. doi:10.1161/01.STR.0000185721.73445.fd
14. Sidhartha JM, Purma AR, Reddy LVPK, et al. Risk factors for medical complications of acute hemorrhagic stroke. *J Acute Dis.* 2015;4:222–225. doi:10.1016/j.joad.2015.07.002
15. Balami JS, Chen RL, Grunwald IQ, et al. Neurological complications of acute ischaemic stroke. *Lancet Neurol.* 2011;10:357–371. doi:10.1016/S1474-4422(10)70313-6
16. Stroke Unit Trialists' Collaboration. Collaborative systematic review of the randomised trials of organised inpatient (stroke unit) care after stroke. *BMJ.* 1997;314:1151–1159. doi:10.1136/bmj.314.7088.1151
17. Govan L, Langhorne P, Weir CJ; Stroke Unit Trialists Collaboration. Does the prevention of complications explain the survival benefit of organized inpatient (stroke unit) care?: further analysis of a systematic review. *Stroke.* 2007;38:2536–2540. doi:10.1161/STROKEAHA.106.478842
18. Akhtar N, Kamran S, Singh R, et al. Prolonged stay of stroke patients in the emergency department may lead to an increased risk of complications, poor recovery, and increased mortality. *J Stroke Cerebrovasc Dis.* 2016;25:672–678. doi:10.1016/j.jstrokecerebrovasdis.2015.10.018

2 Worsening of Cerebral Ischemic Infarction

Hazem Shoirah, Christeena Kurian, Laura Stein, and Johanna T. Fifi

KEY POINTS

- Worsening of cerebral ischemic infarction occurs in up to 25% of stroke patients.
- Mechanism of worsening varies based on the underlying stroke etiology.
- Common mechanisms include recurrent embolization, flow failure, progression of edema, and derangement of metabolic parameters.
- Early recognition, revascularization, secondary prevention, and adequate supportive measures can improve the outcomes of patients at risk of ischemic worsening.

INTRODUCTION

The brain utilizes a constant supply of blood to maintain oxygenation and glucose metabolism, such that approximately 15% to 20% of cardiac output is directed to the brain (1). Compromise in cerebral blood flow, regardless of the cause, potentially places the brain at risk for infarction, and the brain has autoregulatory mechanisms to attempt to preserve blood flow. Worsening of acute cerebral infarction depends on the success of acute therapy, adequacy of compensatory efforts to maintain blood flow, and ability to address the underlying mechanism of infarct with successful secondary prevention. Underlying stroke mechanisms significantly impact the likelihood of neurologic worsening. Among patients with ischemic stroke, 20% to 25% may suffer early neurological deterioration (END), which is often defined as a gain of 4 or more points on the National Institutes of Health Stroke Scale (NIHSS) score (2,3). Approximately 37% of small vessel infarcts and 33% of larger artery occlusive disease strokes worsen, compared to only 7% of patients with embolic stroke (2). An understanding of signs

 DOI: 10.1891/9780826124791.0002

to watch for and requisite investigative workup can potentially avoid progression of infarction.

PATHOPHYSIOLOGY

The pathophysiology of the worsening of ischemic stroke is closely related to the underlying stroke type (Table 2.1). The etiology additionally dictates the strategies that should be implemented to prevent such worsening.

Small Vessel Disease and Lacunar Infarctions

Small vessel lacunar infarcts account for 25% of all ischemic strokes (4). Lacunes are small 1 to 15 mm infarcts located most commonly in the putamen, pallidum, pons, internal capsule, caudate nucleus, thalamus, corona radiata, and, less frequently, in the cerebral peduncles and subcortical white matter (5). Etiologies include arteriosclerosis, typically involving distal penetrating arteries leading to smaller parenchymal island infarcts; parent artery plaque or occlusion by thrombosis or embolus, typically involving proximal penetrating arteries leading to larger infarcts; microemboli; and hereditary disorders such as CADASIL and CARASIL (5–7). Classic syndromes include pure motor, pure sensory, mixed motor sensory, ataxic hemiparesis, and clumsy hand dysarthria.

Table 2.1 Overview of Mechanisms of Ischemic Stroke Worsening

Stroke Type	Mechanism of Worsening
Small vessel disease	Progressive small vessel occlusion, progression of edema
Intracranial atherosclerosis	Recurrent artery-to-artery embolization, small vessel occlusion, flow failure
Extracranial large vessel disease	Recurrent artery-to-artery embolization, flow failure
Intracranial large vessel occlusion	Collateral failure, progression of edema
Centrally embolic sources	Recurrent embolization
Rare causes: vasculitis, infection, hypercoagulable state, genetic disorder, etc.	Recurrent infarction with failure to recognize and address underlying cause
Other considerations	Hyperglycemia, hyperthermia, medical complications, hemorrhagic conversion

As opposed to embolic and large artery strokes, lacunar strokes can have a more gradual onset. This is likely due to involvement of small vessels and terminal branches as well as lack of collateralization. The Harvard Cooperative Stroke Registry noted that 62% of lacunar infarcts fluctuate or progress (2). In another study, 25% of patients with acute lacunar stroke worsened in the first 72 hours from onset, with the majority of worsening within the first 24 hours (8).

Certain risk factors may predispose patients with small vessel strokes to worsen. In one study, diabetes predicted motor progression, and in another, hypertension was independently associated with clinical deterioration in small vessel strokes (9). In contrast, others have suggested that an overall high burden of vascular risk factors, as opposed to a single one, independently predicts symptom progression (10). Leukoaraiosis, or the severity of subcortical ischemic change that likely reflects vascular risk factor burden, has also been reported to have an independent association with symptom progression or neurological deterioration after acute small vessel infarction (10,11). It has been postulated that leukoaraiosis volume predicts infarct growth because of impaired microcirculation and tissue capability to handle ischemia (12). Despite the risk factor profile, the severity of motor deficits on admission and larger infarct size are also associated with neurological deterioration (11,13).

Proposed mechanisms for progression of small vessel stroke include impaired hemodynamics, progressive branch occlusion, and peri-infarct edema (7). It has been suggested that an imbalance between excitatory and inhibitory neurotransmitters, glutamate and GABA, may also play a role in lacunar infarct progression (14).

Intracranial Atherosclerosis

Symptomatic intracranial atherosclerotic disease (ICAD) is one of the leading causes of stroke worldwide, with significant interracial variability. In Caucasians, ICAD is responsible for 8% to 10% of ischemic strokes, whereas in Chinese populations it accounts for 33% to 50% of stroke cases (15,16). Blacks and Hispanics are eight times more likely to have symptomatic ICAD as the etiology of their stroke compared to Caucasians. The mechanism of ICAD-related stroke varies. Artery-to-artery embolization of a destabilized plaque is by far the most common mechanism, accounting for 50% of incident and 70% of recurrent ICAD-related strokes (17). One-quarter of the time, plaque involves the ostium of perforator arteries and lacunar-type strokes also occur. The progressive stenosis caused by an enlarging plaque may result in impaired cerebral perfusion secondary to flow failure. This only occurs in 9% of cases, as these lesions are slowly progressive and pial collateralization develops. However, flow failure can be aggravated by systemic hypotension, hypoxia, or acute plaque destabilization resulting in sudden, severe narrowing or occlusion of the vessel beyond the compensatory capacity of the established collaterals.

Extracranial Vascular Disease

Large artery atherosclerosis (LAA), especially at the carotid bifurcation, is the most common type of extracranial vascular disease. Extracranial vascular disease of the carotid arteries accounts for up to 25% of all acute ischemic strokes (18). Other less common extracranial vascular disease includes stenosis of the vertebral artery, dissection, fibromuscular dysplasia, carotid webs, or embolic occlusion (19–21). LAA primarily causes stroke by artery-to-artery embolization from atheromatous material or thrombotic caps aggregated on acutely ruptured plaques. Up to 13% of patients with emergent large vessel occlusions are found to have tandem cervical carotid occlusion (22). Among all stroke etiologies, LAA carries the highest risk of recurrent embolization if untreated, accounting for up to 37% of recurrent strokes in the first 7 days (23). The 2-year risk of recurrent ischemic events from an acutely symptomatic LAA is 26%, most of which occurs in the first 2 weeks. This risk decreases over time and returns to the baseline risk of asymptomatic carotid stenosis after 6 months to 2 years.

Like ICAD, LAA is slowly progressive, allowing for development of collateral supply. While flow failure is rare, it may be encountered when the anatomy results in isolation of the downstream vasculature (e.g., with incomplete circle of Willis or with occlusion of contralateral carotid artery). Additionally, some nonatherosclerotic pathologies of the carotid artery may result in more acute decompensation (e.g., vessel dissection). Flow failure may be aggravated by systemic hypotension, hypoxia, or other severe metabolic derangements, and result in watershed infarctions with a classic string-of-beads appearance on parenchymal imaging (Figure 2.1).

Intracranial Large Vessel Occlusion

Large vessel occlusion (LVO) is a term that refers to the complete occlusion of an intracranial vessel of a large caliber, typically the intracranial internal carotid artery (in its subterminal segment or the terminus), the proximal segments of the anterior cerebral artery (ACA) or the middle cerebral artery (MCA), the basilar artery, or the

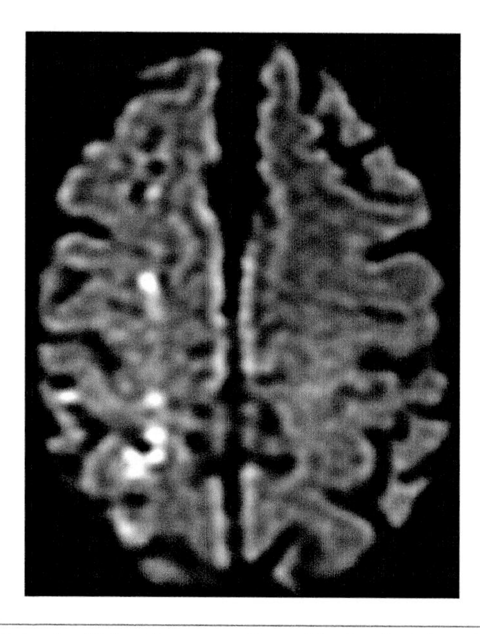

Figure 2.1 Watershed infarction presenting with classic string-of-beads appearance.

proximal posterior cerebral artery. Most LVOs are embolic in origin, although 23% may have underlying ICAD (24). The embolic source is of cardiac origin in most cases, although it may be artery-to-artery in 10% to 15% of cases (25). LVO is generally resistant to systemic thrombolytics, with recanalization rates as low as 20%. The natural history of non-recanalized LVO is very poor with the majority of patients being dead or severely disabled within 90 days of their stroke (26,27). The advent of thrombectomy and its superiority over best medical therapy has dramatically improved outcomes of patients with LVO (22) (Figure 2.2). While the neurological presentation of those strokes is often severe, further neurological worsening can be seen in non-recanalized LVO patients. Acutely, LVO results in a core of irreversibly infarcted tissue with a surrounding region of reduced perfusion or oligemia that may be functionally impaired but still salvageable. This region is called the "penumbra" and is the target of revascularization therapy. Occlusions affecting more proximal vessels, which supply larger territories, are more likely to exhibit worsening compared to more distal vessels (28). The preservation of the penumbra is directly proportionate to the sustainability

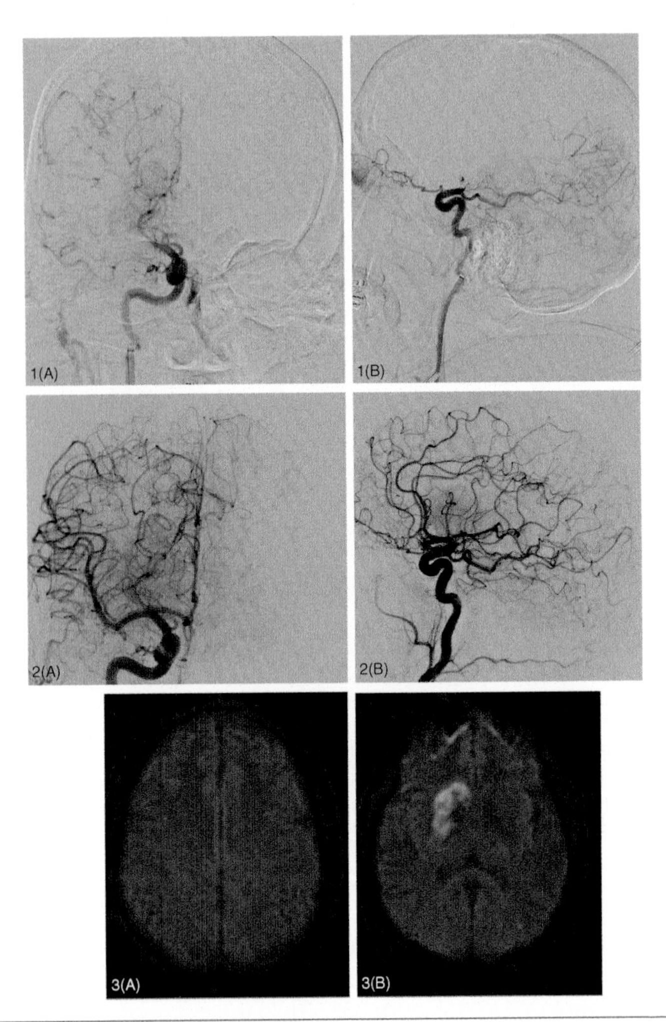

Figure 2.2 Acute occlusion of the right internal carotid artery terminus on anteroposterior (1A) and lateral (1B) angiographic views. After successful thrombectomy, full revascularization is achieved (2A–B). DWI series of MRI reveal minimal ischemic burden (3A–B).

DWI, diffusion-weighted imaging.

of the pial collaterals of the penumbra and the time from the index occlusion. Penumbral progression to infarction occurs rapidly over time, and the benefit of revascularization is reduced by 7% with every hour delay in revascularization (29). The degree of collateral flow varies from one patient to the other. Seventy-two percent of patients with good collateral flow will benefit from thrombectomy performed within 240 minutes from symptom onset, compared to only 15% of patients with poor collateral flow undergoing the procedure in the same time frame (30). Carefully selected patients with good collaterals benefit from thrombectomy up to 24 hours from their last known well time (31,32).

Occasionally, collateral flow maintains good neurological function in the penumbra. In these cases, the presentation of LVO can be deceptively mild. LVO is seen in 7% to 30% of patients who present with minor stroke syndromes or a transient ischemic attack (TIA) (3). These patients are at a significantly higher risk of early neurological worsening in the first 24 hours (33). Rapid recognition and treatment, when appropriate, can prevent such a catastrophic deterioration.

Another mechanism of worsening in LVO is progression of cerebral edema. Patients with occlusion of the proximal MCA who are not candidates for revascularization or who have delayed or incomplete revascularization may develop malignant MCA syndrome. Progression of cerebral edema may lead to progressive midline shift, development of a contralateral ACA, stroke secondary to the impingement of the contralateral ACA, and eventually transtentorial herniation with a high risk of severe morbidity or mortality.

Cardiac and Other Embolic Strokes

In the Harvard Cooperative Stroke Registry, 31% of patients were diagnosed with embolic stroke. Emboli may travel from any more proximal vascular source. The aortic arch is the most proximal source of artery-to-artery embolus and may account for up to 4% of strokes (34). Aortic plaques greater than 4 mm are considered to be at highest risk for subsequent stroke (35). Cardiac risk factors such as atrial fibrillation (AF), recent myocardial infarction, or valvular dysfunction are found in 25% of all stroke patients (2). By modern estimates, cardioembolic strokes account for up to 30% of all acute ischemic strokes (4). The most common cause of cardioembolic stroke is AF, whereby stagnant blood in the left atrial appendage forms clots that embolize. Cardioembolic strokes are often larger, involve superficial and deep structures of the brain, and may involve multiple vascular territories at the same time. As the Framingham Heart Study demonstrated, the prevalence of AF increases with age, and the risk of stroke is almost five times higher in adults with AF (36). Especially prior to the success of endovascular therapy, stroke in patients with AF was associated with almost twofold increase in 30-day mortality than non-AF stroke. Additionally, stroke recurrence rate is significantly higher in patients with AF (37). Aside from AF, patients can have cardioembolic strokes from other arrhythmias, valvular disease, infective and noninfective endocarditis, cardiomyopathies and reduced cardiac output, cardiac tumors, paradoxical emboli via septal defects, and lesions of the myocardium or chambers that embolize.

Rare Causes and General Considerations

Unusual presentations of stroke, such as young age or other systemic disease, may point to a less common etiology, such as infection, vasculitis, or genetic disorders, which have a tendency for progression or worsening course. Optimization of medical care also impacts the progression of cerebral ischemia, irreversible cellular injury, and neurological decline. Hyperthermia may worsen ischemic stroke in 12% to 25% of patients (38,39). While there is preclinical and clinical evidence of the beneficial effects of hypothermia as a neuroprotectant in neurological injury, spontaneous hypothermia at presentation has been linked to early neurological worsening in ischemic patients (28). Hyperglycemia is seen in up to 40% of patients and is also associated with worsening outcomes.

PREVENTION

With an understanding of underlying stroke etiology, worsening of ischemic infarction can be mitigated. The following steps are essential for optimum stroke outcomes: rapid diagnosis, appropriate provision of acute revascularization therapy, close monitoring, supportive care, recognition of etiology, and timely initiation of secondary prevention strategies.

Rapid Diagnosis

Failure to recognize a stroke, either because of transient or ambiguous symptoms, or lack of sufficient expertise, puts the patient at risk of recurrent stroke. Up to 70% of patients presenting with minor stroke or TIA do not undergo vessel imaging in their initial stroke triage phase. Those patients are at risk of early recurrent embolism from a symptomatic intracranial or extracranial stenosis or flow failure from an untreated LVO. Algorithms that prioritize noninvasive parenchymal and vascular imaging (e.g., CT and CT angiography [CTA]) for patients presenting with stroke-like symptoms can assist with identification of consequential findings. Expert neurological clinical assessment remains of paramount importance.

Telestroke consultation can bridge gaps in the timely availability of such expertise (40).

Acute Revascularization Therapy

The timely revascularization of occluded vessels can significantly reduce stroke symptoms and disability. All patients presenting within 4.5 hours from last known well time should be considered for tPA if they have no contraindications to its use. Additionally, all patients with LVO who present within 6 hours from their last known well time should be considered for mechanical thrombectomy. Patients with LVO presenting within 6 to 24 hours from last known well time should undergo perfusion imaging (CT perfusion [CTP] or magnetic resonance perfusion [MRP]) to assess for a sufficiently large penumbra and a relatively small core of ischemia (41). Patients who present with minor stroke symptoms or a TIA and an underlying LVO should be placed in a highly monitored setting. The decision to perform endovascular thrombectomy in these cases is controversial, and studies are ongoing. Thorough assessment of the stability of their collaterals may assist in the decision making and include perfusion imaging or a bedside orthostatic challenge test. Prehospital and emergency department protocols for hyperacute clinical and radiological assessment of stroke should be instated to facilitate the rapid recognition and determination of patient eligibility for time-sensitive treatments.

Patient Monitoring

Stroke patients should be monitored in units with sufficiently trained nursing staff and appropriate monitoring equipment. The admission of patients to dedicated stroke units has been shown to improve outcomes when compared to patients admitted to nonstroke units (42). While frequent neurological assessment is important for all stroke patients, monitoring should be vigilant in the high-risk populations, including patients who have undergone revascularization treatments (systemic thrombolysis or mechanical thrombectomy), have impending flow failure (e.g., flow-limiting stenosis or occlusion), and/or have risk for development of malignant MCA edema.

Supportive Care

Certified stroke centers have evidence-based protocols aimed to reduce common complications and optimize outcomes. Accreditation bodies such as the Joint Commission perform regular assessments to ensure the quality of care in stroke centers around the country. Routine methods for prevention of common sequelae of stroke, such as aspiration pneumonia and deep venous thrombosis, have been established and include screening protocols and order sets. While flat bed rest was found to have no specific benefit for stroke patients in general (43), patients with impending flow failure may benefit from flow augmentation measures that include flat bed rest, supplementation with intravenous fluids, or pharmacological pressure support. Strict control of temperature and prevention of hyperthermia is of clinical benefit. While the prospects of hypothermia as a neuroprotectant are promising, there is no evidence for its routine implementation in clinical care currently. Similarly, management of hyperglycemia is advisable, although the value of aggressive glycemic control is still the subject of investigation.

Recognition of Etiology

Occasionally, the etiology of stroke becomes apparent during the hyperacute triage phase. Cervical vascular disease or ICAD may be seen on CTA or magnetic resonance angiography (MRA) used in hyperacute triage. AF may be detected on initial ECG or cardiac monitoring. However, when the etiology is not immediately identified, further workup should be initiated based on presentation. For example, in a febrile patient with an embolic pattern of infarction, endocarditis is of greater concern and evaluation should include transthoracic echo and blood cultures. While more invasive than transthoracic echocardiography (TTE), transesophageal echocardiography (TEE) identifies a potential cardioembolic source more often (44). Depending on the suspected cardioembolic source, TEE provides better visualization of left atrial appendage thrombi, but the left ventricle is typically visualized best with TTE. Additionally, a bubble study may help identify a septal defect, such as patent foramen ovale (PFO), as a source for paradoxical embolism. TEE also provides the most reliable image of ulcerated aortic plaque (45). Patients with embolic-appearing stroke of unknown source (ESUS) should undergo extensive workup to identify the source of emboli. Paroxysmal AF is identified in 16% to 18% of such patients and should be thoroughly investigated (46,47). Prolonged, implantable cardiac monitors are more sensitive in the detection of paroxysmal AF compared to standard monitoring.

High-resolution MRA performed on 3T machines and modalities of vessel wall imaging can reveal mural plaque without stenosis and identify high-risk features like plaque hemorrhage or destabilization (48). Vessel wall imaging is also helpful in evaluation of vasculitic pathologies and can differentiate between vasculitis and other pathologies (49). Though invasive, catheter-based angiography can provide valuable information regarding stroke etiology when the etiology is not clear with less invasive testing. It is most helpful for full evaluation of vasculitis or ICAD.

When one suspects flow failure as the mechanism of stroke in symptomatic ICAD, cerebrovascular reserve of the affected territory can be assessed by an acetazolamide challenge perfusion study (50). Patients with impaired cerebrovascular reserve are at higher risk of flow failure related recurrence. B-mode ultrasound can help detect unstable, ulcerated carotid plaques, and fat suppressed MRA can aid in detecting dissection. Genetic testing should always be considered when there is concern for inherited stroke syndromes such as CADASIL, CARASIL, or MELAS.

Secondary Prevention Strategies

Measures of secondary prevention include the timely initiation of antithrombotic therapy. Patients with mild, nondisabling strokes or high-risk TIAs may benefit from brief periods of dual antiplatelets (51,52). A regimen of dual antiplatelet therapy in combination with high potency lipid lowering agents like HMG-CoA reductase inhibitors (statins) has also become the standard of care in the management of acutely symptomatic ICAD. This regimen of maximum medical therapy for 3 months duration has been found to result in lower risk of recurrent stroke compared to endovascular intracranial stenting (53). Angioplasty, with or without intracranial stenting, remains a treatment option for patients who have recurrent stroke in spite of maximum medical therapy.

Prevention of further AF-related stroke with anticoagulation is essential. Depending on the size of infarct, anticoagulation may be initially held to decrease the chance of hemorrhagic conversion with systemic anticoagulation. With small strokes anticoagulation can at times be started 24 hours after the infarct, whereas large strokes can require up to 2 weeks without anticoagulation (54). There are now many choices of medication for systemic anticoagulation in addition to warfarin including the factor Xa inhibitors rivaroxaban, apixaban, and edoxaban, as well as the direct thrombin inhibitor dabigatran (55–57). While many patients with ESUS will be found to have underlying paroxysmal AF, there is currently no evidence to support the routine use of anticoagulants in those patients before a diagnosis of AF is made (58). Patients with ESUS and an underlying PFO may benefit from closure, particularly if they have large interatrial shunts or atrial septal aneurysms (59–61).

Patients with symptomatic carotid stenosis should be considered for timely revascularization with carotid artery stenting (CAS) or carotid endarterectomy (CEA). Given the high recurrence rate of stroke in these patients, revascularization should occur as early as safely possible. The benefit of revascularization declines rapidly over time, as does the risk of recurrence. Patients with 50% to 69% stenosis, for example, mostly benefit if revascularization is performed within 2 weeks from the index event (62). This benefit rapidly declines thereafter, especially in women. The number needed to treat after 4 weeks is three times that of patients treated in the first 2 weeks. For patients with large hemispheric strokes, however, delayed carotid revascularization may be reasonable. For patients with less common etiologies of stroke, secondary prevention should be tailored to the underlying condition. Discovery of an infectious vegetation, for instance, requires intravenous antibiotics, while discovery of an atrial myxoma might necessitate surgery. Patients with emboli from prosthetic valve or left ventricular assist device typically warrant earlier anticoagulation despite a risk for hemorrhagic conversion given the high risk for further emboli. Aortic plaques are treated with antiplatelet or anticoagulant agents, depending on size, morphology, and response. The Aortic Arch Related Cerebral Hazard (ARCH) Trial failed to show superiority of aspirin plus clopidogrel over warfarin (63). However, in those patients with larger, mobile atheroma, or who fail antiplatelet agents, anticoagulation is more commonly used. In patients diagnosed with vasculitis, evaluation for immunosuppression therapy should be quickly initiated.

CONCLUSION

Acute ischemic stroke worsening is a common and serious condition affecting up to 25% of stroke patients. Risk varies based on underlying stroke mechanism, with specific clinical scenarios carrying significantly higher risk of worsening. Strategies aimed at early diagnosis and identification of stroke etiology can help identify high-risk patients. Appropriate rapid revascularization, supportive care in monitored stroke units, and treatment of the underlying disease with implementation of secondary prevention vastly improve stroke outcomes.

REFERENCES

1. Markus HS. Cerebral perfusion and stroke. *J Neurol Neurosurg Psychiatry*. 2004;75(3):353–361. doi:10.1136/jnnp.2003.025825

2. Mohr JP, Caplan LR, Melski JW, et al. The Harvard Cooperative Stroke Registry: a prospective registry. *Neurology.* 1978;28(8):754–762. doi:10.1212/WNL.28.8.754
3. Kim J-T, Heo S-H, Yoon W, et al. Clinical outcomes of patients with acute minor stroke receiving rescue IA therapy following early neurological deterioration. *J Neurointerv Surg.* 2016;8(5):461–465. doi:10.1136/neurintsurg-2015-011690
4. Kolominsky-Rabas PL, Weber M, Gefeller O, et al. Epidemiology of ischemic stroke subtypes according to TOAST criteria: incidence, recurrence, and long-term survival in ischemic stroke subtypes: a population-based study. *Stroke.* 2001;32(12):2735–2740. doi:10.1161/hs1201.100209
5. Caplan LR. *Caplan's Stroke: a clinical approach.* Cambridge, UK: Cambridge University Press; 2016.
6. Mohr JP, Grotta JC, Wolf PA. *Stroke: Pathophysiology, diagnosis, and management.* 6th ed. Amsterdam, Netherlands: Elsevier; 2004.
7. Del Bene A, Palumbo V, Lamassa M, et al. Progressive lacunar stroke: review of mechanisms, prognostic features, and putative treatments. *Int J Stroke.* 2012;7(4):321–329. doi:10.1111/j.1747-4949.2012.00789.x
8. Audebert HJ, Pellkofer TS, Wimmer ML, et al. Progression in lacunar stroke is related to elevated acute phase parameters. *Eur Neurol.* 2004;51(3):125–131. doi:10.1159/000077012
9. Yamamoto H, Bogousslavsky J, van Melle G. Different predictors of neurological worsening in different causes of stroke. *Arch Neurol.* 1998;55(4):481–486. doi:10.1001/archneur.55.4.481
10. Nannoni S, Del Bene A, Palumbo V, et al. Predictors of progression in patients presenting with minor subcortical stroke. *Acta Neurol Scand.* 2015;132(5):304–309. doi:10.1111/ane.12399
11. Feng C, Tan Y, Wu Y-F, et al. Leukoaraiosis correlates with the neurologic deterioration after small subcortical infarction. *J Stroke Cerebrovasc Dis.* 2014;23(6):1513–1518. doi:10.1016/j.jstrokecerebrovasdis.2013.12.032
12. Ay H, Arsava EM, Rosand J, et al. Severity of leukoaraiosis and susceptibility to infarct growth in acute stroke. *Stroke.* 2008;39(5):1409–1413. doi:10.1161/STROKEAHA.107.501932
13. Takase K-I, Murai H, Tasaki R, et al. Initial MRI findings predict progressive lacunar infarction in the territory of the lenticulostriate artery. *Eur Neurol.* 2011;65(6):355–360. doi:10.1159/000327980
14. Serena J, Leira R, Castillo J, et al. Neurological deterioration in acute lacunar infarctions: the role of excitatory and inhibitory neurotransmitters. *Stroke.* 2001;32(5):1154–1161. doi:10.1161/01.STR.32.5.1154
15. Wong KS, Huang YN, Gao S, et al. Intracranial stenosis in Chinese patients with acute stroke. *Neurology.* 1998;50(3):812–813. doi:10.1212/WNL.50.3.812

16. Sacco RL, Kargman DE, Gu Q, et al. Race-ethnicity and determinants of intracranial atherosclerotic cerebral infarction. The Northern Manhattan Stroke Study. *Stroke*. 1995;26(1):14–20. doi:10.1161/01.STR.26.1.14
17. Lopez-Cancio E, Matheus MG, Romano JG, et al. Infarct patterns, collaterals and likely causative mechanisms of stroke in symptomatic intracranial atherosclerosis. *Cerebrovasc Dis*. 2014;37(6):417–422. doi:10.1159/000362922
18. Petty GW, Brown RD, Whisnant JP, et al. Ischemic stroke subtypes: a population-based study of incidence and risk factors. *Stroke*. 1999;30(12):2513–2516. doi:10.1161/01.STR.30.12.2513
19. Béjot Y, Daubail B, Debette S, et al. Incidence and outcome of cerebrovascular events related to cervical artery dissection: the Dijon Stroke Registry. *Int J Stroke*. 2014;9(7):879–882. doi:10.1111/ijs.12154
20. Olin JW, Froehlich J, Gu X, et al. The United States Registry for Fibromuscular Dysplasia: results in the first 447 patients. *Circulation*. 2012;125(25):3182–3190. doi:10.1161/CIRCULATIONAHA.112.091223
21. Choi PMC, Singh D, Trivedi A, et al. Carotid webs and recurrent ischemic strokes in the era of CT angiography. *AJNR Am J Neuroradiol*. 2015;36(11):2134–2139. doi:10.3174/ajnr.A4431
22. Goyal M, Menon BK, van Zwam WH, et al. Endovascular thrombectomy after large-vessel ischaemic stroke: a meta-analysis of individual patient data from five randomised trials. *Lancet*. 2016;387(10029):1723–1731. doi:10.1016/S0140-6736(16)00163-X
23. Lovett JK, Coull AJ, Rothwell PM. Early risk of recurrence by subtype of ischemic stroke in population-based incidence studies. *Neurology*. 2004;62(4):569–573. doi:10.1212/01.WNL.0000110311.09970.83
24. Yoon W, Kim SK, Park M-S, et al. Endovascular treatment and the outcomes of atherosclerotic intracranial stenosis in patients with hyperacute stroke. *Neurosurgery*. 2015;76(6):680–686. doi:10.1227/NEU.0000000000000694
25. Goyal M, Demchuk AM, Menon BK, et al. Randomized assessment of rapid endovascular treatment of ischemic stroke. *N Engl J Med*. 2015;372(11):1019–1030. doi:10.1056/NEJMoa1414905
26. Mozaffarian D, Benjamin EJ, Go AS, et al. Heart disease and stroke statistics—2015 update: a report from the American Heart Association. *Circulation*. 2015;131(4):e29–e322. doi:10.1161/CIR.0000000000000152
27. Bhatia R, Hill MD, Shobha N, et al. Low rates of acute recanalization with intravenous recombinant tissue plasminogen activator in ischemic stroke: real-world experience and a call for action. *Stroke*. 2010;41(10):2254–2258. doi:10.1161/STROKEAHA.110.592535
28. Nacu A, Bringeland GH, Khanevski A, et al. Early neurological worsening in acute ischaemic stroke patients. *Acta Neurol Scand*. 2015;133(1):25–29. doi:10.1111/ane.12418

29. Saver JL, Goyal M, van der Lugt A, et al. Time to treatment with endovascular thrombectomy and outcomes from ischemic stroke: a meta-analysis. *JAMA*. 2016;316(12):1279–1289. doi:10.1001/jama.2016.13647
30. Sallustio F, Motta C, Pizzuto S, et al. CT angiography-based collateral flow and time to reperfusion are strong predictors of outcome in endovascular treatment of patients with stroke. *J Neurointerv Surg*. 2016;9(10):940–943. doi:10.1136/neurintsurg–2016–012628
31. Nogueira RG, Jadhav AP, Haussen DC, et al. Thrombectomy 6 to 24 hours after stroke with a mismatch between deficit and infarct. *N Engl J Med*. 2018;378(1):11–21. doi:10.1056/NEJMoa1706442
32. Albers GW, Marks MP, Kemp S, et al. Thrombectomy for stroke at 6 to 16 hours with selection by perfusion imaging. *N Engl J Med*. 2018;378(8):708–718. doi:10.1056/NEJMoa1713973
33. Kim J-T, Park M-S, Chang J, et al. Proximal arterial occlusion in acute ischemic stroke with low NIHSS scores should not be considered as mild stroke. *PLoS One*. 2013;8(8):e70996. doi:10.1371/journal.pone.0070996
34. Tunick PA, Culliford AT, Lamparello PJ, et al. Atheromatosis of the aortic arch as an occult source of multiple systemic emboli. *Ann Intern Med*. 1991;114(5):391–392. doi:10.7326/0003-4819-114-5-391
35. Di Tullio MR, Sacco RL, Homma S. Atherosclerotic disease of the aortic arch as a risk factor for recurrent ischemic stroke. *N Engl J Med*. 1996;335(19):1464–1465. doi:10.1056/nejm199611073351913
36. Wolf PA, Abbott RD, Kannel WB. Atrial fibrillation as an independent risk factor for stroke: the Framingham Study. *Stroke*. 1991;22(8):983–988. doi:10.1161/01.STR.22.8.983
37. Lin HJ, Wolf PA, Kelly-Hayes M, et al. Stroke severity in atrial fibrillation. The Framingham Study. *Stroke*. 1996;27(10):1760–1764. doi:10.1161/01.STR.27.10.1760
38. Wang Y, Lim LL, Levi C, et al. Influence of admission body temperature on stroke mortality. *Stroke*. 2000;31(2):404–409. doi:10.1161/01.STR.31.2.404
39. Reith J, Jørgensen HS, Pedersen PM, et al. Body temperature in acute stroke: relation to stroke severity, infarct size, mortality, and outcome. *Lancet*. 1996;347(8999):422–425. doi:10.1016/S0140-6736(96)90008-2
40. Wechsler LR, Demaerschalk BM, Schwamm LH, et al. Telemedicine quality and outcomes in stroke: a scientific statement for healthcare professionals from the American Heart Association/American Stroke Association. *Stroke*. 2016;48(1):e3–e25. doi:10.1161/str.0000000000000114
41. Powers WJ, Rabinstein AA, Ackerson T, et al. 2018 Guidelines for the early management of patients with acute ischemic stroke: a guideline for healthcare professionals from the American Heart Association/American Stroke Association. *Stroke*. 2018;49:e46–e110. doi:10.1161/STR.0000000000000158

42. Stroke Unit Trialists' Collaboration. Organised inpatient (stroke unit) care for stroke. *Cochrane Database Syst Rev.* 2013;23 Suppl 2(9):CD000197.
43. Anderson CS, Arima H, Lavados P, et al. Cluster-randomized, crossover trial of head positioning in acute stroke. *N Engl J Med.* 2017;376(25):2437–2447. doi:10.1056/NEJMoa1615715
44. Pearson AC, Labovitz AJ, Tatineni S, et al. Superiority of transesophageal echocardiography in detecting cardiac source of embolism in patients with cerebral ischemia of uncertain etiology. *J Am Coll Cardiol.* 1991;17(1):66–72. doi:10.1016/0735-1097(91)90705-E
45. Horowitz DR, Tuhrim S, Budd J, et al. Aortic plaque in patients with brain ischemia: diagnosis by transesophageal echocardiography. *Neurology.* 1992;42(8):1602–1604. doi:10.1212/WNL.42.8.1602
46. Gladstone DJ, Spring M, Dorian P, et al. Atrial fibrillation in patients with cryptogenic stroke. *N Engl J Med.* 2014;370(26):2467–2477. doi:10.1056/NEJMoa1311376
47. Higgins P, MacFarlane PW, Dawson J, et al. Noninvasive cardiac event monitoring to detect atrial fibrillation after ischemic stroke: a randomized, controlled trial. *Stroke.* 2013;44(9):2525–2531. doi:10.1161/STROKEAHA.113.001927
48. Klein IF, Lavallée PC, Touboul PJ, et al. In vivo middle cerebral artery plaque imaging by high-resolution MRI. *Neurology.* 2006;67(2):327–329. doi:10.1212/01.wnl.0000225074.47396.71
49. Cao W, Cheng X, Li H, et al. Evaluation of cerebrovascular reserve using xenon-enhanced CT scanning in patients with symptomatic middle cerebral artery stenosis. *J Clin Neurosci.* 2014;21(2):293–297. doi:10.1016/j.jocn.2013.04.038
50. Obusez EC, Hui F, Hajj-Ali RA, et al. High-resolution MRI vessel wall imaging: spatial and temporal patterns of reversible cerebral vasoconstriction syndrome and central nervous system vasculitis. *AJNR Am J Neuroradiol.* 2014;35(8):1527–1532. doi:10.3174/ajnr.A3909
51. Wang Y, Wang Y, Zhao X, et al. Clopidogrel with aspirin in acute minor stroke or transient ischemic attack. *N Engl J Med.* 2013;369(1):11–19. doi:10.1056/NEJMoa1215340
52. Johnston SC, Easton JD, Farrant M, et al. Clopidogrel and aspirin in acute ischemic stroke and high-risk TIA. *N Engl J Med.* 2018;379(3):215–225. doi:10.1056/NEJMoa1800410
53. Derdeyn CP, Chimowitz MI, Lynn MJ, et al. Aggressive medical treatment with or without stenting in high-risk patients with intracranial artery stenosis (SAMMPRIS): the final results of a randomised trial. *Lancet.* 2014;383(9914):333–341. doi:10.1016/S0140-6736(13)62038-3
54. Immediate anticoagulation of embolic stroke: brain hemorrhage and management options. Cerebral Embolism Study Group. *Stroke.* 1984;15(5):779–789. doi:10.1161/01.STR.15.5.779

55. Granger CB, Alexander JH, McMurray JJV, et al. Apixaban versus warfarin in patients with atrial fibrillation. *N Engl J Med.* 2011;365(11):981–992. doi:10.1056/NEJMoa1107039
56. Eikelboom JW, Connolly SJ, Brueckmann M, et al. Dabigatran versus warfarin in patients with mechanical heart valves. *N Engl J Med.* 2013;369(13):1206–1214. doi:10.1056/NEJMoa1300615
57. Patel MR, Mahaffey KW, Garg J, et al. Rivaroxaban versus warfarin in nonvalvular atrial fibrillation. *N Engl J Med.* 2011;365(10):883–891. doi:10.1056/NEJMoa1009638
58. Hart RG, Sharma M, Mundl H, et al. Rivaroxaban for stroke prevention after embolic stroke of undetermined source. *N Engl J Med.* 2018;378(23):2191–2201. doi:10.1056/NEJMoa1802686
59. Mas J-L, Derumeaux G, Guillon B, et al. Patent foramen ovale closure or anticoagulation vs. antiplatelets after stroke. *N Engl J Med.* 2017;377(11):1011–1021. doi:10.1056/NEJMoa1705915
60. Saver JL, Carroll JD, Thaler DE, et al. Long-term outcomes of patent foramen ovale closure or medical therapy after stroke. *N Engl J Med.* 2017;377(11):1022–1032. doi:10.1056/NEJMoa1610057
61. Søndergaard L, Kasner SE, Rhodes JF, et al. Patent foramen ovale closure or antiplatelet therapy for cryptogenic stroke. *N Engl J Med.* 2017;377(11):1033–1042. doi:10.1056/NEJMoa1707404
62. Rothwell PM, Eliasziw M, Gutnikov SA, et al. Sex difference in the effect of time from symptoms to surgery on benefit from carotid endarterectomy for transient ischemic attack and nondisabling stroke. *Stroke.* 2004;35(12):2855–2861. doi:10.1161/01.STR.0000147040.20446.f6
63. Amarenco P, Davis S, Jones EF, et al. Clopidogrel plus aspirin versus warfarin in patients with stroke and aortic arch plaques. *Stroke.* 2014;45(5):1248–1257. doi:10.1161/STROKEAHA.113.004251

3 Expansion of Intracerebral Hemorrhage

Vignan Yogendrakumar, Joshua N. Goldstein, and Dar Dowlatshahi

KEY POINTS

- Hematoma expansion that follows spontaneous intracerebral hemorrhage is predictive of poor long-term functioning.
- Numerous definitions of hematoma expansion are currently in use (≥3 mL, ≥6 mL, ≥12.5 mL, ≥26%, ≥33%).
- Time to CT and anticoagulant use are two clinical factors that are consistently associated with hematoma expansion.
- Large hemorrhage volume, irregular shape, and hematoma heterogeneity are major noncontrast predictors of expansion.
- Spot sign is a major predictor of subsequent expansion. Sensitivity of spot sign can be improved with dynamic imaging.
- Treatment options attempting to restrict and prevent hematoma expansion are limited

INTRODUCTION

Spontaneous intracerebral hemorrhage is the most devastating stroke subtype and is a major cause of morbidity and mortality across the world (1). This nontraumatic rupture of cerebral blood vessels is the second most common form of stroke and accounts for approximately 10% to 30% of first ever stroke presentations (2). Intracerebral hemorrhage has a 1-month mortality ranging from 30% to 55%, and approximately 75% of survivors continue to suffer severe disability long term (2,3).

The annual incidence of hemorrhage is reported to be 10 to 30 per 100,000 (1). In contrast to ischemic stroke, intracerebral hemorrhage has not significantly changed in the past 40 years (4).

 DOI: 10.1891/9780826124791.0003

While individual countries have reported varying changes in hemorrhage rates, a large meta-analysis of more than 8,000 patients assessed from 1980 to 2008 reported an overall incidence worldwide of 24.6 per 100,000 person years (95% confidence interval [CI]: 19.7–30.7) (4,5). Intracerebral hemorrhage is increasingly seen with age and may relate to the increased use of anticoagulation in older adults and the higher prevalence of amyloid angiopathy and hypertension (1). Earlier studies have previously suggested an increased rate of hemorrhage in men; however, more recent work by Gokhale et al. has not shown significant differences between sexes (5). The only exception to this is in Japanese men, where there is a significantly higher occurrence of intracerebral hemorrhage (4). Certain ethnicities are also associated with higher rates of intracerebral hemorrhage, including East and Southeast Asians, Latin Americans, Blacks, and Native Americans (1,4). Within ethnic groups, geographical differences in intracerebral hemorrhage incidence have also been noted. There is a higher rate of hemorrhage in those living in Asia versus Asian migrants living in North America (4). Black New Yorkers have a higher rate of hemorrhage occurrence compared to those living outside of the United States (4). Overall, however, there is a lower incidence in higher income countries (6). Environmental factors, such as cardiovascular risk control, socioeconomic status, and appropriate healthcare access are clearly influential in the incidence of intracerebral hemorrhage.

Intracerebral hemorrhage is a major public health issue. Due to limited treatment options and our aging population, hospital admissions for intracerebral hemorrhage increased by 18% from 1990 to 2000 (1) and are projected to increase further. Care of patients with intracerebral hemorrhage is further complicated by the dynamic nature of the disease. Patients are often subject to rapid changes in their clinical status within the first few hours to days of symptom onset (7). These changes are often associated with complications that can lead to clinical deterioration and include fever, seizure, intraventricular extension, and hematoma expansion (8,9). Early deterioration is a known predictor of poor long-term outcome (10).

Hematoma expansion after arrival stands as one of the most critical and frequent contributors to poor outcome. It occurs early in the presentation and is the proposed therapeutic target of treatment trials, both past and present. An improved understanding of this process can ultimately lead to treatments that are successful at preventing it. This chapter focuses specifically on our current understandings of hematoma expansion: how we define it, how it occurs, what best predicts it, and how we may treat it in the future.

DEFINING HEMATOMA EXPANSION

Formally, hematoma expansion is simply defined as an enlargement in hematoma volume when comparing a baseline scan to subsequent imaging. Yet, the amount of expansion required to be deemed significant has been a subject of continued debate. Moreover, the frequency and occurrence of hematoma expansion vary depending on the definition used (3).

Hematoma expansion has been an area of active investigation over the past 30 years as brain imaging has become more accessible. Early expansion definitions first used in the late 1980s were varied, largely arbitrary, and without statistical basis. Using the ABC/2 approximation method, common definitions included absolute volume enlargements of greater than 2 mL or greater than 20 mL and relative volume increases of 50% or more (11,12). The first attempt to derive a statistically based definition of hematoma expansion was conducted in the mid-1990s by Kazui et al. Using a consensus of five readers as a gold standard, changes in hematoma volume over a mean time course of 35 (±31.1) hours were assessed via a receiver operating characteristic (ROC) curve. A mathematically optimal cut point was calculated to be at 12.5 mL and 40% (11). Thus, the absolute definition of ≥12.5 mL may represent significant hematoma expansion, has since been used in a number of studies, and continues to be actively used today. In contrast, the definition of 40% was not widely adopted. A relative definition of greater than 33% was introduced by Brott et al. (13). The rationale proposed to use 33% was twofold. First, a change in hematoma volume of at least 33% relative to the baseline correlates with a 10% change in the diameter of a hematoma. Brott et al. argued that this would be easy to detect by a physician during an acute assessment (13). Second, it was deemed that a change of 33% or greater would represent true growth and not variability secondary to imaging technique. Since its introduction in 1997, this definition has been adopted widely and used for a number of subsequent studies (14). Another definition of ≥6 mL was loosely based on expansion definitions used in neurotrauma and neurosurgical circles to evaluate traumatic intraparenchymal hemorrhages and has also been used by several subsequent studies (14,15).

These definitions were all formally reevaluated by Dowlatshahi et al. in 2011. Changes in hematoma volume over the course of 24 hours (in patients presenting under 6 hours of symptom onset) were compared to poor clinical outcome of a 90-day modified Rankin Scale (mRS) score of 4 or higher. All definitions (≥3 mL, ≥6 mL, ≥12.5 mL, ≥26%, ≥33%) were independently predictive of poor outcome (Table 3.1) (14). Of note, specificity increased with higher threshold definitions but at the cost of decreased sensitivity. Additional analysis also showed that absolute definitions were slightly more predictive of poor outcome than relative definitions, especially when severe disability or death (mRS 5–6) was assessed. Similar findings (using definitions: ≤5 mL, 5.1–12.5 mL, >12.5 mL, ≤33%, 34%–50%, >50%) were reported in a concurrent study by Delcourt et al. (16). Hematoma expansion is an independent determinant of mortality and outcome. For every 10% of hematoma growth there is a 5% increased hazard of death and a 16% likelihood of a 1-point increase in a patient's baseline mRS score (17).

Regardless of the definition used, the definition must be greater than the minimal detectable difference of the measuring technique used. Brott et al. had used a sufficiently large threshold in order to ensure enlargement was detectable by the human eye (13). This may be valid when dealing with moderately sized hematomas, but may not be sensitive in very small hematomas, such as those under 5 mL. Indeed, the minimal detectable difference of commonly used planimetric volume assessment program exceeds 33% in hematomas less than 15 mL in volume (18). Conversely, the minimal detectable differences become very large, and larger than the absolute thresholds of 6 mL, as

Table 3.1 Sensitivity and Specificity of Various Definitions for Prediction of Poor Outcome (Modified Rankin Score 4–6)

Definition	Sensitivity (%)	Specificity (%)	PPV (%)	NPV (%)	aOR	95% CI
≥3 mL	46	81	70	60	2.99	1.88–4.77
≥6 mL	35	88	74	58	3.11	1.84–5.26
≥12.5 mL	22	95	81	55	3.98	1.94–8.18
≥26%	40	79	65	57	2.59	1.63–4.10
≥33%	37	83	68	57	2.73	1.70–4.39

aOR, adjusted odds ratio; CI, confidence interval; NPV, negative predictive value; PPV, positive predictive value.

Source: From Dowlatshahi D, Demchuk AM, Flaherty ML, et al. Defining hematoma expansion in intracerebral hemorrhage. *Neurology.* 2011;76(14):1238–1244. doi:10.1212/WNL.0b013e3182143317

hematoma volume increases, or when anatomical boundaries are altered or compressed (19).

The timing of both baseline imaging and subsequent reimaging are equally important (Table 3.2). Kazui et al. first commented on this, noting that patients presenting under 3 hours of symptom onset had a higher frequency of hematoma expansion (11). This frequency declined with patients who presented in later time windows. Similar findings were noted by Brott et al. (13). Based on numerous studies, the frequency of hematoma expansion ranges from 18% to 38% (2). The reasons for this wide range of incidence are due to the practical complications of assessing hematoma expansion. Serial imaging is required to provide more accurate information but is impractical due to the unacceptable amount of radiation exposure. One study was able to overcome this obstacle with the use of transcranial B ultrasound. Forty-four patients with new intracerebral hemorrhage were prospectively assessed with serial ultrasounds (every 30 min

Table 3.2 Expansion by Time

	Frequency of Hematoma Expansion
Kazui et al. (11): ≥12.5 mL or ≥40% Follow-up imaging: 120 hours from symptom onset	
≤3 hours	27/74 (36%)
3–6 hours	7/45 (16%)
6–12 hours	5/33 (15%)
12–24 hours	2/34 (6%)
24–48 hours	0/18 (0%)
Brott et al. (13): >33% Follow-up imaging: 20 hours from baseline CT	
≤3 hours	39/103 (38%)
Brouwers et al. (114): >6 mL or >33% Follow-up imaging: 11–25 hours from baseline CT	
≤6 hours	89/156 (79%)
>6 hours	24/156 (21%)
Yao et al. (21): >6 mL or >33% Follow-up imaging: 72 hours from baseline CT	
<3 hours	47/74 (63%)

for the first 6 hours). By the 12-hour mark, 20% of patients exhibited hematoma expansion with the majority of expansion occurring in the first 6 hours following baseline imaging (20).

Ultimately, any growth is detrimental, irrespective of definition. Looking at the most recent observational and treatment trials, the most common definitions used are: ≥6 mL, ≥12.5 mL, and ≥33%. Although there are several factors that influence the frequency of patients meeting the criteria for hematoma expansion, the most important is time to imaging. Given that most hematoma stabilization approaches target early presentations, it is reasonable to estimate that one-third of patients presenting within 6 hours are undergoing active hematoma expansion.

PATHOPHYSIOLOGY

The exact mechanisms that underlie hematoma formation and expansion are complex and not fully clear. Hematoma formation and expansion is a heterogeneous process with multiple events occurring in parallel. Pathological studies and translational models have advanced our understanding of hematoma pathology. The pathophysiologic events of an intracerebral hemorrhage occur in four major phases: vessel rupture, baseline hematoma formation, hematoma expansion, and edema formation (the latter is not a primary focus of this chapter) (22).

The mechanisms leading to vessel rupture vary widely based on pathology. Intracerebral hemorrhage is broadly divided into primary and secondary forms. Primary intracerebral hemorrhages result from changes in cerebral vasculature brought on by hypertension and cerebral amyloid angiopathy. In hypertension, smooth muscle cells can proliferate and undergo necrosis concurrently, resulting in collagen deposition and vessel stiffening. In addition, end vessels exposed to chronically high pressures can also develop Charcot–Bouchard aneurysms. This results in brittle and stiff vessels, which can rupture spontaneously when exposed to high enough pressure (6). In contrast, beta-amyloid deposition in small- and mid-sized cortical blood vessels is the hallmark feature of cerebral amyloid angiopathy. Beta-amyloid deposition results in microaneurysm formations, fibrinoid necrosis, smooth muscle cell replacement, and perivascular leakage. Secondary intracerebral hemorrhages are caused by a variety of pathologies including brain tumors, aneurysms, and vascular malformations (6).

Initial hematoma development is rapid. The forming hematoma faces little counterpressure from the surrounding tissue initially. This is believed to result in the sudden onset of symptoms seen in the majority of clinical cases. As bleeding continues in the hyperacute phase (within the first hour), counterpressure from the tissue increases. Cessation of baseline hematoma formation is believed to occur when the counterpressure from the adjacent brain tissue overcomes the force of the blood leaving the vessel (6). The force at which blood exits a vessel has been found to be especially important in baseline hematoma volume determination. A surrogate measure of force was suggested by Rodriguez-Luna et al. to be baseline hemorrhage volume divided by onset-to-imaging time, termed as ultraearly hematoma growth (23), where rapid ultraearly growth rates were associated with larger final hemorrhage volumes.

Hematoma expansion was originally hypothesized to be caused by a single vessel that bursts, causing the original hemorrhage event, which then continues to bleed, resulting in expansion (3). However, no direct pathological evidence has been found to support this notion, and expansion can occur many hours after an initial bleed event. This makes the concept of a single vessel bursting and then continuing to actively bleed less likely (3,24). Our most current understanding of expansion originates from the pathological studies of hemorrhage by CM Fisher (25). In a seminal publication from 1971, Fisher microscopically examined hemorrhages as a whole. Most notable in his observations was the presence of multiple sites of arterial bleeding located at the periphery of the primary hematoma. These additional sites appeared to be smaller arterioles adjacent to the primary hematoma that were mechanically disrupted, resulting in sources of secondary bleeding. Fisher described these sources of additional bleeding to occur in an "avalanche fashion" (25). Studies have since provided increasing support to Fisher's avalanche theory of hematoma expansion. Hematomas have been observed to change the axial direction of growth over time and are commonly noted to exhibit irregular shapes as they grow and expand (6,26). Even computational models designed to test the avalanche theory were able to reliably recreate models that carried characteristics similar to clinically observed hemorrhage events. These include asymmetric bleed patterns, a bimodal distribution of hematoma volume, and increased final volume in models that were designed to simulate anticoagulation use (27).

Ultimately, hematoma expansion appears to be a heterogeneous process. In addition to flow dynamics discussed previously, numerous biochemical changes are also noted during the acute expansion period. There is evidence of hemostasis pathway dysregulation with plasma protein induction and secondary inflammation related to clotting proteins (2). Blood–brain barrier breakdown has been noted to occur during initial hematoma formation and is of particular importance as several studies have seen an association between resultant perihematomal edema and hematoma growth (22). Using CT perfusion technology, we can now observe an increased permeability in patients undergoing hemorrhagic transformation following acute stroke (28).

Irrespective of the underlying pathophysiology, the goal of hemorrhage treatment has largely been to mitigate expansion, thereby preventing further deterioration and improving outcomes. The priority is to investigate these pathophysiological changes in the context of attempting to identify biomarkers (clinical, biochemical, or radiological) predictive of hematoma expansion. It is the hope that with acute identification of expansion risk factors we can try to mitigate the risk of these various components and ultimately prevent hematoma enlargement.

RADIOLOGICAL PREDICTORS

Given that the diagnosis of intracerebral hemorrhage is confirmed with imaging, the bulk of expansion predictors are radiological. Imaging biomarkers are divided broadly into two categories based on the presence or absence of contrast use. Noncontrast imaging markers involve assessing the characteristics of the hematoma and include baseline volume, margin irregularity, and heterogeneity. Contrast biomarkers are associated with the presence of contrast extravasation during CT angiography (CTA).

Noncontrast Predictors

Volume

Baseline hematoma volume is a consistent predictor of hematoma expansion (3,29–32). Independent of the time to CT and other confounders, large volume hemorrhages are at increased risk of expansion. There is no particular threshold of baseline volume that is predictive of hematoma expansion; however, hemorrhage volumes greater than 10 mL are more likely to expand (29). In contrast, small volume hemorrhages are often stable and less prone to expansion. Hemorrhages with baseline volumes less than 10 mL have a low likelihood of subsequent growth and are associated with good long-term outcomes (30).

Shape and Margin Irregularity

The shape of a hematoma is influenced by the nature of adjacent tissue and potential for secondary vessel rupture. As such, hemorrhage shapes are not necessarily spheroid or ellipsoid. Irregular margins are commonly observed and are associated with hematoma expansion. Fuji et al. (33) first categorized hematoma shape into three broad forms: spherical with smooth margins, irregular shaped with irregular margins, and separated with fluid levels. Hemorrhages with irregular margins were associated with expansion in this study of 419 patients (33). Later work by Barras et al. graded the degree of margin irregularity with a 1 to 5 scale (29). Hemorrhages could range from category 1, smooth with no irregular margins, to category 5, multiple irregular nodularities, with each nodular irregularity increasing the score by 1. Blacquiere et al. used this scale to associate margin irregularity with hematoma expansion (sensitivity: 69% [95% CI: 59–78], specificity 46% [95% CI: 40–53] for grades 4 and 5) (34). It has since been suggested that irregular margins may reflect ongoing secondary vessel rupture and therefore, represent an "intermediate stage of maturity" as the bleed continues to its final volume (35).

Heterogeneity: The Swirl, Black Hole, Blend, Island, and Satellite Signs

As a hemorrhage forms and evolves, it becomes increasingly hyperdense relative to the surrounding tissue. Heterogeneity, a mixture of hypo- and hyperattenuation within a hematoma, is often observed and has been studied extensively (Figure 3.1). First noted during the 1980s in extra-axial hematomas, the "swirl sign" is defined as an area of low attenuation within an extra-axial bleed (i.e., an epidural hematoma) (36). This area of low attenuation, often isoattenuating relative to brain tissue, is thought to represent extravasating blood and correlates with areas of active bleeding seen during surgical evacuations (36). Work by Selariu et al. attempted to adapt the swirl sign to intracerebral hemorrhage patients (37). In a retrospective study of 203 patients, swirl signs were observed in 30%. These individuals had larger baseline hematoma volumes, midline shift, and increased intraventricular involvement. The presence of the swirl sign was an independent predictor of death and poor outcome. Hematoma expansion, however, was not explicitly assessed. A smaller study conducted by Kim et al. in 2008 did not find an association between swirl sign and expansion (38).

In 2016, Li et al. introduced the "black hole" sign (39) is described as a region of relative hypoattenuation that is encapsulated within the hematoma and does not connect with adjacent brain tissue. In an attempt to create a degree of objectivity to hematoma heterogeneity, the authors stipulated that a Hounsfield difference of greater

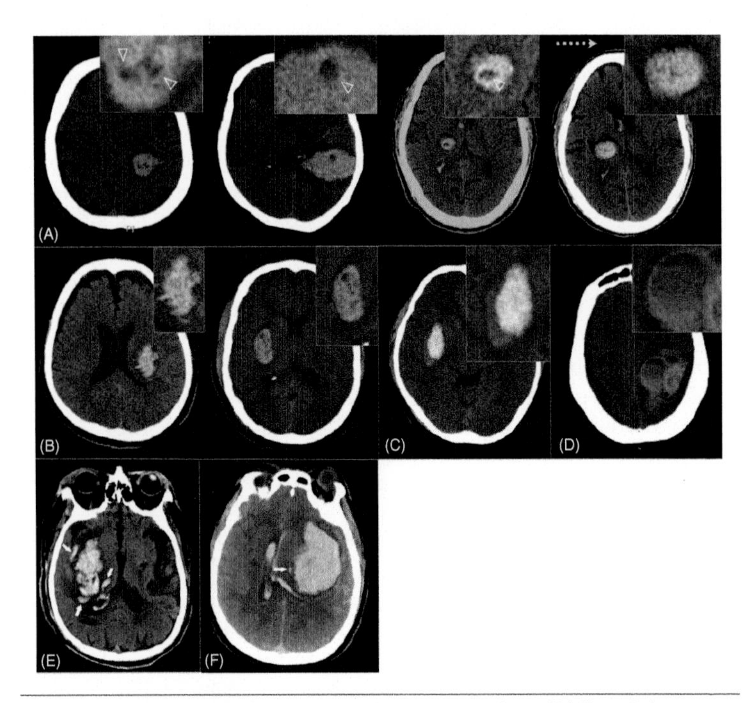

Figure 3.1 Multipanel of noncontrast hemorrhage signs. (A) From left to right, swirl sign, black hole sign, and a central hypodensity demonstrating significant expansion on repeat CT. (B) Hemorrhage with irregular margins and hemorrhage with heterogeneous density. (C) Blend sign. (D) Fluid level. (E) Island Sign. (F) Satellite Sign.

Source: From Boulouis G, Morotti A, Brouwers HB, et al. Noncontrast computed tomography hypodensities predict poor outcome in intracerebral hemorrhage patients. *Stroke.* 2016;47(10):2511–2516. doi:10.1161/STROKEAHA.116.014425 (Panels A-D); Li Q, Liu QJ, Yang WS, et al. Island sign: an imaging predictor for early hematoma expansion and poor outcome in patients with intracerebral hemorrhage. *Stroke.* 2017;48(11):3019–3025. doi:10.1161/STROKEAHA.117.017985 (Panel E); Yu Z, Zheng J, Ali H, et al. Significance of satellite sign and spot sign in predicting hematoma expansion in spontaneous intracerebral hemorrhage. *Clin Neurol Neurosurg.* 2017;162:67–71. doi:10.1016/j.clineuro.2017.09.008 (Panel F).

than 28 units be observed between the region of hypoattenuation and the rest of the hematoma. In a single center, prospective study (n = 206), the black hole sign was observed in 30 patients. Similar to the swirl sign, the black hole sign was associated with larger baseline volumes and was independently associated with expansion (>12.5 mL or >33%) when adjusted for baseline volume and time to CT (39). The same authors have also looked at hypoattenuation surrounding a hematoma and adjacent to brain tissue. This concept, termed the "blend sign," is seen in approximately 17% of hemorrhage patients and was independently associated with hematoma expansion in a retrospective analysis of 172 patients that adjusted for baseline volume and time to CT (40). In the past year, two signs based on the presence of smaller hemorrhages adjacent to the primary hematoma have been developed: island sign, defined as ≥3 (when completely separate) or ≥4 (when some or all are linked) smaller bleeds scattered adjacently to the primary hematoma (41), and satellite sign, defined as a single smaller hemorrhage (diameter <10 mm) located 1 to 20 mm from the primary hematoma (42).

There are a limited number of direct head-to-head comparisons between the patterns of heterogeneity described earlier. Sporns et al. compared blend and black hole signs to each other and to spot sign in a single center retrospective cohort study (43). Predicting for poor outcome (mRS 4–6 at time of discharge), both signs reported low sensitivities, high specificities, and high positive predictive values. All three signs were predictive of poor outcome in univariate analysis; however, both heterogeneous markers were not statistically significant in logistic regression (43). Further comparisons have largely been with spot sign specifically. In separate retrospective cohorts, blend sign and satellite sign were predictive of hematoma expansion, even after adjusting for spot sign. In both these studies however, spot sign was found to be more accurate and had greater predictability overall (44,45).

Although each sign shows individual promise, the baseline prevalence is highly variable, and the replication of findings has not been consistent (Table 3.3) (35,46,47). Predictive scores have not yet implemented heterogeneity into their respective models due to a lack of standardization and arguably, difficulty in implementation given the precise definitions used in each sign. This creates the argument that rather than specific signs, perhaps the presence or absence of heterogeneity in any form is sufficient to predict expansion (35). Work by Boulouis et al. assessed this concept in a large cohort of 1,029 patients (30). Heterogeneity, simply defined as observing hypoattenuation and/or fluid levels within a hematoma, was observed in 28.3% of a developmental cohort (n = 784) and 40.4% of a replication cohort (n = 245). More than 50% of patients with hypoattenuation were associated with hematoma expansion and independent of baseline volume, time to CT, warfarin use, and spot sign (adjusted odds ratio [aOR] 3.42 [2.21–5.31]).

Table 3.3 Predictive Capabilities of Noncontrast Imaging Signs

	Definition	Sensitivity (%)	Specificity (%)	PPV (%)	NPV (%)	aOR	95% CI
Black Hole Sign							
Li et al. (39)	>33% or >12.5 mL	31.9	94.1	73.3	73.2	4.12	1.44–11.77
Yu et al. (46)	>33% or >12.5 mL	43.75	84.54	42.28	82.00	4.09	1.52–11.00
Blend Sign							
Li et al. (40)	>33% or >12.5 mL	39.3	95.5	82.7	74.1	20.23	5.13–79.77
Zheng et al. (44)	>33% or >12.5 mL	42.86	88.51	54.55	82.80	6.50	1.89–22.33
Island Sign							
Li et al. (41)	>33% or >6 mL	44.7	98.2	92.7	77.7	31.89	8.67–117.29
Satellite Sign							
Yu et al. (45)	>33% or >12.5 mL	59.46	68.97	37.93	84.21	3.75	1.28–11.05

aOR, adjusted odds ratio; CI, confidence interval; NPV, negative predictive value; PPV, positive predictive value.

Overall, baseline volume, margin irregularity, and hematoma heterogeneity are all strongly associated and recognized predictors of expansion. Both baseline volume and hematoma hypodensity have been recently incorporated into expansion scores; such expansion scores have the potential for use as clinical prediction rules in emerging clinical trials.

Contrast Predictors

Contrast manifests in intracerebral hemorrhage as an area of hyperdensity seen within a hematoma during CTA (48). It is hypothesized that the presence of these hyperdensities is representative of contrast extravasation from blood vessels and may represent ongoing bleeding (49).

The original concept of contrast extravasating from blood vessels during an acute hemorrhage was first observed in formal angiography studies throughout the 1970s and early 1990s (50). Becker et al. and Murai et al. were the first to investigate the use of iodinated contrast in hemorrhage and found an association between contrast hyperdensity presence and mortality (51,52). With CTA gaining prominence in clinical practice, Goldstein et al. and Kim et al. noted an association between contrast presence and hematoma expansion (38,50). Subsequent studies have had similar findings, albeit each of these studies used differing descriptions and definitions of contrast presence (48). The term "spot sign" was first introduced by Wada et al. in 2007. Spot sign is formally defined as "1 or more 1- to 2-mm foci of enhancement within the hematoma on CTA source images" (53). Subsequent studies have adopted Wada's definition and spot sign was formally tested in the PREDICT observational cohort study (54) (Figure 3.2). Looking at patients presenting less than 6 hours from multiple centers, patients were provided baseline CT, CTA, follow-up imaging at 24 hours, and clinical follow-up at 90 days. Adjusting for relevant covariates, spot sign was found to be independently predictive of hematoma expansion (defined in this case as >6 mL or >33%). PREDICT reported a sensitivity and specificity of 51% (39–63) and 85% (78–90), respectively. An association between spot sign and mortality was also observed (54). Spot sign has since become the dominant representation of contrast extravasation.

Subsequent studies have since focused on better understanding the properties of spot sign and increasing the sensitivity/specificity and predictive values of this biomarker. Small hemorrhages are less likely to be spot sign positive (55). A higher rate of contrast extravasation is associated with a higher degree of hematoma

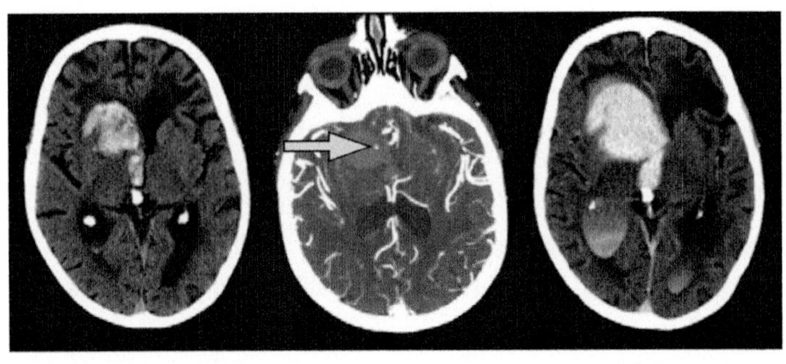

Baseline noncontrast CT (total hematoma volume 19.6 mL) | Baseline CTA (single spot sign positive) | 24 h follow-up noncontrast CT (total hematoma volume 110.8 mL)

Figure 3.2 Spot sign on CT angiography in a patient with intracerebral hemorrhage. The spot sign (arrow) has a density of 173 Hounsfield units. The spot sign is located within the hematoma. There is no connection to any outside vessel.

CTA, CT angiography.

Source: From Demchuk AM, Dowlatshahi D, Rodriguez-Luna D, et al. Prediction of haematoma growth and outcome in patients with intracerebral haemorrhage using the CT-angiography spot sign (PREDICT): a prospective observational study. *Lancet Neurol.* 2012;11(4):307–314. doi:10.1016/S1474-4422(12)70038-8 (Panel).

expansion (56). Increasing CT tube current improves the accuracy of the spot sign, and perhaps most important, the timing of CTA has also emerged as a major factor in increasing the sensitivity of spot sign. The majority of initial contrast biomarker studies, including PREDICT, used first-pass CTA technology. These studies had an overall sensitivity and specificity of 53% (95% CI: 49–57) and 88% (95% CI: 86–89), respectively (48). When combined with other CT imaging modalities, such as postcontrast CT and dynamic CTA, a pooled meta-analysis showed increases in the sensitivity (73% [95% CI: 67–79]) (48). Further studies have shown that performing a "delayed CTA," a second CTA, 90 seconds following the first-pass scan, could also increase the sensitivity of spot signs (57). The degree of delay has been tested up to 5 minutes ("the leakage sign") and continue to show increases in sensitivity/specificity (58). However, while the frequency of spot sign can be improved with dynamic and delayed imaging, this does not always correlate with significant hematoma expansion. An assessment of spot sign acquisition during arterial and venous phases showed that while the spot sign was more frequently seen in the venous phase, total hematoma enlargement was significantly larger in patients who were spot sign positive during the arterial phase of imaging acquisition (59).

Radiological markers appear to be very promising as predictors of hematoma expansion. However, clinical variables, such as concomitant antithrombotic use and time of presentation, also play a role in influencing expansion. These factors have been extensively explored in an attempt to develop better predictive models.

CLINICAL PREDICTORS

As previously noted, initial definition studies commented on an association between early time to CT and hematoma expansion. This finding has since been reported in numerous observation and intervention studies (55,60–62). The time to CT is one of the most consistently associated clinical predictors of expansion (60,63,64). Anticoagulant use, in particular warfarin, is another clinical factor strongly associated with hematoma expansion (21,62).

Studies looking at additional clinical markers have yielded inconsistent findings. Baseline Glasgow Coma Scale (GCS), National Institutes of Health Stroke Scale (NIHSS) scores, C-reactive protein (CRP), D-dimer, and increased serum creatinine have all been linked with expansion, albeit replication of these findings is limited and conflicting (2,63,65). Associations between reduced platelet activity and expansion have been observed in a single center prospective study (66); however, links between the use of antiplatelet drugs and expansion are conflicting (62,67).

The relationships between blood pressure and hemorrhage are intuitive and have been studied extensively. Patients with an acute hemorrhage often exhibit an increased blood pressure on presentation to the emergency room. There is concern that increased blood pressure may increase the risk of hematoma expansion. Studies in which patients had serial blood pressure measurements found associations between maximal systolic pressure and expansion (68). Furthermore, findings from the SAMURAI-ICH (69) study show that patients with elevated blood pressure, even after antihypertensive treatment, have an increased risk of poor long-term outcome. However, associations between blood pressure and expansion are present in some studies but absent in others. This is likely due to the confounding elements of treatment and the inherent difficulty of recording blood pressure in observational studies when the assessment of blood pressure is not the primary goal. Ultimately, while observational studies have shown links between blood pressure and expansion, subsequent intervention studies have not shown causation (70,71).

GENETIC PREDICTORS

The understanding of the potential links between our genetics and the predisposition for hemorrhage and expansion is limited, but several associations have been observed. In 2012, Brouwers et al. identified certain alleles of the apolipoprotein E (APOE) genotype as a potentially new risk factor for hematoma expansion (72). The APOE genotype, well known for its involvement in Alzheimer's disease comes in three forms: ε2, ε3, and ε4. The ε3 allele is seen in 50% to 90% of the population. Variants ε2 and ε4 are seen in 1% to 5% and 5% to 35%, respectively. Based on pathological studies, the ε4 allele increases amyloid deposition within cerebral vasculature (73). The ε2 allele induces vasculopathic changes that increase the risk of vessel rupture and may also be associated with local coagulation inhibition. Hence, it was postulated that ε2 allele carriers may carry an increased risk of intracerebral hemorrhage and hematoma expansion (73).

In a single center, retrospective study of hemorrhage patients greater than 55 years, Brouwers et al. showed an association between hematoma expansion in lobar hemorrhage and APOE ε2 (72). An increased number of copies of the ε2 allele gene increased the risk of bleeding. The presence of spot sign was also associated with APOE ε2 (74). A subgroup analysis of patients categorized as having probable or definite cerebral amyloid angiopathy (based on the Boston criteria) also showed an association between expansion and ε2. The applicability of the work by Brouwers et al., however, is limited as the study of the APOE genotype included only those of European ancestry and was retrospective. Nevertheless, it is a compelling finding that may help further our understanding of the underlying pathophysiology of hematoma expansion.

MANAGEMENT

There is no widely accepted therapy for intracerebral hemorrhage. Treatment is largely supportive, and outcomes are often poor. In contrast to ischemic stroke, where therapies can reverse ongoing ischemia, the primary event of blood extravasation from a vessel cannot be reversed. Treatment is therefore aimed toward preventing further clinical worsening, and hematoma expansion has become a major target of ongoing trials. Management options are varied and diverse, ranging from blood pressure control to the use of hemostatic agents such as factor VIIa and tranexamic acid. Attempts at mitigating hematoma expansion have yielded conflicting results thus far. The majority of options described in the following are still under ongoing study.

Blood Pressure Control

Increases in blood pressure are often observed during the acute presentation of intracerebral hemorrhage. These increases are thought to worsen hematoma expansion and clinical outcomes. As such, there is active investigation into whether acute blood pressure lowering may limit expansion and effectively "turn off the tap." The INTERACT study was the first randomized controlled trial to assess blood pressure management in the context of acute hemorrhage (70). Patients with elevated systolic pressures ranging from 150 to 220 mmHg were randomized to either intensive (target systolic <140) or consensus guided (<180 mmHg) blood pressure reduction. Agents used in this study include: urapidil, nimodipine, nicardipine, labetalol, nitroglycerin, furosemide, hydralazine, and nitroprusside. Intensive blood pressure reduction was associated with decreases in proportional hemorrhage growth; however, these findings were not statistically significant when adjusted for baseline hemorrhage volume or time to CT (70). A follow-up study of the INTERACT cohort showed that intensive blood pressure reduction was significant in those with an earlier time to randomization. That is, early blood pressure reduction within 3 hours was effective in reducing hemorrhage growth (75). A subsequent study (INTERACT-2) did not show statistically significant differences in death between intensive and traditional treatment arms; however, a reduction in disability was seen in the intensive treatment arm (76). Although not statistically significant by our conventional standards, the reduction in death trended favorably toward intensive management (odds ratio [OR] 0.87 [95% CI: 0.75–1.01], $p = .06$). Furthermore, due to the logistics of trial enrollment, the median time from symptom onset to achieving target blood pressure was in excess of 6 hours, which likely missed the optimal timeline to mitigate hematoma expansion.

A parallel series of studies (ATACH/ATACH-2) also assessed intensive (target range: 110–139 mmHg) versus consensus (target range: 140–179 mmHg) guided blood pressure management in patients presenting under 4.5 hours from symptom onset, particularly with the use of nicardipine (77,78). The chief findings of ATACH-2 were similar to that of INTERACT-2: intensive blood pressure reduction did not prevent death (aOR 1.04 [95% CI: 0.85–1.27], $p = .84$) or hematoma expansion (aOR 0.78 [95% CI: 0.58–1.03], $p = .08$) to a significant degree. When adjusted for age, baseline GCS, and intraventricular hemorrhage, patients treated intensively reported a higher rate of adverse outcomes (aOR: 1.3 [95% CI: 1.00–1.69], $p = .05$) (78). Of note, patients in both arms exhibited large reductions in systolic pressure, more than expected. In the intensive arm, patients had a mean systolic pressure of 128.9 ± 16 mmHg by 2 hours while those in the conventional arm had a mean systolic pressure of 141.1 ± 14.8 mmHg. In effect, the "control" arm of ATACH-2 was comparable to the "intensive" arm of INTERACT-2. So while the study was ultimately negative for the primary and secondary outcomes, the reason for this may be due to the fact that the intended comparisons could not be actually made, and the results may reflect a type II error.

There is also ongoing debate regarding the effects that aggressive blood pressure management can have on cerebral perfusion pressure. The concern is that aggressive blood pressure lowering can inadvertently lower cerebral perfusion pressure resulting in potential ischemia. While initial studies assessing cerebral blood flow have found no major relationships with intensive blood pressure reduction, further investigations are ongoing (79,80). At this time, the evidence for aggressive blood pressure reduction is mixed. We would thereby encourage a graded approach of reduction based on the systolic blood pressure seen on presentation. It is likely safe to reduce systolic pressures between 140 and 180 mmHg to a target of less than 140 mmHg acutely. Systolic pressures greater than 180 mmHg warrant reduction, but individuals may want to consider an interim reduction target of less than 160 mmHg within the first 24 hours, followed by targeting less than 140 mmHg by 48 hours.

Anticoagulant Reversal

Spontaneous hemorrhage associated with anticoagulants is at a markedly elevated risk of mortality (21). Anticoagulant hemorrhages are larger at baseline and inherently more prone to expansion (81). Reversing the effects of anticoagulation is critical and is shown to have a positive effect on outcomes if performed acutely (82).

The rapid reversal of warfarin involves the use of multiple agents such as vitamin K, fresh frozen plasma, and prothrombin complex concentrate (83). Vitamin K activates the coagulation cascade and through this process is converted to an oxidized form (84). Warfarin prevents the conversion of oxidized vitamin K back to its reduced form and thus, any further activation of the coagulation pathway through the vitamin. Administering high doses of vitamin K (5–10 mg, slow intravenous [IV] administration to reduce risk of anaphylaxis) results in the reversal of this effect. However, full international normalized ratio (INR) correction can take 6 to 24 hours (84). As such, secondary agents that can quickly reverse INR transiently, such as fresh frozen plasma and prothrombin complex concentrates, are often coadministered alongside vitamin K (81,84). Fresh frozen plasma is affordable and widely used in clinical practice; however, each dose can take up to an hour to administer. Because approximately eight doses are required for anticoagulation reversal, the window to prevent hematoma expansion can be missed (85). Prothrombin complex concentrate is made up of factors II, VII, IX, X (4-factor variant has more factor VII compared to 3-factor), protein C and S, and low amounts of heparin (86). Prothrombin complex concentrates can rapidly reverse INR within 15 minutes of administration but are significantly more expensive and may be less available (83,87). A comparison between fresh frozen plasma and 4-factor prothrombin complex concentrates in patients presenting with warfarin associated hemorrhage (INCH trial, n = 50) showed significantly faster reversals of INR (INR <1.2 within 3 hours: 9% vs. 67%, $p < .0003$) and reduced hematoma expansion (mean expansion at 24 hours: 22.1 mL vs. 8.3 mL, $p < .018$) in the prothrombin concentrate cohort (88). When available, we recommend the use of prothrombin complex concentrate with vitamin K in the reversal of warfarin associated hemorrhage.

The use of direct oral anticoagulants, such as dabigatran, apixaban, and rivaroxaban, continues to increase due to their relative ease of use and reduced side effect profiles (89–91). Treatment options vary on the anticoagulant.

Idarucizumab (Praxbind, Boehringer Ingelheim) is a monoclonal antibody fragment that binds specifically to dabigatran. Rapid reversal of anticoagulant activity occurs within minutes of administration (92,93). The drug is traditionally administered in two doses, albeit the REVERSE-AD study showed that a single 5 g dose was adequate in 98% of treated patients (92). If unavailable, alternatives include activated prothrombin complex concentrate (FEIBA) or 4-factor prothrombin complex concentrate. If the medication is taken within 2 hours of hemorrhage development, oral activated charcoal can also be used to prevent any further absorption from the gastrointestinal tract (94). In contrast to dabigatran, specific reversal antidotes are not yet currently available for apixaban or rivaroxaban. In these scenarios, 4-factor prothrombin complex concentrates can be used, and oral activated charcoal is also an option (apixaban: within 6 hours, rivaroxaban: within 8 hours) (95). A reversal agent for direct Xa inhibitors, andexanet alfa (Portola Pharmaceuticals), is currently in development (96). The use of recombinant factor VIIa is not recommended for the correction of anticoagulant-related hemorrhage.

Antiplatelet Reversal

As highlighted before, the effects of antiplatelet therapy on hemorrhage growth are unclear. The need to reverse antiplatelet effect via platelet transfusion was evaluated through the PATCH trial (97). Patients (n = 190) presenting with hemorrhage under 6 hours and either on acetyl salicylic acid (ASA), clopidogrel, or dipyridamole were randomized to platelet transfusion or the standard of care. No major benefits in either clinical outcome or hemorrhage growth were seen in the platelet transfusion group. In fact, those given a platelet transfusion had poorer outcomes compared to controls. The exact reasons for this finding are not clear. As such, reversal of antiplatelet therapy through transfusion is not recommended. Desmopressin has shown potential as a therapeutic agent in hemorrhage patients with reduced platelet activity by increasing the release of von Willebrand factor (98). While some studies have found desmopressin to be successful in correcting platelet activity and reducing the extent of hematoma growth (98), others have found no significant benefit (99). Further study is required before this approach can be recommended.

Recombinant Factor VIIA

Factor VII acts at the sites of vascular rupture and endothelial damage to induce hemostasis (100). It binds with exposed tissue factor to convert factor X to its active form, accelerating the formation of a downstream fibrin clot (101). Approximately 1% of factor VII that circulates within the body is in its active form (101). Recombinant factor VIIa (NovoSeven, Novo Nordisk) is thought to increase the activity of the exposed tissue-factor coagulation pathway. It is delivered as a single IV dose given over 2 minutes. Originally developed for the treatment of hemophilia, the off-label use of recombinant factor VIIa has grown and includes the treatment of von Willebrand disease, perioperative blood loss, and acute intracerebral hemorrhage (102,103). The risk of thromboembolism is the primary safety concern with the majority of reported thrombotic risks associated with the drug's off-label uses. The drug is tolerated well in hemophilia populations, who at baseline are often younger and possess less cardiovascular risk factors.

A phase II trial by Mayer et al. was the first major evaluation of recombinant factor VIIa and intracerebral hemorrhage (103). A double-blind randomized controlled trial with four treatment arms, patients presenting with hemorrhage under 3 hours, were randomized to placebo, 40, 80, or 160 mcg/kg doses of treatment drug. Nonsignificant reductions in hematoma volume were observed in the 40 and 80 mcg/kg treatment arms. A treating dose of 160 mcg/kg had a significant reduction in hematoma growth compared to placebo (mean absolute increase of 2.9 mL, 98.3% CI: –0.8–6.6, $p < .008$) (103). Both 80 and 160 mcg/kg treatment arms also reported an increased number of favorable outcomes (mRS 0–3; 80 mcg/kg: 51% vs. 31%, $p = .008$; 160 mcg/kg: 46% vs. 31%, $p = .02$). However, arterial thrombotic events (stroke, myocardial infarction) were significantly more frequent in the intervention arms. A pooled analysis of dose escalation and placebo-controlled trials indicated that the increased risk of arterial events was associated primarily with higher doses of the medication (120 and 160 mcg/kg) (102). Lower doses were therefore selected in a subsequent phase III trial.

The FAST trial was a placebo-controlled trial with factor VIIa 20 and 80 mcg/kg treatment arms. Although the 80 mcg/kg treatment arm was associated with a significant reduction in hematoma growth, no improvements in long-term outcome were observed. Again, thrombotic events were significantly higher in the intervention arms compared to placebo (104). However, subanalysis of FAST did provide evidence that a certain subgroup of patients, those presenting under 70 years, with onset-to-treatment times under 2.5 hours and with baseline intracerebral and intraventricular volumes less than 60 and 5 mL, respectively, benefited from 80 mcg/kg factor VIIa treatment (105). These findings were replicated in the phase II data and have led to the argument that proper patient selection is crucial to treatment success. The current thought is that only a proportion of patients with intracerebral hemorrhage will benefit from treatment, but all hemorrhage patients are at risk of potential harm. As such, the positive effect of treatment was effectively diluted in the FAST trial, but improved patient selection could prevent this issue in the future. The SPOTLIGHT (NCT01359202) and STOP-IT (NCT00810888) trials attempted to improve patient selection by using the spot sign as a way of identifying patients most at risk of hematoma expansion. In both studies patients presenting under 6 hours with hemorrhage and a positive spot sign were randomized to 80 mcg/kg or placebo. Due to difficulties with patient recruitment, both trials pooled their data together. A pooled analysis of SPOTLIGHT/STOP-IT showed no significant reduction in hematoma growth (presented at the International Stroke Conference 2017, Houston, Texas). Further details are forthcoming as at the time of writing, the pooled analysis of SPOTLIGHT/STOP-IT has not been published (115). Citing a mixed degree of benefit and ongoing thromboembolic risk, recombinant factor VIIa is not presently recommended for the treatment of intracerebral hemorrhage.

Tranexamic Acid

Tranexamic acid is a synthetic derivative of lysine. First developed in the 1960s, it is used extensively in a variety of surgical and trauma environments to reduce active bleeding (106). It acts by blocking native lysine binding sites on plasminogen, preventing fibrinolysis in the process. The drug has an estimated half-life of 80 minutes with 90% clearance by 24 hours (106). Tranexamic acid does cross the placenta, albeit no teratogenic effects have been identified. The drug can be delivered intravenously or orally with peak concentrations at 1 and 3 hours, respectively (106). Dosing of tranexamic acid varies on the clinical context.

Its wide use in a varying number of clinical scenarios can be attributed to its overall effectiveness and low thrombogenic side effect profile. The CRASH-2 trial (n = 20,211) demonstrated both reduced bleeding deaths and vascular occlusive events (myocardial infarction, stroke) in acute trauma patients given tranexamic acid compared against placebo (107). A meta-analysis of orthopedic surgeries showed no increased incidence of venous-thromboembolism and a separate meta-analysis of spinal surgeries (n = 411) showed reduced bleeding with no episodes of thromboembolism (106).

There is intense interest in tranexamic acid and its potential use in intracranial hemorrhage. A nested study within the CRASH-2 cohort focused on traumatic brain injury patients with intracerebral hemorrhage (108). In 270 patients, mean total hemorrhage growth was reduced in the tranexamic acid cohort compared to placebo (5.9 mL vs. 8.1 mL, $p = .33$). A second study in brain injury patients also showed a nonsignificant reduction in hemorrhage growth (109). A pilot trial evaluating the feasibility of tranexamic acid in primary intracerebral hemorrhage was performed by Sprigg et al. (110) in 2011 that led to the development of TICH-2, a double-blind randomized control trial evaluating tranexamic acid against placebo in patients presenting under 8 hours (111). In a study population of 2,325 patients, tranexamic acid was found to significantly reduce hematoma expansion (>6 mL or >33%, adjusted binary OR 0.88 [0.66-0.98]). However, no benefit to functional outcome was observed. It remains to be seen if the subset of patients presenting early in this trial experienced a clinical benefit (116). The STOP-AUST trial is actively recruiting to evaluate the efficacy of tranexamic acid versus placebo, focusing on hemorrhage patients presenting under 4.5 hours who are also spot sign positive (112). Within China, active recruitment is ongoing for the TRAIGE trial, a placebo-controlled randomized trial looking at spot sign positive patients presenting under 8 hours (113). All three trials are dosing tranexamic acid in two phases: (a) a loading dose of 1 g given over 10 to 30 minutes and (b) a second 1 g dose delivered as an infusion over 8 hours, similar to that used in CRASH-2 (107,108,111–113).

CONCLUSION

Hematoma expansion is a dynamic process and a potential target for therapeutic intervention. Our understanding of its pathophysiology remains limited with unanswered fundamental questions in terms of how we define and predict it. Numerous clinical and radiological variables are associated with expansion and offer the opportunity to develop clinical prediction rules. Such prediction rules and risk scores will help risk-stratify patients for clinical trials and may eventually help guide clinical management.

REFERENCES

1. Qureshi AI, Mendelow AD, Hanley DF. Intracerebral haemorrhage. *Lancet (London, England)*. 2009;373(9675):1632–1644. doi:10.1016/S0140-6736(09)60371-8
2. Balami JS, Buchan AM. Complications of intracerebral haemorrhage. *Lancet Neurol*. 2012;11(1):101–118. doi:10.1016/S1474-4422(11)70264-2
3. Brouwers HB, Greenberg SM. Hematoma expansion following acute intracerebral hemorrhage. *Cerebrovasc Dis*. 2013;35(3):195–201. doi:10.1159/000346599
4. van Asch CJ, Luitse MJ, Rinkel GJ, et al. Incidence, case fatality, and functional outcome of intracerebral haemorrhage over time, according to age, sex, and ethnic origin: a systematic review and meta-analysis. *Lancet Neurol*. 2010;9(2):167–176. doi:10.1016/S1474-4422(09)70340-0
5. Gokhale S, Caplan LR, James ML. Sex differences in incidence, pathophysiology, and outcome of primary intracerebral hemorrhage. *Stroke*. 2015;46(3):886–892. doi:10.1161/STROKEAHA.114.007682
6. Schlunk F, Greenberg SM. The pathophysiology of intracerebral hemorrhage formation and expansion. *Transl Stroke Res*. 2015;6(4):257–263. doi:10.1007/s12975-015-0410-1
7. Ovesen C, Christensen AF, Havsteen I, et al. Prediction and prognostication of neurological deterioration in patients with acute ICH: a hospital-based cohort study. *BMJ Open*. 2015;5(7):e008563. doi:10.1136/bmjopen-2015-008563
8. Fan J-S, Huang H-H, Chen Y-C, et al. Emergency department neurologic deterioration in patients with spontaneous intracerebral hemorrhage: incidence, predictors, and prognostic significance. *Acad Emerg Med*. 2012;19(2):133–138. doi:10.1111/j.1553-2712.2011.01285.x

9. Leira R, Dávalos A, Silva Y, et al. Early neurologic deterioration in intracerebral hemorrhage: predictors and associated factors. *Neurology*. 2004;63(3):461–467. http://www.ncbi.nlm.nih.gov/pubmed/15304576
10. Yogendrakumar V, Smith EE, Demchuk AM, et al. Lack of early improvement predicts poor outcome following acute intracerebral hemorrhage. *Crit Care Med*. 2018;46:e310–e317. doi:10.1097/CCM.0000000000002962
11. Kazui S, Naritomi H, Yamamoto H, et al. Enlargement of spontaneous intracerebral hemorrhage. Incidence and time course. *Stroke*. 1996;27(10):1783–1787. http://www.ncbi.nlm.nih.gov/pubmed/8841330
12. Newman GC. Clarification of abc/2 rule for ICH volume. *Stroke*. 2007;38(3):862. doi:10.1161/01.STR.0000257309.50643.0a
13. Brott T, Broderick J, Kothari R, et al. Early hemorrhage growth in patients with intracerebral hemorrhage. *Stroke*. 1997;28(1):1–5. http://www.ncbi.nlm.nih.gov/pubmed/8996478
14. Dowlatshahi D, Demchuk AM, Flaherty ML, et al. Defining hematoma expansion in intracerebral hemorrhage: relationship with patient outcomes. *Neurology*. 2011;76(14):1238–1244. doi:10.1212/WNL.0b013e3182143317
15. Chang EF, Meeker M, Holland MC. Acute traumatic intraparenchymal hemorrhage: risk factors for progression in the early post-injury period. *Neurosurgery*. 2006;58(4):647–656. doi:10.1227/01.NEU.0000197101.68538.E6
16. Delcourt C, Huang Y, Arima H, et al. Hematoma growth and outcomes in intracerebral hemorrhage: the INTERACT1 study. *Neurology*. 2012;79(4):314–319. doi:10.1212/WNL.0b013e318260cbba
17. Davis SM, Broderick J, Hennerici M, et al. Hematoma growth is a determinant of mortality and poor outcome after intracerebral hemorrhage. *Neurology*. 2006;66(8):1175–1181. doi:10.1212/01.wnl.0000208408.98482.99
18. Rodriguez-Luna D, Boyko M, Subramaniam S, et al. Magnitude of hematoma volume measurement error in intracerebral hemorrhage. *Stroke*. 2016;47(4):1124–1126. doi:10.1161/STROKEAHA.115.012170
19. Kosior JC, Idris S, Dowlatshahi D, et al. Quantomo: validation of a computer-assisted methodology for the volumetric analysis of intracerebral haemorrhage. *Int J Stroke*. 2011;6(4):302–305. doi:10.1111/j.1747-4949.2010.00579.x
20. Ovesen C, Christensen AF, Krieger DW, et al. Time course of early postadmission hematoma expansion in spontaneous intracerebral hemorrhage. *Stroke*. 2014;45(4):994–999. doi:10.1161/STROKEAHA.113.003608
21. Flibotte JJ, Hagan N, O'Donnell J, et al. Warfarin, hematoma expansion, and outcome of intracerebral hemorrhage. *Neurology*. 2004;63(6):1059–1064. http://www.ncbi.nlm.nih.gov/pubmed/15452298
22. Lim-Hing K, Rincon F. Secondary hematoma expansion and perihemorrhagic edema after intracerebral hemorrhage: from bench work to practical aspects. *Front Neurol*. 2017;8:74. doi:10.3389/fneur.2017.00074

23. Rodriguez-Luna D, Rubiera M, Ribo M, et al. Ultraearly hematoma growth predicts poor outcome after acute intracerebral hemorrhage. *Neurology*.2011;77(17):1599–1604.doi:10.1212/WNL.0b013e3182343387
24. Brouwers HB, Falcone GJ, McNamara KA, et al. CTA spot sign predicts hematoma expansion in patients with delayed presentation after intracerebral hemorrhage. *Neurocrit Care*. 2012;17(3):421–428. doi:10.1007/s12028-012-9765-2
25. Fisher CM. Pathological observations in hypertensive cerebral hemorrhage. *J Neuropathol Exp Neurol*. 1971;30(3):536–550. http://www.ncbi.nlm.nih.gov/pubmed/4105427
26. Greenberg SM, Nandigam RNK, Delgado P, et al. Microbleeds versus macrobleeds: evidence for distinct entities. *Stroke*. 2009;40(7):2382–2386. doi:10.1161/STROKEAHA.109.548974
27. Greenberg CH, Frosch MP, Goldstein JN, et al. Modeling intracerebral hemorrhage growth and response to anticoagulation. *PLoS One*. 2012;7(10):e48458. doi:10.1371/journal.pone.0048458
28. Aviv RI, D'Esterre CD, Murphy BD, et al. Hemorrhagic transformation of ischemic stroke: prediction with CT perfusion. *Radiology*. 2009;250(3):867–877. doi:10.1148/radiol.2503080257
29. Barras CD, Tress BM, Christensen S, et al. Density and shape as CT predictors of intracerebral hemorrhage growth. *Stroke*. 2009;40(4):1325–1331. doi:10.1161/STROKEAHA.108.536888
30. Boulouis G, Morotti A, Brouwers HB, et al. Noncontrast computed tomography hypodensities predict poor outcome in intracerebral hemorrhage patients. *Stroke*. 2016;47(10):2511–2516. doi:10.1161/STROKEAHA.116.014425
31. Dowlatshahi D, Smith EE, Flaherty ML, et al. Small intracerebral haemorrhages are associated with less haematoma expansion and better outcomes. *Int J Stroke*. 2011;6(3):201–206. doi:10.1111/j.1747-4949.2010.00563.x
32. Broderick JP, Brott TG, Duldner JE, et al. Volume of intracerebral hemorrhage. A powerful and easy-to-use predictor of 30-day mortality. *Stroke*. 1993;24(7):987–993.
33. Fujii Y, Tanaka R, Takeuchi S, et al. Hematoma enlargement in spontaneous intracerebral hemorrhage. *J Neurosurg*. 1994;80(1):51–57. doi:10.3171/jns.1994.80.1.0051
34. Blacquiere D, Demchuk AM, Al-Hazzaa M, et al. Intracerebral hematoma morphologic appearance on noncontrast computed tomography predicts significant hematoma expansion. *Stroke*. 2015;46(11):3111–3116. doi:10.1161/STROKEAHA.115.010566
35. Boulouis G, Morotti A, Charidimou A, et al. Noncontrast computed tomography markers of intracerebral hemorrhage expansion. *Stroke*. 2017;48(4):1120–1125. doi:10.1161/STROKEAHA.116.015062
36. Al-Nakshabandi NA. The swirl sign. *Radiology*. 2001;218(2):433. doi:10.1148/radiology.218.2.r01fe09433

37. Selariu E, Zia E, Brizzi M, et al. Swirl sign in intracerebral haemorrhage: definition, prevalence, reliability and prognostic value. *BMC Neurol.* 2012;12(1):109. doi:10.1186/1471-2377-12-109
38. Kim J, Smith A, Hemphill JC, et al. Contrast extravasation on CT predicts mortality in primary intracerebral hemorrhage. *Am J Neuroradiol.* 2008;29:520–525. doi:10.3174/ajnr.A0859
39. Li Q, Zhang G, Xiong X, et al. Black hole sign: novel imaging marker that predicts hematoma growth in patients with intracerebral hemorrhage. *Stroke.* 2016;47(7):1777–1781. doi:10.1161/STROKEAHA.116.013186
40. Li Q, Zhang G, Huang Y-J, et al. Blend sign on computed tomography: novel and reliable predictor for early hematoma growth in patients with intracerebral hemorrhage. *Stroke.* 2015;46(8):2119–2123. doi:10.1161/STROKEAHA.115.009185
41. Li Q, Liu Q-J, Yang W-S, et al. Island sign: an imaging predictor for early hematoma expansion and poor outcome in patients with intracerebral hemorrhage. *Stroke.* 2017;48(11):3019–3025. doi:10.1161/STROKEAHA.117.017985
42. Shimoda Y, Ohtomo S, Arai H, et al. Satellite sign: a poor outcome predictor in intracerebral hemorrhage. *Cerebrovasc Dis.* 2017;44(3–4):105–112. doi:10.1159/000477179
43. Sporns PB, Schwake M, Kemmling A, et al. Comparison of spot sign, blend sign and black hole sign for outcome prediction in patients with intracerebral hemorrhage. *J Stroke.* 2017;19(3):333–339. doi:10.5853/jos.2016.02061
44. Zheng J, Yu Z, Xu Z, et al. The accuracy of the spot sign and the blend sign for predicting hematoma expansion in patients with spontaneous intracerebral hemorrhage. *Med Sci Monit.* 2017;23:2250–2257. http://www.ncbi.nlm.nih.gov/pubmed/28498827
45. Yu Z, Zheng J, Ali H, et al. Significance of satellite sign and spot sign in predicting hematoma expansion in spontaneous intracerebral hemorrhage. *Clin Neurol Neurosurg.* 2017;162:67–71. doi:10.1016/j.clineuro.2017.09.008
46. Yu Z, Zheng J, Ma L, et al. The predictive accuracy of the black hole sign and the spot sign for hematoma expansion in patients with spontaneous intracerebral hemorrhage. *Neurol Sci.* 2017;38:1591–1597. doi:10.1007/s10072-017-3006-6
47. Morotti A, Boulouis G, Romero JM, et al. Blood pressure reduction and noncontrast CT markers of intracerebral hemorrhage expansion. *Neurology.* 2017;89(6):548–554. doi:10.1212/WNL.0000000000004210
48. Du F-Z, Jiang R, Gu M, et al. The accuracy of spot sign in predicting hematoma expansion after intracerebral hemorrhage: a systematic review and meta-analysis. *PLoS One.* 2014;9(12):e115777. doi:10.1371/journal.pone.0115777

49. Dowlatshahi D, Wasserman JK, Momoli F, et al. Evolution of computed tomography angiography spot sign is consistent with a site of active hemorrhage in acute intracerebral hemorrhage. *Stroke*. 2014;45(1):277–280. doi:10.1161/STROKEAHA.113.003387
50. Goldstein J, Fazen L, Snider R, et al. Contrast extravasation on CT angiography predicts hematoma expansion in intracerebral hemorrhage. *Neurology*. 2007;68(12):889–894. doi:10.1212/01.wnl.0000257087.22852.21
51. Becker KJ, Baxter AB, Bybee HM, et al. Extravasation of radiographic contrast is an independent predictor of death in primary intracerebral hemorrhage. *Stroke*. 1999;30(10):2025–2032. http://www.ncbi.nlm.nih.gov/pubmed/10512902
52. Murai Y, Takagi R, Ikeda Y, et al. Three-dimensional computerized tomography angiography in patients with hyperacute intracerebral hemorrhage. *J Neurosurg*. 1999;91(3):424–431. doi:10.3171/jns.1999.91.3.0424
53. Wada R, Aviv RI, Fox AJ, et al. CT angiography "spot sign" predicts hematoma expansion in acute intracerebral hemorrhage. *Stroke*. 2007;38:1257–1262. doi:10.1161/01.STR.0000259633.59404.f3
54. Demchuk AM, Dowlatshahi D, Rodriguez-Luna D, et al. Prediction of haematoma growth and outcome in patients with intracerebral haemorrhage using the CT-angiography spot sign (PREDICT): a prospective observational study. *Lancet Neurol*. 2012;11(4):307–314. doi:10.1016/S1474-4422(12)70038-8
55. Dowlatshahi D, Yogendrakumar V, Aviv RI, et al. Small intracerebral hemorrhages have a low spot sign prevalence and are less likely to expand. *Int J Stroke*. 2016;11(2):191–197. doi:10.1177/1747493015616635
56. Brouwers HB, Battey TWK, Musial HH, et al. Rate of contrast extravasation on computed tomographic angiography predicts hematoma expansion and mortality in primary intracerebral hemorrhage. *Stroke*. 2015;46(9):2498–2503. doi:10.1161/STROKEAHA.115.009659
57. Ciura VA, Brouwers HB, Pizzolato R, et al. Spot sign on 90-second delayed computed tomography angiography improves sensitivity for hematoma expansion and mortality: prospective study. *Stroke*. 2014;45(11):3293–3297. doi:10.1161/STROKEAHA.114.005570
58. Orito K, Hirohata M, Nakamura Y, et al. Leakage sign for primary intracerebral hemorrhage. *Stroke*. 2016;47(4):958–963. doi:10.1161/STROKEAHA.115.011578
59. Rodriguez-Luna D, Dowlatshahi D, Aviv RI, et al. Venous phase of computed tomography angiography increases spot sign detection, but intracerebral hemorrhage expansion is greater in spot signs detected in arterial phase. *Stroke*. 2014;45(3):734–739. doi:10.1161/STROKEAHA.113.003007

60. Falcone GJ, Biffi A, Brouwers HB, et al. Predictors of hematoma volume in deep and lobar supratentorial intracerebral hemorrhage. *JAMA Neurol.* 2013;70:988. doi:10.1001/jamaneurol.2013.98
61. Broderick JP, Diringer MN, Hill MD, et al. Determinants of intracerebral hemorrhage growth: an exploratory analysis. *Stroke.* 2007;38(3):1072–1075. doi:10.1161/01.STR.0000258078.35316.30
62. Cucchiara B, Messe S, Sansing L, et al. Hematoma growth in oral anticoagulant related intracerebral hemorrhage. *Stroke.* 2008;39(11):2993–2996. doi:10.1161/STROKEAHA.108.520668
63. Huynh TJ, Aviv RI, Dowlatshahi D, et al. Validation of the 9-point and 24-point hematoma expansion prediction scores and derivation of the PREDICT A/B scores. *Stroke.* 2015;46(11):3105–3110. doi:10.1161/STROKEAHA.115.009893
64. Yao X, Xu Y, Siwila-Sackman E, et al. The HEP score: a nomogram-derived hematoma expansion prediction scale. *Neurocrit Care.* 2015;23(2):179–187. doi:10.1007/s12028-015-0147-4
65. Di Napoli M, Parry-Jones AR, Smith CJ, et al. C-reactive protein predicts hematoma growth in intracerebral hemorrhage. *Stroke.* 2014;45(1):59–65. doi:10.1161/STROKEAHA.113.001721
66. Naidech AM, Jovanovic B, Liebling S, et al. Reduced platelet activity is associated with early clot growth and worse 3-month outcome after intracerebral hemorrhage. *Stroke.* 2009;40(7):2398–2401. doi:10.1161/STROKEAHA.109.550939
67. Sansing LH, Messe SR, Cucchiara BL, et al. Prior antiplatelet use does not affect hemorrhage growth or outcome after ICH. *Neurology.* 2009;72(16):1397–1402. doi:10.1212/01.wnl.0000342709.31341.88
68. Ohwaki K, Yano E, Nagashima H, et al. Blood pressure management in acute intracerebral hemorrhage: relationship between elevated blood pressure and hematoma enlargement. *Stroke.* 2004;35(6):1364–1367. doi:10.1161/01.STR.0000128795.38283.4b
69. Sakamoto Y, Koga M, Yamagami H, et al. Systolic blood pressure after intravenous antihypertensive treatment and clinical outcomes in hyperacute intracerebral hemorrhage: the stroke acute management with urgent risk-factor assessment and improvement-intracerebral hemorrhage study. *Stroke.* 2013;44(7):1846–1851. doi:10.1161/STROKEAHA.113.001212
70. Anderson CS, Huang Y, Wang JG, et al. Intensive blood pressure reduction in acute cerebral haemorrhage trial (INTERACT): a randomised pilot trial. *Lancet Neurol.* 2008;7(5):391–399. doi:10.1016/S1474-4422(08)70069-3
71. Qureshi AI, Palesch YY, Barsan WG, et al. Intensive blood-pressure lowering in patients with acute cerebral hemorrhage. *N Engl J Med.* 2016;375(11):1033–1043. doi:10.1056/NEJMoa1603460
72. Brouwers HB, Biffi A, Ayres AM, et al. Apolipoprotein e genotype predicts hematoma expansion in lobar intracerebral hemorrhage. *Stroke.* 2012;43(6):1490–1495. doi:10.1161/STROKEAHA.111.643262

73. Brunkhorst R, Foerch C. What causes hematoma enlargement in lobar intracerebral hemorrhage?: novel insights from a genetic study. *Stroke*. 2012;43(6):1458–1459. doi:10.1161/STROKEAHA.112.651976
74. Brouwers HB, Biffi A, McNamara KA, et al. Apolipoprotein E genotype is associated with CT angiography spot sign in lobar intracerebral hemorrhage. *Stroke*. 2012;43(8):2120–2125. doi:10.1161/STROKEAHA.112.659094
75. Arima H, Huang Y, Wang JG, et al. Earlier blood pressure-lowering and greater attenuation of hematoma growth in acute intracerebral hemorrhage: INTERACT pilot phase. *Stroke*. 2012;43(8):2236–2238. doi:10.1161/STROKEAHA.112.651422
76. Anderson CS, Heeley E, Huang Y, et al. Rapid blood-pressure lowering in patients with acute intracerebral hemorrhage. *N Engl J Med*. 2013;368(25):2355–2365. doi:10.1056/NEJMoa1214609
77. Antihypertensive Treatment of Acute Cerebral Hemorrhage (ATACH) investigators. Antihypertensive treatment of acute cerebral hemorrhage. *Crit Care Med*. 2010;38(2):637–648. doi:10.1097/CCM.0b013e3181b9e1a5
78. Qureshi AI, Palesch YY, Barsan WG, et al. Intensive blood-pressure lowering in patients with acute cerebral hemorrhage. *N Engl J Med*. 2016;375(11):1033–1043. doi:10.1056/NEJMoa1603460
79. Butcher KS, Jeerakathil T, Hill M, et al. The intracerebral hemorrhage acutely decreasing arterial pressure trial. *Stroke*. 2013;44(3):620–626. doi:10.1161/STROKEAHA.111.000188
80. Gioia L, Klahr A, Kate M, et al. The intracerebral hemorrhage acutely decreasing arterial pressure trial II (ICH ADAPT II) protocol. *BMC Neurol*. 2017;17(1):100. doi:10.1186/s12883-017-0884-4
81. Huttner HB, Schellinger PD, Hartmann M, et al. Hematoma growth and outcome in treated neurocritical care patients with intracerebral hemorrhage related to oral anticoagulant therapy: comparison of acute treatment strategies using vitamin K, fresh frozen plasma, and prothrombin complex concentrates. *Stroke*. 2006;37(6):1465–1470. doi:10.1161/01.STR.0000221786.81354.d6
82. Kuramatsu JB, Gerner ST, Schellinger PD, et al. Anticoagulant reversal, blood pressure levels, and anticoagulant resumption in patients with anticoagulation-related intracerebral hemorrhage. *JAMA*. 2015;313(8):824–836. doi:10.1001/jama.2015.0846
83. Aguilar MI, Hart RG, Kase CS, et al. Treatment of warfarin-associated intracerebral hemorrhage: literature review and expert opinion. *Mayo Clin Proc*. 2007;82(1):82–92. doi:10.4065/82.1.82
84. Steiner T, Rosand J, Diringer M. Intracerebral hemorrhage associated with oral anticoagulant therapy: current practices and unresolved questions. *Stroke*. 2006;37(1):256–262. doi:10.1161/01.STR.0000196989.09900.f8

85. Lee SB, Manno EM, Layton KF, et al. Progression of warfarin-associated intracerebral hemorrhage after INR normalization with FFP. *Neurology*. 2006;67(7):1272–1274. doi:10.1212/01.wnl.0000238104.75563.2f
86. Bershad EM, Suarez JI. Prothrombin complex concentrates for oral anticoagulant therapy-related intracranial hemorrhage: a review of the literature. *Neurocrit Care*. 2010;12(3):403–413. doi:10.1007/s12028-009-9310-0
87. Pabinger I, Brenner B, Kalina U, et al. Prothrombin complex concentrate (Beriplex P/N) for emergency anticoagulation reversal: a prospective multinational clinical trial. *J Thromb Haemost*. 2008;6(4):622–631. doi:10.1111/j.1538-7836.2008.02904.x
88. Steiner T, Poli S, Griebe M, et al. Fresh frozen plasma versus prothrombin complex concentrate in patients with intracranial haemorrhage related to vitamin K antagonists (INCH): a randomised trial. *Lancet Neurol*. 2016;15(6):566–573. doi:10.1016/S1474-4422(16)00110-1
89. Patel MR, Mahaffey KW, Garg J, et al. Rivaroxaban versus warfarin in nonvalvular atrial fibrillation. *N Engl J Med*. 2011;365(10):883–891. doi:10.1056/NEJMoa1009638
90. Granger CB, Alexander JH, McMurray JJ V, et al. Apixaban versus warfarin in patients with atrial fibrillation. *N Engl J Med*. 2011;365(11):981–992. doi:10.1056/NEJMoa1107039
91. Connolly SJ, Ezekowitz MD, Yusuf S, et al. Dabigatran versus warfarin in patients with atrial fibrillation. *N Engl J Med*. 2009;361(12):1139–1151. doi:10.1056/NEJMoa0905561
92. Pollack C V, Reilly PA, van Ryn J, et al. Idarucizumab for dabigatran reversal—full cohort analysis. *N Engl J Med*. 2017;377(5):431–441. doi:10.1056/NEJMoa1707278
93. Pollack C V, Reilly PA, Eikelboom J, et al. Idarucizumab for dabigatran reversal. *N Engl J Med*. 2015;373(6):511–520. doi:10.1056/NEJMoa1502000
94. Pradaxa (dabigatran) [product monograph]. Burlington, Ontario, Canada: Boehringer Ingelheim Canada Ltd. 2017.
95. Company B-MS. Eliquis [package insert]. 2017.
96. Connolly SJ, Milling TJ, Eikelboom JW, et al. Andexanet alfa for acute major bleeding associated with factor Xa inhibitors. *N Engl J Med*. 2016;375(12):1131–1141. doi:10.1056/NEJMoa1607887
97. Baharoglu MI, Cordonnier C, Al-Shahi Salman R, et al. Platelet transfusion versus standard care after acute stroke due to spontaneous cerebral haemorrhage associated with antiplatelet therapy (PATCH): a randomised, open-label, phase 3 trial. *Lancet (London, England)*. 2016;387(10038):2605–2613. doi:10.1016/S0140-6736(16)30392-0
98. Naidech AM, Maas MB, Levasseur-Franklin KE, et al. Desmopressin improves platelet activity in acute intracerebral hemorrhage. *Stroke*. 2014;45(8):2451–2453. doi:10.1161/STROKEAHA.114.006061

99. Mappus J, Fellows S, Anand S, et al. The use of desmopressin acetate in patients presenting with intracranial hemorrhage: a review. *Trauma*. 2017;19(1):3–10. doi:10.1177/1460408616669745
100. Mayer SA, Brun NC, Broderick J, et al. Safety and feasibility of recombinant factor VIIa for acute intracerebral hemorrhage. *Stroke*. 2005;36(1):74–79. doi:10.1161/01.STR.0000149628.80251.b8
101. Mayer SA. Ultra-early hemostatic therapy for intracerebral hemorrhage. *Stroke*. 2003;34(1):224–229. http://www.ncbi.nlm.nih.gov/pubmed/12511778
102. Diringer MN, Skolnick BE, Mayer SA, et al. Risk of thromboembolic events in controlled trials of rFVIIa in spontaneous intracerebral hemorrhage. *Stroke*. 2008;39(3):850–856. doi:10.1161/STROKEAHA.107.493601
103. Mayer SA, Brun NC, Begtrup K, et al. Recombinant activated factor VII for acute intracerebral hemorrhage. *N Engl J Med*. 2005;352(8):777–785. doi:10.1056/NEJMoa042991
104. Mayer SA, Brun NC, Begtrup K, et al. Efficacy and safety of recombinant activated factor VII for acute intracerebral hemorrhage. *N Engl J Med*. 2008;358(20):2127–2137. doi:10.1056/NEJMoa0707534
105. Mayer SA, Davis SM, Skolnick BE, et al. Can a subset of intracerebral hemorrhage patients benefit from hemostatic therapy with recombinant activated factor VII? *Stroke*. 2009;40(3):833–840. doi:10.1161/STROKEAHA.108.524470
106. Tengborn L, Blombäck M, Berntorp E. Tranexamic acid--an old drug still going strong and making a revival. *Thromb Res*. 2015;135(2):231–242. doi:10.1016/j.thromres.2014.11.012
107. CRASH-2 trial collaborators, Shakur H, Roberts I, et al. Effects of tranexamic acid on death, vascular occlusive events, and blood transfusion in trauma patients with significant haemorrhage (CRASH-2): a randomised, placebo-controlled trial. *Lancet (London, England)*. 2010;376(9734):23–32. doi:10.1016/S0140-6736(10)60835-5
108. CRASH-2 Collaborators IBS. Effect of tranexamic acid in traumatic brain injury: a nested randomised, placebo controlled trial (CRASH-2 Intracranial Bleeding Study). *BMJ*. 2011;343:d3795. http://www.ncbi.nlm.nih.gov/pubmed/21724564
109. Zehtabchi S, Abdel Baki SG, Falzon L, et al. Tranexamic acid for traumatic brain injury: a systematic review and meta-analysis. *Am J Emerg Med*. 2014;32(12):1503–1509. doi:10.1016/j.ajem.2014.09.023
110. Sprigg N, Renton CJ, Dineen RA, et al. Tranexamic acid for spontaneous intracerebral hemorrhage: a randomized controlled pilot trial (ISRCTN50867461). *J Stroke Cerebrovasc Dis*. 2014;23(6):1312–1318. doi:10.1016/j.jstrokecerebrovasdis.2013.11.007
111. Sprigg N, Robson K, Bath P, et al. Intravenous tranexamic acid for hyperacute primary intracerebral hemorrhage: protocol for a randomized, placebo-controlled trial. *Int J Stroke*. 2016;11(6):683–694. doi:10.1177/1747493016641960

112. Meretoja A, Churilov L, Campbell BC, et al. The spot sign and tranexamic acid on preventing ICH growth–AUStralasia Trial (STOP-AUST): protocol of a phase II randomized, placebo-controlled, double-blind, multicenter trial. *Int J Stroke.* 2014;9(4):519–524. doi:10.1111/ijs.12132

113. Liu L, Wang Y, Meng X, et al. Tranexamic acid for acute intracerebral hemorrhage growth predicted by spot sign trial: rationale and design. *Int J Stroke.* 2017;12(3):326–331. doi:10.1177/1747493017694394

114. Brouwers HB, Chang Y, Falcone G, et al. Predicting hematoma expansion after primary intracerebral hemorrhage. *JAMA Neurol.* 2014;71(2):158–164. doi:10.1001/jamaneurol.2013.5433

115. Gladstone D, Aviv RI, Demchuk AM, et al. Randomized Trial of HemostaticTherapy for 'Spot Sign' Positive Intracerebral Hemorrhage: Primary Results From the SPOTLIGHT/STOP-IT Study Collaboration. *Stroke.* 2007;38(2).

116. Sprigg N, Flaherty K, Appleton JP, et al. Tranexamic acid for hyperacute primary IntraCerebral Haemorrhage (TICH-2): an international randomised, placebo-controlled, phase 3 superiority trial. *The Lancet.* 2018;391(10135):2107–2115. doi:10.1016/s0140-6736(18)31033-x

4 Cerebral Edema in Stroke

Niraj A. Arora and Kristine H. O'Phelan

KEY POINTS

- Cerebral edema development in ischemic and hemorrhagic stroke has prognostic significance.
- Ischemic and hemorrhagic stroke can lead to the development of cerebral edema through different mechanisms.
- The role of sulfonylurea 1-transient receptor potential melastatin 4 (SUR1-TRPM-4) receptors in the brain has generated interest in the development of preventive therapies for ischemic cerebral edema. Though a number of targets have been studied to prevent cerebral edema after hemorrhagic stroke, the role of these therapies in clinical practice is still limited.
- Prompt recognition and early treatment of worsening clinical features including signs of herniation is the key to limiting secondary injury caused by cerebral edema.
- Decompressive surgery is the treatment of choice for cerebral edema after ischemic stroke compared to medical therapy for selected patient populations.
- Clinical trials are ongoing to determine the role of minimally invasive surgery (MIS) for early hematoma evacuation for cerebral edema after hemorrhagic stroke.

INTRODUCTION

Stroke is the fifth major cause of death in the United States. Eighty-seven percent of strokes are ischemic and thirteen percent are hemorrhagic (1). The incidence of cerebral edema in ischemic stroke is reported to be about 10% to 15% in large retrospective case studies (2). It is most commonly seen in internal carotid artery (ICA) and middle cerebral artery (MCA) main stem and cerebellar strokes where it carries a mortality of about 50% to 80% (3–5). The risk factors for development of cerebral edema in ischemic stroke are

 DOI: 10.1891/9780826124791.0004

history of hypertension or heart failure, increased baseline white blood cell count, major early CT hypodensity involving greater than 50% of the MCA territory, and involvement of additional vascular territories (5). The development of cerebral edema after intracerebral hemorrhage (ICH) is related to perihematomal edema in the first 24 hours, which peaks around 5 to 6 days and lasts up to 14 days (6). Morbidity and mortality is highest in the first 24 hours after ICH and approaches close to 50% (1). Although clinical risk factors have not been proven to predict the degree of cerebral edema after hemorrhagic stroke, certain causes such as vasogenic factors, inflammation, thrombin activation, red blood cell (RBC) lysis, and hemoglobin toxicity likely lead to brain edema after ICH (7). Factors contributing to poor prognosis in the initial phase after hemorrhagic stroke are hematoma size, early hematoma growth, and presence of additional intraventricular hemorrhage (IVH) (8).

PATHOPHYSIOLOGY

Ischemic Stroke

Cerebral edema develops within 24 to 48 hours of initial insult and reaches maximum by 3 to 5 days (Figure 4.1) (2).

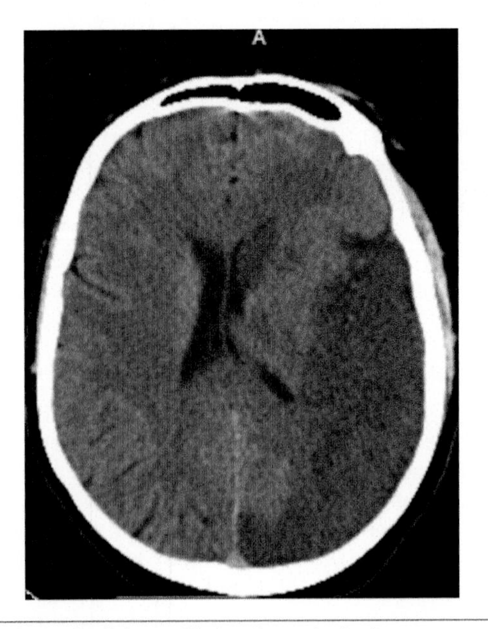

Figure 4.1 Pathophysiology of ischemic cerebral edema.

A series of events happen simultaneously in the absence of oxygen, glucose, and adenosine triphosphate (ATP). There is increased production of lactic acid due to anaerobic metabolism and decreased production of ATP. This leads to failure of the Na^+–K^+-ATPase pump, which normally takes three Na^+ ions out of the cell, while pulling two K^+ ions into the cell, causing net negativity. In the absence of ATP this pump fails, leading to excess Na^+ within the cell and accumulation of water molecules within the cell. This causes cellular swelling or cytotoxic (intracellular) edema. This develops within a few minutes of ischemia (9,10). There is failure of the Na^+–Ca^{2+}-ATPase pump, which normally brings sodium inside the cell and removes Ca^{2+} out of the cell. Failure of this pump causes Ca^{2+} buildup within the cell, which in turn causes excitotoxicity through increased glutamate release within the central nervous system, increased activation of proteases and lipase, which breaks down proteins within the cell and neuron cell membrane respectively. Increased Ca^{2+} activates the generation of free radicals and reactive oxygen species, which also damages the neurons (Figure 4.2) (9).

Recently, the role of the SUR1-TRPM-4 receptor has been highlighted. These receptors are a type of Ca-ATPase receptor, which are expressed in the brain during conditions of ischemia, hypoxia, or trauma. Unregulated opening of these channels leads to edema and oncotic cell death (11). Lack of ATP also causes mitochondrial dysfunction, which releases apoptotic factors and causes neuronal death (7,10). Within 4 to 6 hours of ischemic injury, there is disruption of the blood–brain barrier (BBB) causing movement of proteins and fluids from the intravascular to the interstitial space. This is called vasogenic (extracellular) edema. Several mediators have been identified that cause BBB disruption. These include aquaporins, free radicals, proteases such as matrix metalloproteases, inflammatory cells and their mediators; bradykinin, vascular endothelial growth factor, and nitric oxide synthase (10).

Reperfusion and Cerebral Edema

If reperfusion is induced in already irreversibly damaged brain tissues, it leads to increased vascular permeability and vasogenic edema. Also, late restoration of blood flow may prompt further ischemic damage by increasing reactive oxygen species, calcium influx, and excitatory amino acids and worsening cerebral edema. This phenomenon is frequent (28%) among thrombolysis-treated ischemic stroke patients, occurring in severe forms in 10% (2,12) and is called by the misnomer "luxury perfusion" during conventional angiography.

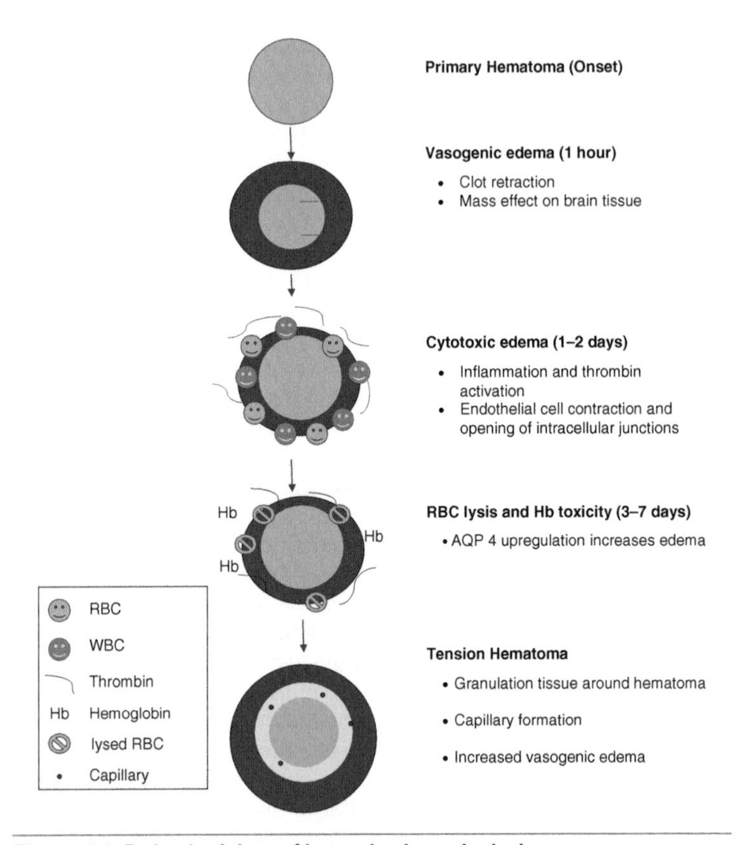

Figure 4.2 Pathophysiology of hemorrhagic cerebral edema.

RBC, red blood cell; WBC, white blood cell.

Hemorrhagic Stroke

The development of spontaneous ICH is related to chronic microvascular changes, which cause rupture of blood vessels within the brain. The main risk factors include age, hypertension (50%–70%), cerebral amyloid angiopathy, hematologic disorders (8%), and vessel abnormalities including vascular malformations (13). Within an hour there is formation of a hematoma, which causes destruction of surrounding brain tissue by direct mass effect. Hematomas also cause neuronal and glial cell death due to apoptosis, breakdown of BBB, and vasogenic edema (13,14). The highest risk for hematoma expansion occurs within 1 to 6 hours, which causes more tissue damage and worsened clinical manifestations. It is related to persistent bleeding and/or rebleeding from single arteriolar rupture or bleeding into the perihemorrhage penumbra zone. Although there is low blood flow around acute hematomas, there is no convincing evidence of significant tissue ischemia. Cerebral edema develops in perihemorrhagic areas or intrahematoma regions within 24 hours, peaks in 7 days, and starts to decrease by 9 to 14 days (Figure 4.3) (15). Clot formation is followed by clot retraction which leads to a decrease in hydrostatic pressure and an increase in oncotic pressure around the hematoma leading to extravasation of plasma proteins causing vasogenic edema (16). There is an inflammatory cell infiltrate (leucocytes and macrophages) and microglial activation after spontaneous ICH, which leads to a cascade of events causing cellular swelling and BBB disruption. The coagulation cascade is activated as blood flows within the brain tissue (17). Thrombin is activated and causes endothelial cell contraction and activation of protease activated receptors (MMP9, MMP2). This in turn leads to opening of intracellular junctions. Src kinase phosphorylation causing injury of the brain microvascular endothelial cell (BMVEC) and perivascular astrocytes, results in the disruption of the BBB and formation of edema. ICH leads to

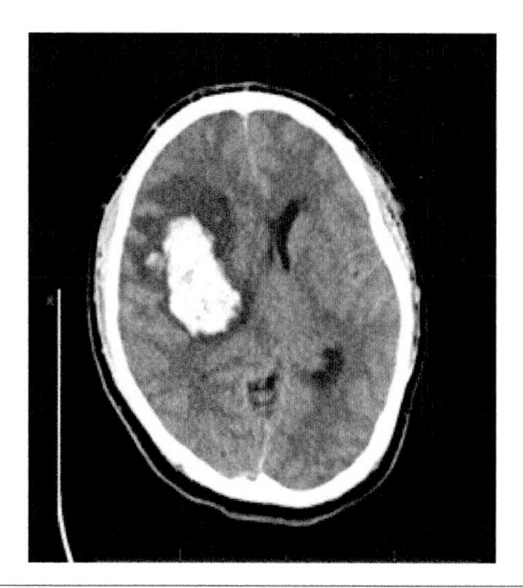

Figure 4.3 Head CT scan showing perihemorrhagic edema in patient with ICH.

ICH, intracerebral hemorrhage.

rupture of RBCs, which begins within 24 hours of hemorrhage. Finally, hemoglobin, heme, and iron accumulation leads to AQP4 upregulation and increases BBB permeability and delayed brain edema (3–7 days) (17).

PREVENTION

Prevention of Cerebral Edema After Ischemic Stroke

SUR1-TRPM4 receptors are overexpressed in ischemic regions of brain. This leads to increased channel opening, which is triggered by depletion of ATP resulting in the unregulated flow of ions, brain edema, and oncotic cell death. The SUR1-TRPM4 receptors can be blocked by the antidiabetic medication, glyburide. The potential neuroprotective effect of glyburide has been the basis of a recent clinical trial GAMES-RP. This is a phase II trial that evaluated intravenous glyburide (RP-1127) for prevention of cerebral edema in ischemic stroke. It has been hypothesized that RP-1127 treatment will lead to decreased midline shift and better clinical outcomes. At the time of this publication, intravenous glyburide safety has been established in hemispheric stroke patients with a high risk of cerebral edema development (11). Phase III studies with efficacy end points are being planned.

Prevention of Cerebral Edema After Hemorrhagic Stroke

Cerebral edema after ICH is thought to be related to toxicity directly from the hematoma itself. Medical management may include the use of hyperosmolar therapies such as mannitol and hypertonic saline. These agents, however, have not been adequately studied to show benefit in ICH. Early surgical therapy to remove hematoma, on the other hand, has been studied in multiple, randomized clinical trials and reveals trends toward better clinical outcomes for patients with spontaneous supratentorial ICH. The Surgical Trial in Intracerebral Hemorrhage (STICH) trials I and II studied subjects with acute ICH without intraventricular extension operated within 8 to 12 hours of event and found a small but potential clinically significant survival advantage. This has formed the foundation for further surgical trials (18–20).

MIS may reduce primary and secondary brain injury after supratentorial ICH patients. A recent meta-analysis of MIS studies found potential clinical benefit in noncomatose patients with superficial hematoma (volume 25–40 mL) and surgery within 72 hours after symptom onset (21).

For cerebellar hemorrhages, preventive treatment depends on the size of the cerebellar hematoma, the degree of compression of the fourth ventricle, and clinical and brainstem function. Patients with Glasgow Coma Scale (GCS) score ≥14 and hematoma less than 3 cm diameter are usually treated conservatively. If the fourth ventricle is obliterated then urgent clot removal should be undertaken before deterioration. If the hematoma size exceeds 3 cm in diameter but the fourth ventricle is not completely obliterated, surgery may not be required and ventricular drainage alone may be sufficient. If the hematoma exceeds 3 cm in diameter or brainstem compression results in disturbance in consciousness (GCS score ≤13), clot removal is recommended before condition of the patient deteriorates (22–24).

IDENTIFICATION

Clinical Features

There is a considerable degree of variation in the clinical features and presentation among individuals with stroke. Cerebral edema is the final common pathway of either ischemic or hemorrhagic stroke, which can present as raised intracranial pressure. There could be focal deficits (hemiplegia, global or expressive aphasia, severe dysarthria, neglect, gaze preference, and a visual field defect) from direct insults to the cortex or subcortical areas (4). However, a decline in the level of consciousness related to the shifting of the thalamus and brainstem due to cerebral edema is the most specific alarming sign of potentially life-threatening cerebral edema (25). It should be differentiated from eyelid apraxia, which occurs in patients with right hemispheric involvement even though it may appear de novo in deteriorating patients (26). Nausea and vomiting, dizziness, headache, and blurred vision are some of the early symptoms of cerebral edema. New anisocoria greater than 1 mm, dilated pupils, lateral rectus palsy (false localizing sign), and worsened weakness or ataxia are additional signs. One should be watchful about the early signs of herniation, which are mentioned in Table 4.1.

Imaging

Ischemic Stroke

Noncontrast CT scans are performed in ischemic stroke patients to rule out intracranial hemorrhage. However, early signs of infarct include loss of the insular cortical ribbon, sulcal effacement, and loss of the gray–white junction differentiation with blurring of the basal ganglia nuclei differentiation. Hypodensity more than 50% of MCA artery distribution or other territorial distribution is a risk factor for the development of malignant cerebral edema. Cerebral imaging with CT also plays an important role in confirming the

Table 4.1 Herniation Syndromes

Clinical Features	Uncal Herniation (Lateral Transtentorial) Stages			Central Transtentorial Herniation Stages			
	Early Third Nerve	Late Third Nerve	Midbrain–Pons	Diencephalic	Midbrain–Upper Pons	Lower Pons–Upper Medulla	Medulla
Consciousness	May be normal. Not a reliable sign	Stupor or coma		Altered (agitation, stupor, or coma)	Comatose	Comatose	Comatose
Pupils	Ipsilateral dilating pupil (may be sluggish)	Ipsilateral dilated	Contralateral pupil dilated and then bilateral pupil dilated (5–6 mm)	Small (1–3 mm) but reactive	Midposition (3–5 mm), fixed	Midposition (3–5 mm), fixed	Dilated (>5 mm)
Oculomotor	Doll's eyes: normal or dysconjugate. CWC: slow ipsilateral deviation	External oculomotor ophthalmoplegia	External oculomotor ophthalmoplegia	Doll's eyes: conjugate. CWC: positive. May develop Parinaud's syndrome	Dysconjugate eye movements, impaired doll's eyes, and CWC	Absent: doll's eyes and CWC	Absent: doll's eyes and CWC

(*continued*)

Table 4.1 Herniation Syndromes (*continued*)

Clinical Features	Uncal Herniation (Lateral Transtentorial) Stages			Central Transtentorial Herniation Stages			
Respirations	Normal	Hyperpnea (CNH)	Hyperpnea (CNH)	Sighs, yawns, and later Cheyne–Stokes	Cheyne–Stokes or sustained tachypnea	Tachypnea but shallow breathing	Ataxic breathing
Motor	Appropriate response. Contralateral Babinski positive	Contralateral hemiplegia. May develop ipsilateral hemiplegia (Kernohan's phenomenon) and then bilateral decerebration	Bilateral decerebrate posturing	Early: appropriate motor response, upper motor neuron signs. Later: motionless and then decorticate posturing	Decorticate and then bilateral decerebrate	Flaccid. Occasional triple flexion to pain	No response. Occasional triple flexion to pain

CNH, central neurogenic hyperventilation; CWC, cold water calorics.

findings objectively when clinical deterioration occurs. Noncontrast brain MRI is the preferred imaging modality in patients with ischemic stroke. Diffusion lesion volume of more than 82 mL within 6 hours of stroke onset is a high specific diffusion-weighted imaging (DWI) threshold for prediction of life-threatening cerebral edema (27). Additionally, a simple scoring system for early detection of malignant cerebral edema has been developed based on baseline National Institutes of Health Stroke Scale (NIHSS), Alberta Stroke Program Early CT Score (ASPECTS), Collateral Score, and revascularization status (28).

Hemorrhagic Stroke

Noncontrast CT scan of brain is considered the gold standard for detection of acute intracranial hemorrhage. Blood is visualized as hyperdense compared to brain tissue. Perihemorrhagic edema (PHE) is detected as hypodense areas around the hemorrhage (Figure 4.3). MRI imaging can also be used in ICH to detect acute as well as chronic hemorrhage. Gradient echo and T2* susceptibility weighted MRI are very sensitive for detection of acute hemorrhage and identification of prior hemorrhage.

MANAGEMENT

Medical Treatment

Table 4.2 shows nonsurgical strategies in the treatment of cerebral edema common to ischemic and hemorrhagic stroke. Medication doses for the most common drugs used in the management of cerebral edema are listed in Table 4.3.

Surgical Treatment

Ischemic Cerebral Edema

For patients with massive anterior territory stroke, surgery is potentially lifesaving. Three European randomized controlled trials have been conducted comparing medical management to early surgical treatment. These include HAMLET (Hemicraniectomy After Middle cerebral artery infarction with Life-threatening Edema Trial), DECIMAL (DEcompressive Craniectomy In MALignant middle cerebral artery infarction), and DESTINY (DEcompressive Surgery for the Treatment of malignant INfarction of the middle cerebral arterY) (40,41)

Pooled analysis of these trials comparing decompressive hemicraniectomy with best medical management showed clinical benefit of surgery specifically in patients from 18 to 60 years old with an NIHSS score greater than 15, decreased level of consciousness

Table 4.2 Nonsurgical Strategies in the Management of Cerebral Edema in Stroke

Measures	Method	Rationale
Position	30–45 degree HOB elevation	Increases venous return outflow from cranial vault and also reduces mean carotid pressure but no net change in CBF (29)
Neck position	Keep neck straight, avoid tight ties around neck	Avoid constriction of jugular venous outflow
Maintain airway and adequate oxygenation	Goal PaO_2 >60 mmHg or O_2 saturation >90%	Hypoxia causes further ischemic brain injury
Temperature modulation (goal 36°C–37°C)	Acetaminophen Cooling measures	Maintain normothermia Fever increases metabolic demand and increases CBF and ICP, which in turn exacerbates cerebral edema (30)
Sedation, analgesia with or without paralytics	Combination of short-acting opioid (fentanyl or remifentanil), propofol +/– vecuronium/ rocuronium	Reduce agitation, which decreases metabolic demand, improves ventilator synchrony, decreases sympathetic responses (hypertension and tachycardia)
Hyperventilation	Mechanical ventilation with goal $PaCO_2$ 30–35 mmHg	Lowers ICP by reducing $PaCO_2$, which causes cerebral vasoconstriction thus reducing the CBV and CBF (31) Use briefly for clinical evidence of raised ICP (neurologic deterioration) or chronically for documented raised ICP unresponsive to other measures
Osmotic therapy (goal serum osmolality up to 320 mmol/l)	Mannitol Hypertonic saline (3%, 23%)	Expands plasma volume, improves rheologic properties of blood, causes fluid shift into intravascular space via osmotic gradient

(*continued*)

Table 4.2 Nonsurgical Strategies in the Management of Cerebral Edema in Stroke (*continued*)

Measures	Method	Rationale
Glucose control (goal 140–180 mg%)	Insulin therapy	Hyperglycemia causes increased oxidative load, cerebral edema, and hemorrhagic transformation of ischemic stroke and inflammation (32,33) Hyperglycemia exacerbates cerebral edema and perihematomal cell death in ICH, which leads to worse clinical outcomes (34)
Antiepileptic therapy	Antiepileptic drugs	Decrease cortical irritability in high-risk injuries
Treatment of hypotension (goal SBP > 90 mmHg)	Norepinephrine, phenylephrine, epinephrine	Normalize intravascular volume and maintain euvolemia
Treatment of malignant hypertension	Labetalol, nicardipine, hydralazine	Ischemic cerebral edema: Severe arterial HTN aggravates cerebral edema and causes hemorrhagic transformation of ischemic tissue. Treatment is required if DBP > 120 mmHg, or SBP > 220 mmHg during the first 24 hours (24,35,36) Hemorrhagic cerebral edema: Lowering of systolic blood pressure to 140–160 mmHg is safe and may improve functional outcome (37–39)
Medical coma	Pentobarbital	Decrease metabolic rate and CBV and hence ICP reduction

CBF, cerebral blood flow; CBV, cerebral blood volume; DBP, diastolic blood pressure; HOB, head of bed; HTN, hypertension; ICH, intracerebral hemorrhage; ICP, intracranial pressure; SBP, systolic blood pressure.

Table 4.3 Medication and Doses Used in the Treatment of Edema in Stroke

Medication/Route/ Duration	Dose	Side Effects/ Complications
Mannitol/Peripheral access/90 min–6 hours	1 g/kg over 5–15 min followed by 0.5 g/kg q4–6 hours	Dehydration Hypotension Acute kidney injury Rebound ICP elevation Electrolyte disturbances
Hypertonic saline/ Central access/90 min–4 hours	3%–5 mL/kg bolus over 5–20 min 23%–30 mL over 5–10 min	Pulmonary edema Heart failure Acute kidney injury Hypernatremia Osmotic demyelination with rapid sodium increase
Pentobarbital/Central or peripheral/Long acting	3–7 mg/kg bolus followed by 1–5 mg/kg/hr continuous infusion	Hypotension Inability to follow neurological examination Respiratory depression and mucus plugging

ICP, intracranial pressure.

without bilaterally fixed or dilated pupils and with a hypodensity involving at least 50% of the MCA territory on CT. A maximum time window of 48 hours from stroke onset to surgical decompression was adopted based on these studies. The case fatality rate was substantially lower in the surgical decompression group (28% vs. 78% in the conservative arm), with an absolute risk reduction of 50%. Favorable outcome as defined by modified Rankin Scale (mRS) of 1 to 4 was found in 75% patients treated with decompression surgery compared to 24% patients treated with conservative medical management. This represents a mortality benefit but may not always represent a functional outcome benefit.

Cerebellar Ischemic Stroke

Posterior fossa ischemic stroke is relatively rare compared to anterior circulation stroke. Eighty percent of patients developing signs of brainstem compression will die (42,43), usually within hours to days. Therefore no randomized controlled trials are available so far for the management of cerebellar infarction with worsening edema (43). Close monitoring is the key to detect early evidence of brainstem compression (altered level of consciousness, gaze paresis, decerebrate posturing, extensor plantar responses, progressive cranial nerve deficits) or hydrocephalus (vomiting, altered level of consciousness, pinpoint pupils, extensor plantar responses) (44,45).

Serial CT scans are helpful for the assessment during rapid deterioration. Brainstem compression is usually not responsive to medical treatment alone and requires surgical decompression and placement of a ventriculostomy drain (43,44). Table 4.4 lists surgical methods in stroke with increasing edema and their rationale.

Hemorrhagic Cerebral Edema

There are surgical interventions that have been shown to be of benefit for cerebral edema complicating ICH. In patients with ICH with IVH developing obstructive hydrocephalus, management with external ventricular drain (EVD) placement helps to decrease the intracranial pressure and thus decrease cerebral edema. Early clot removal as studied in the STICH trials may be of benefit in certain populations. Subgroup analysis showed that patients with hematomas less than 1 cm from the cortical surface were more likely to have favorable outcomes since surgical risks may outweigh the benefits from damage to deeper neural structures and more

Table 4.4 Surgical Treatment for Ischemic Cerebral Edema

Surgery	Methods	Rationale
Decompressive surgery in ICA stroke	Hemicraniectomy and duraplasty	Provides edematous tissue to expand outside the cranial vault, reducing tissue shifts and pressure within the intracranial compartment, thereby restoring cerebral perfusion and minimizing derangements in oxygenation of noninfarcted tissue
Decompressive surgery in cerebellar stroke	Suboccipital craniectomy	Rapid decompression of the fourth ventricle and decreases brainstem compression (44)

ICA, internal carotid artery.

bleeding in patients with deeper hemorrhages. The STICH II trial results confirmed that early surgery does not increase the rate of death or disability at 6 months and might have a small but clinically relevant survival advantage for patients with spontaneous superficial ICH without IVH (20). The Minimally Invasive Surgery plus alTeplase in Intracerebral hemorrhage Evacuation (MISTIE) trial found that hematoma evacuation was associated with significant reduction in PHE as compared to medical therapy alone. PHE does not appear to be exacerbated by alteplase when the drug is delivered to an intracranial clot. Currently, the MISTIE III trial has completed planned enrollment of 500 patients and continues with ongoing follow-up. Its primary end point is to evaluate the functional outcome at 180 and 365 days after stroke. The study is funded by NINDS and is a multicenter randomized trial. Recently, a feasibility study of Image-Guided BrainPath-Mediated Transsulcul Hematoma Evacuation was published, which included 39 patients with symptomatic supratentorial hemorrhage, with minimal or no intraventricular extension, who were deemed medically stable for surgery. The median time duration from onset of ICH to surgery was 24.5 hours (interquartile range 16–66 hours). This approach had a high rate of clot evacuation and may provide functional independence (46). This is being studied in the ongoing ENRICH trial, a phase III, randomized, multicenter trial comparing standard medical management to early surgical hematoma evacuation using minimally invasive parafascicular surgery (MIPS) in the treatment of ICH. Patients with cerebellar hemorrhages of more than 3 cm in diameter with evidence of signs of obstructive hydrocephalus and mass effect may benefit from emergent evacuation. However, if there is loss of brainstem reflexes and extensor posturing, surgery may be of no benefit in regard to functional outcome (47). Table 4.5 shows the stage wise approach to the management of ICH (48–56).

CONCLUSION

Cerebral edema in ischemic and hemorrhagic stroke remains a significant complication/sequel of the underlying disease and prompt diagnosis and management remains of utmost importance. Time tested medical management has not changed significantly over the past two decades. However, the use of MIS could change the paradigm for the surgical management for ICH. The use of hemicraniectomy for malignant MCA infarcts complicated by life-threatening edema remains the best treatment in selected patients. More research is needed to explore the role of potential molecular targets for the management of cerebral edema in patients after acute stroke.

Table 4.5 Stage Wise Approach to the Management of ICH

Stage	Treatment strategy and rationale
Hematoma	**1.** Surgical Evacuation–Decrease mass effect and hematoma induced injury **2.** BP reduction–(Goal SBP less than 140 mmHg is safe) (24) **3.** Temperature modulation
Vasogenic Edema	Osmotherapy–Mannitol, HTS, Furosemide
Inflammation	**1.** Neutrophil depletion by using anti-PMN antibodies → reduce BBB permeability, MMP-9 expression, perihematomal axonal injury and the astrocytic and microglia/macrophage responses → provide a better outcome after ICH (48,49) **2.** MMP inhibitor (GM6001), ROS scavengers or TNF-alpha neutralizing antibody can decrease the neurotoxicity caused by PMNs, and then protect neurons from injury (50) **3.** Microglia activation inhibition: Minocycline (51,52) **4.** Immunomodulators: Fingolimod (53), Dexamethasone (54)
Thrombin activation	Thrombin inhibitor: Hirudin, argatroban or cycloheximide. No effect on hematoma volume or brain edema after ICH but prevent ICH induced neuron loss (55).
RBC lysis	Iron chelator: Desferrioxamine Basis for Intracerebral Hemorrhage Deferoxamine (iDEF) Trial Hematoma resolution: PPAR Gamma agonist (56)

BBB, blood–brain barrier; HTS, hypertonic saline; ICH, intracerebral hemorrhage; MMP-9, matrix metallopeptidase-9; PMN, polymorphonuclear cells; RBC, red blood cell; ROS, reactive oxygen species; SBP, systolic blood pressure; TNF, tumor necrosis factor.

REFERENCES

1. Babi MA, James ML. Peri-Hemorrhagic edema and secondary hematoma expansion after intracerebral hemorrhage: from benchwork to practical aspects. *Front Neurol.* 2017;8:4. doi:10.3389/fneur.2017.00004
2. Dostovic Z, Dostovic E, Smajlovic D, et al. Brain edema after ischaemic stroke. *Med Arch.* 2016;70(5):339–341. doi:10.5455/medarh.2016.70.339-341

3. Ropper AH, Shafran B. Brain edema after stroke. Clinical syndrome and intracranial pressure. *Arch Neurol.* 1984;41(1):26–29. doi:10.1001/archneur.1984.04050130032017
4. Hacke W, Schwab S, Horn M, et al. 'Malignant' middle cerebral artery territory infarction: clinical course and prognostic signs. *Arch Neurol.* 1996;53(4):309–315. doi:10.1001/archneur.1996.00550040037012
5. Kasner SE, Demchuk AM, Berrouschot J, et al. Predictors of fatal brain edema in massive hemispheric ischemic stroke. *Stroke.* 2001;32(9):2117–2123. doi:10.1161/hs0901.095719
6. Qureshi AI, Mendelow AD, Hanley DF. Intracerebral haemorrhage. *Lancet.* 2009;373(9675):1632–1644. doi:10.1016/s0140-6736(09)60371-8
7. Zheng H, Chen C, Zhang J, et al. Mechanism and therapy of brain edema after intracerebral hemorrhage. *Cerebrovasc Dis.* 2016;42(3–4):155–169. doi:10.1159/000445170
8. Staykov D, Wagner I, Volbers B, et al. Natural course of perihemorrhagic edema after intracerebral hemorrhage. *Stroke.* 2011;42(9):2625–2629. doi:10.1161/strokeaha.111.618611
9. Michinaga S, Koyama Y. Pathogenesis of brain edema and investigation into anti-edema drugs. *Int J Mol Sci.* 2015;16(5):9949–9975. doi:10.3390/ijms16059949
10. Stokum JA, Gerzanich V, Simard JM. Molecular pathophysiology of cerebral edema. *J Cereb Blood Flow Metab.* 2016;36(3):513–538. doi:10.1177/0271678x15617172
11. Sheth KN, Elm JJ, Molyneaux BJ, et al. Safety and efficacy of intravenous glyburide on brain swelling after large hemispheric infarction (GAMES-RP): a randomised, double-blind, placebo-controlled phase 2 trial. *Lancet Neurol.* 2016;15(11):1160–1169. doi:10.1016/s1474-4422(16)30196-x
12. Strbian D, Meretoja A, Putaala J, et al. Cerebral edema in acute ischemic stroke patients treated with intravenous thrombolysis. *Int J Stroke.* 2013;8(7):529–534. doi:10.1111/j.1747-4949.2012.00781.x
13. Rincon F, Mayer SA. Novel therapies for intracerebral hemorrhage. *Curr Opin Crit Care.* 2004;10(2):94–100. doi:10.1097/00075198-200404000-00003
14. Hua Y., Keep RF, Hoff JT, et al. Brain injury after intracerebral hemorrhage: the role of thrombin and iron. *Stroke.* 2007;38(2 Suppl):759–762. doi:10.1161/01.str.0000247868.97078.10
15. Venkatasubramanian, C, Mlynash M, Finley-Caulfield A, et al. Natural history of perihematomal edema after intracerebral hemorrhage measured by serial magnetic resonance imaging. *Stroke.* 2011;42(1):73–80. doi:10.1161/strokeaha.110.590646
16. Wagner KR, Xi G, Hua Y, et al. Lobar intracerebral hemorrhage model in pigs: rapid edema development in perihematomal white matter. *Stroke.* 1996;27(3):490–497. doi:10.1161/01.str.27.3.490
17. Ziai WC. Hematology and inflammatory signaling of intracerebral hemorrhage. *Stroke.* 2013;44(6 Suppl 1):S74–S78. doi:10.1161/strokeaha.111.000662

18. Gregson BA, Broderick JP, Auer LM, et al. Individual patient data subgroup meta-analysis of surgery for spontaneous supratentorial intracerebral hemorrhage. *Stroke*. 2012;43(6):1496–1504. doi:10.1161/strokeaha.111.640284
19. Mendelow AD, Gregson B, Fernandes H, et al. Early surgery versus initial conservative treatment in patients with spontaneous supratentorial intracerebral haematomas in the International Surgical Trial in Intracerebral Haemorrhage (STICH): a randomised trial. *Lancet*. 2005;365(9457):387–397. doi:10.1016/s0140-6736(05)70233-6
20. Mendelow AD, Gregson BA, Rowan EN, et al. Early surgery versus initial conservative treatment in patients with spontaneous supratentorial lobar intracerebral haematomas (STICH II): a randomised trial. *Lancet*. 2013;382(9890):397–408. doi:10.1016/s0140-6736(13)60986-1
21. Zhou X, Chen J, Li Q, et al. Minimally invasive surgery for spontaneous supratentorial intracerebral hemorrhage: a meta-analysis of randomized controlled trials. *Stroke*. 2012;43(11):2923–2930. doi:10.1161/strokeaha.112.667535
22. Kirollos RW, Tyagi AK, Ross SA, et al. Management of spontaneous cerebellar hematomas: a prospective treatment protocol. *Neurosurg*. 2001;49(6):1378–1386; discussion 1386–1387. doi:10.1097/00006123-200112000-00015
23. Kobayashi S, Sato A, Kageyama Y, et al. Treatment of hypertensive cerebellar hemorrhage—surgical or conservative management? *Neurosurg*. 1994;34(2):246–250; discussion 250–251. doi:10.1097/00006123-199402000-00006
24. Hemphill JC 3rd, Greenberg SM, Anderson CS, et al. Guidelines for the management of spontaneous intracerebral hemorrhage: a guideline for healthcare professionals from the American Heart Association/American Stroke Association. *Stroke*. 2015;46(7):2032–2060. doi:10.1161/str.0000000000000069
25. Frank JI. Large hemispheric infarction, deterioration, and intracranial pressure. *Neurol*. 1995;45(7):1286–1290. doi:10.1212/wnl.45.7.1286
26. Averbuch-Heller L, Leigh RJ, Mermelstein V, et al. Ptosis in patients with hemispheric strokes. *Neurol*. 2002;58(4):620–624. doi:10.1212/wnl.58.4.620
27. Thomalla G, Hartmann F, Juettler E, et al. Prediction of malignant middle cerebral artery infarction by magnetic resonance imaging within 6 hours of symptom onset: a prospective multicenter observational study. *Ann Neurol*. 2010;68(4):435–445. doi:10.1002/ana.22125
28. Jo K, Bajgur SS, Kim H, et al. A simple prediction score system for malignant brain edema progression in large hemispheric infarction. *PLoS One*. 2017;12(2):e0171425. doi:10.1371/journal.pone.0171425
29. Durward QJ, Maestro RFD, Amacher AL, et al. The influence of systemic arterial pressure and intracranial pressure on the development of cerebral vasogenic edema. *J Neurosurg*. 1983;59(5):803–809. doi:10.3171/jns.1983.59.5.0803

30. Rossi S, Zanier ER, Mauri I, et al. Brain temperature, body core temperature, and intracranial pressure in acute cerebral damage. *J Neurol Neurosurg Psychiatry*. 2001;71(4):448–454. doi:10.1136/jnnp.71.4.448
31. Grubb RL Jr, Raichle ME, Eichling JO, et al. The effects of changes in $PaCO_2$ on cerebral blood volume, blood flow, and vascular mean transit time. *Stroke*. 1974;5(5):630–639. doi:10.1161/01.str.5.5.630
32. Bruno A, Liebeskind D, Hao Q, et al. Diabetes mellitus, acute hyperglycemia, and ischemic stroke. *Curr Treat Options Neurol*. 2010;12(6):492–503. doi:10.1007/s11940-010-0093-6
33. Schiffner L. Glucose management in critically ill medical and surgical patients. *Dimens Crit Care Nurs*. 2014;33(2):70–77. doi:10.1097/dcc.0000000000000025
34. Goldstein JN, Gilson AJ. Critical care management of acute intracerebral hemorrhage. *Curr Treat Options Neurol*. 2011;13(2):204–216. doi:10.1007/s11940-010-0109-2
35. de Courten-Myers GM, Kleinholz M, Holm P, et al. Hemorrhagic infarct conversion in experimental stroke. *Ann Emerg Med*. 1992;21(2):120–126. doi:10.1016/s0196-0644(05)80144-1
36. Jauch EC, Saver JL, Adams HP, et al. Guidelines for the early management of patients with acute ischemic stroke: a guideline for healthcare professionals from the American Heart Association/American Stroke Association. *Stroke*. 2013;44(3):870–947. doi:10.1161/str.0b013e318284056a
37. Vemmos KN, Tsivgoulis G, Spengos K, et al. U-Shaped relationship between mortality and admission blood pressure in patients with acute stroke. *J Intern Med*. 2004;255(2):257–265. doi:10.1046/j.1365-2796.2003.01291.x
38. Anderson CS, Heeley E, Huang Y, et al. Rapid blood-pressure lowering in patients with acute intracerebral hemorrhage. *N Engl J Med*. 2013;368(25):2355–2365. doi:10.1056/nejmoa1214609
39. Qureshi AI, Palesch YY, Barsan WG, et al. Intensive blood-pressure lowering in patients with acute cerebral hemorrhage. *N Engl J Med*. 2016;375(11):1033–1043. doi:10.1056/nejmoa1603460
40. Vahedi K, Hofmeijer J, Juettler E, et al. Early decompressive surgery in malignant infarction of the middle cerebral artery: a pooled analysis of three randomised controlled trials. *Lancet Neurol*. 2007;6(3):215–222.
41. Singh V, Edwards NJ. Advances in the critical care management of ischemic stroke. *Stroke Res Treat*. 2013;2013:1–7. doi:10.1155/2013/510481
42. Heros RC. Cerebellar hemorrhage and infarction. *Stroke*. 1982;13(1):106–109. doi:10.1161/01.str.13.1.106
43. Sypert GW, Lvord EC. Cerebellar infarction. A clinicopathological study. *Arch Neurol*. 1975;32(6):357–363. doi:10.1001/archneur.1975.00490480023001
44. Heros RC. Surgical treatment of cerebellar infarction. *Stroke*. 1992;23(7):937–938. doi:10.1161/01.str.23.7.937

45. Wijdicks EF, Sheth KN, Carter BS, et al. Recommendations for the management of cerebral and cerebellar infarction with swelling: a statement for healthcare professionals from the American Heart Association/American Stroke Association. *Stroke.* 2014;45(4):1222–1238. doi:10.1161/01.str.0000441965.15164.d6
46. Labib MA, Shah M, Kassam AB, et al. The safety and feasibility of image-guided brainpath-mediated transsulcul hematoma evacuation: a multicenter study. *Neurosurg.* 2017;80(4):515–524. doi:10.1227/neu.0000000000001316
47. Rabinstein AA, Atkinson JL, Wijdicks EF. Emergency craniotomy in patients worsening due to expanded cerebral hematoma: to what purpose? *Neurol.* 2002;58(9):1367–1372. doi:10.1212/wnl.58.9.1367
48. Moxon-Emre I, Schlichter LC. Neutrophil depletion reduces blood-brain barrier breakdown, axon injury, and inflammation after intracerebral hemorrhage. *J Neuropathol Exp Neurol.* 2011;70(3):218–235. doi:10.1097/nen.0b013e31820d94a5
49. Sansing LH, HarrisTH, Kasner SE, et al. Neutrophil depletion diminishes monocyte infiltration and improves functional outcome after experimental intracerebral hemorrhage. *Acta Neurochir Suppl.* 2011;111:173–178. doi:10.1007/978-3-7091-0693-8_29
50. Nguyen HX, O'Barr TJ, Anderson AJ. Polymorphonuclear leukocytes promote neurotoxicity through release of matrix metalloproteinases, reactive oxygen species, andTNF-alpha. *J Neurochem.* 2007;102(3):900–912. doi:10.1111/j.1471-4159.2007.04643.x
51. Wasserman JK, Schlichter LC. Minocycline protects the blood-brain barrier and reduces edema following intracerebral hemorrhage in the rat. *Exp Neurol.* 2007;207(2):227–237. doi:10.1016/j.expneurol.2007.06.025
52. Wang J, Tsirka SE. Tuftsin fragment 1–3 is beneficial when delivered after the induction of intracerebral hemorrhage. *Stroke.* 2005;36(3):613–618. doi:10.1161/01.str.0000155729.12931.8f
53. Rolland WB, Lekic T, Krafft PR, et al. Fingolimod reduces cerebral lymphocyte infiltration in experimental models of rodent intracerebral hemorrhage. *Exp Neurol.* 2013;241:45–55. doi:10.1016/j.expneurol.2012.12.009
54. Yang JT, Lee T-H, Lee I-N, et al. Dexamethasone inhibits ICAM-1 and MMP-9 expression and reduces brain edema in intracerebral hemorrhagic rats. *Acta Neurochir (Wien).* 2011;153(11):2197–2203. doi:10.1007/s00701-011-1122-2
55. Fujimoto S, Katsuki H, Ohnishi M, et al. Plasminogen potentiates thrombin cytotoxicity and contributes to pathology of intracerebral hemorrhage in rats. *J Cereb Blood Flow Metab.* 2008;28(3):506–515. doi:10.1038/sj.jcbfm.9600547
56. Zhao X, Sun G, Zhang J, et al. Hematoma resolution as a target for intracerebral hemorrhage treatment: role for peroxisome proliferator-activated receptor gamma in microglia/macrophages. *Ann Neurol.* 2007;61(4):352–362. doi:10.1002/ana.21097

5 Post-Thrombolysis Hemorrhage and Hemorrhagic Transformation of Cerebral Infarction

Juan Jose Goyanes and Lucas Elijovich

KEY POINTS

- Define the physiopathology, epidemiology, classification, and risk factors involved in the incidence of hemorrhagic transformation (HT) of acute ischemic stroke (AIS) after thrombolytic therapy.
- Discuss the different predictive tools using imaging, clinical scores (based on combination of risk factors), and blood markers currently under research that will be able to predict the risk of symptomatic intracerebral bleeding after thrombolytic therapy.
- Establish the recognition and management of symptomatic intracerebral bleeding after thrombolytic therapy.

INTRODUCTION

Every year, more than 795,000 people in the United States have a stroke. Approximately 87% of all strokes are ischemic strokes (1). Intravenous (IV) thrombolytic reperfusion therapy with alteplase (recombinant tissue plasminogen activator or IV r-tPA) is the cornerstone treatment for AIS when it is given to qualifying stroke patients within 3 hours of onset of neurological symptoms, and to a more selective group of qualifying patients within 4.5 hours of neurological symptoms (2). Only 7% of all AISs in the United States are treated with IV r-tPA, largely due to a delay in presentation (1). The main goal of reperfusion therapy is to reestablish cerebral blood flow (CBF) to the ischemic penumbra to preserve at-risk, noninfarcted regions (2–9). A feared complication of thrombolytic therapy is symptomatic intracerebral hemorrhage (sICH).

It is important to differentiate between spontaneous and secondary intracerebral hemorrhage (ICH), such as post-thrombolytic sICH, due to the different pathophysiology, etiologies, and subsequent treatment paradigms that they each require. Spontaneous

 DOI: 10.1891/9780826124791.0005

ICH occurs in the absence of an underlying lesion and has been related to, but not limited to, hypertension, cerebral amyloid angiopathy, sympathomimetic drugs (cocaine, amphetamines), and advanced age (10). Despite the high frequency of these risk factors in the general population, only a small fraction of these patients experience ICH (10). Secondary ICH occurs in the setting of cerebral tumor, vascular malformation, focal or global ischemic injury, or other underlying lesions. The occurrence of secondary ICH is more predictable than spontaneous ICH, especially in the setting of underlying focal ischemic injury with HT of AIS (10). HT is a frequent, spontaneous, and natural consequence of infarction and reperfusion. The incidence of HT ranges from 38% to 71% in autopsy studies and from 13% to 43% in CT studies (11,12). The pathophysiology is characterized by ischemia-related blood extravasation due to a robust inflammatory response and disruption of the blood–brain barrier (BBB) occurring principally within 2 weeks of ischemic stroke (3). Clinically, HT ranges from subtle petechial hemorrhage within infarcted tissue that is asymptomatic to deadly large volume hematoma with mass effect extending beyond the borders of the infarction.

PATHOPHYSIOLOGY

Ischemic stroke, reperfusion injury, and HT all involve disruption of the BBB (3). The BBB is composed of endothelial cells, pericytes, astrocytes, neurons, and the extracellular matrix, which are collectively known as the neurovascular unit. BBB endothelial cells lack fenestrations, have tight junctions (TJs), have minimal pinocytotic activity, and express a number of proteases capable of degrading both harmful and therapeutic molecules (3). Recombinant tissue plasminogen activator is an endogenously synthesized extracellular protease and is also a signaling molecule in the brain (3,13). It mediates matrix remodeling during brain development and plasticity. HT seen with r-tPA may be an effect of not only its thrombolytic action, but also the increase in BBB permeability during ischemia (Figure 5.1) (3,13).

One of the major events of cerebral ischemia is energy failure due to lactic acidosis and lack of glucose and oxygen (3,13–15). Lactic acidosis directly contributes to swelling of endothelial cells, neurons, and astrocytes. Deprivation of oxygen and glucose caused by hypoperfusion has been shown to induce cellular death (3,13–15). Adenosine triphosphate (ATP) derived from mitochondria plays a crucial role in determining cellular survival. Mitochondrial dysfunction during and after cerebral ischemia can lead to the pathogenesis

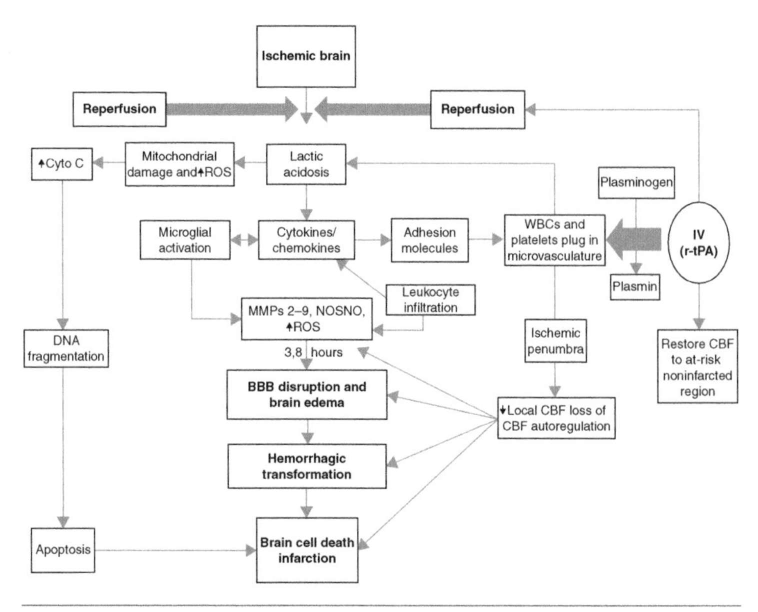

Figure 5.1 Pathophysiology of acute ischemic stroke, BBB disruption, and HT. Loss of CBF autoregulation leads to hypoperfusion secondary to vasoconstriction and decrease in CBF, which leads to energy failure due to lactic acidosis and lack of glucose and oxygen. Mitochondrial dysfunction during and after cerebral ischemia can lead to the pathogenesis of apoptotic cell death in the brain due to activation of cytochrome C. Reperfusion is essential for brain tissue survival; however, it contributes to further tissue damage and possible development of HT. Reperfusion injury includes activation of endothelium, excess production of oxygen free radicals (ROS), inflammatory responses and leukocyte recruitment, increase in cytokine production, and edema formation. These alterations cause deregulated extracellular proteolysis by elevated levels of MMPs (MMP-9 and MMP-2), induced production of nitric oxide (INOS, NO, NOX) and ROS including peroxynitrate formation resulting in BBB breakdown and HT. The median time estimate of BBB disruption from onset of ischemia was proposed to be 3.8 hours. IV r-tPA produces local thrombolysis by converting plasminogen into plasmin, which in turn degrades fibrin into fibrin split products, restoring CBF to at-risk noninfarcted regions during the ischemic penumbra when it is given within 4.5 hours from symptom onset. Paradoxically, IV r-tPA may amplify reperfusion injury and hence HT.

BBB, blood–brain barrier; CBF, cerebral blood flow; HT, hemorrhagic transformation; IV, intravenous; MMP, matrix metalloproteinase; ROS, reactive oxygen species; r-tPA, recombinant tissue plasminogen activator; WBC, white blood cell.

of necrotic or apoptotic cell death in the brain. In particular, depletion of ATP during ischemia inhibits the sodium–potassium ATPase pump leading to an imbalance of ion gradients (3,13–15). The ionic imbalance caused by cerebral ischemia further induces plasma membrane depolarization to trigger massive glutamate release from presynaptic nerve terminals. All of these events contribute to the disruption of the BBB and increased paracellular permeability that results from decreased zonula occludens along the TJ (3,13). Additionally, induction of proteases (e.g., r-tPA, matrix metalloproteinases, cathepsins, and heparanases) contributes to degradation of the BBB extracellular membrane (3,13). Moreover, the induced production of nitric oxide during cerebral ischemia contributes to peroxynitrate formation and BBB breakdown (Figure 5.1) (3,13–15).

Reperfusion is essential for brain tissue survival; however, it can contribute to further tissue damage and possible development of HT (3,13,14). Reperfusion injury includes activation of endothelium, excess production of oxygen free radicals, inflammatory responses and leukocyte recruitment, increase in cytokine production, and edema formation (Figure 5.1) (3,13,14). There are three stages of paracellular permeability after reperfusion, which include reactive hyperemia, hypoperfusion, and biphasic response (3,13,14). Stage 1 is reactive hyperemia, which results from loss of cerebral autoregulation and vasodilation. It leads to an increase in CBF, BBB permeability, and ultimately, cytotoxic edema. Stage 2 is hypoperfusion secondary to vasoconstriction and decrease in CBF. This stage leads to nutritional deficiency in brain tissue and enhances neutrophil adhesion with subsequent inflammatory activity. Stage 3 is due to vasogenic edema, which is associated with alterations in BBB TJs and results in increased permeability to macromolecules (3,13,14). These alterations result in deregulated extracellular proteolysis by elevated levels of matrix metalloproteinases (MMP-9 and MMP-2), cellular fibronectin, and caveolin-1 that independently have predicted HT in clinical trials (3,16–20). By interacting with the NMDA-type glutamate receptor, r-tPA may amplify potentially excitotoxic calcium currents (3,13). In addition, r-tPA increases matrix metalloproteinase degradation after stroke and increases the risks of neurovascular cell death, BBB leakage, edema, and hemorrhage (3,13,14). In animal models, the incidence of sICH can be significantly reduced with inhibition of MMP-2 and MMP-9 activation, which avoids lysis of the BBB (3,20). In one of these models, closure of the BBB with MMP inhibitor (BB-94) given before r-tPA treatment reduced mortality and suggests that this treatment might protect against HT during the early stage of cerebral ischemia and reperfusion (3,20).

Imaging studies with MRI using HARM (**H**yperintense **A**cute **R**eperfusion **M**arker) modality in humans reported an estimated median time of 3.8 hours from ischemia onset to BBB disruption. This time window is consistent with current IV r-tPA clinical practice and likely minimizes complications associated with acute thrombolytic therapy while optimizing clinical outcomes (3,21). Physicians selecting any treatment aimed at preventing or ameliorating the consequences of sICH should consider not only the coagulopathy caused by thrombolysis but also the integrity of the BBB (3,21,22).

IV r-tPA produces local thrombolysis by converting plasminogen into plasmin, which in turn degrades fibrin into fibrin split products (22,23). This results in a transient coagulopathy that peaks 1 to 4 hours after administration with 80% cleared 10 minutes after cessation of the infusion (22,23). Despite rapid clearance, the effect of r-tPA on the coagulation profile may last 24 hours or more from the infusion time and result in prolongation of the prothrombin time (PT) and partial thromboplastin time (PTT) as well as a reduction in fibrinogen levels (22,23). The occurrence of sICH appears to be higher 6 hours after treatment when there is a reduction in fibrinogen less than 200 mg/dL (2,22,23).

CLASSIFICATION AND EPIDEMIOLOGY

HT is a natural consequence of ischemic BBB breakdown that occurs mainly within 2 weeks of ischemic stroke (2,3,9,24). Because r-tPA has a short half-life and other reperfusion therapies including mechanical thrombectomy (MT) have a relatively rapid effect, ICHs within 24 hours of treatment are likely to be related to reperfusion therapy. On the other hand, the majority of ICHs after 1 week of treatment are likely to be the pathophysiologic consequence of ischemic stroke. Despite the increased risk of HT and ICH after thrombolytic therapy, the National Institute of Neurological Disorders and Stroke (NINDS) trial clearly demonstrated that IV r-tPA is safe and effective in achieving improved neurologic outcomes accepting an approximately 6.2% risk of sICH (22,23).

The NINDS definition of sICH includes any HT temporally related to any neurologic worsening, which may be overly inclusive because it captures small petechial hemorrhages associated with minimal neurologic deterioration that are unlikely to have altered long-term functional outcome (25–27). In contrast, the European Cooperative Acute Stroke Study (ECASS) and Safe Implementation of Thrombolysis in Stroke-Monitoring Study (SITS-MOST) definitions include only hemorrhage associated with substantial clinical worsening of ≥4 points on the National Institutes of Health Stroke

Scale (NIHSS) and may be more predictive of ICH that adversely affects long-term outcome (25,26,28).

In previous years, the ECASS II/III classification was used to report sICH and divided it into hemorrhagic infarction (HI) and parenchymal hematoma (PH). HI is a heterogeneous hyperdensity occupying a portion of an ischemic infarct zone on CT, whereas PH refers to a more homogeneous, dense hematoma with mass effect. HI and PH are classified into two subtypes (Table 5.1 and Figure 5.2). The rate of HI is higher than PH (9% vs. 3% respectively). PH 2 with a lesion volume of greater than 30% is the only subtype of HT that

Table 5.1 Heidelberg and ECASS Radiologic Classification Schemes for Post-Thrombolysis Intracranial Hemorrhage

Heidelberg Bleeding Classification	ECASS II-III Classification	Definition
1		Hemorrhagic transformation of infarcted tissue
1a	HI 1	Small petechial hemorrhage without space-occupying effect
1b	HI 2	More confluent petechial hemorrhage without space-occupying effect
1c	PH 1	Hematoma within infarcted tissue, occupying <30%, no substantive mass effect
2	PH 2	Intracerebral hemorrhage within and beyond infarcted tissue Hematoma occupying >30% of the infarcted area with significant space-occupying effect
3		Intracerebral hemorrhage outside the infarcted brain tissue or intracranial–extracerebral hemorrhage
3a		PH remote from infarcted brain tissue
3b		Intraventricular hemorrhage
3c		Subarachnoid hemorrhage
3d		Subdural hemorrhage

ECASS, European Cooperative Acute Stroke Study; HI, hemorrhagic infarction; PH, parenchymal hematoma.

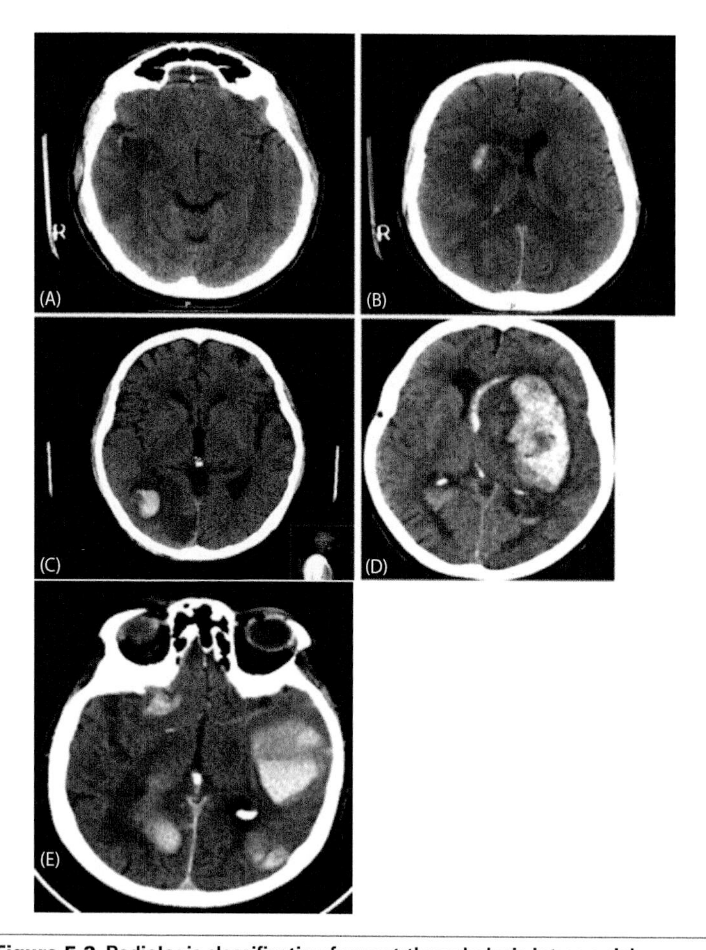

Figure 5.2 Radiologic classification for post-thrombolysis intracranial hemorrhage. (A) CT with hemorrhagic infarction ECASS HI 1/HBC 1a of right temporal lobe and basal ganglia. (B) CT with ECASS HI 2/HBC 1b of right striatum. (C) CT with PH type 1 in right posterior cerebral artery territory. (D) CT with extended ECASS PH 2/HBC 2 of left basal ganglia and insula with additional blood in both lateral ventricles HBC 3b and mass effect causing a shift of midline structures to the right. (E) Bilateral PHs (remote PH) with fluid level in the left PH ECASS PH 2/HBC 3a–3b indicating coagulation disorder.

ECASS, European Cooperative Acute Stroke Study; HI, hemorrhagic infarction; HBC, Heidelberg Bleeding Classification; PH, parenchymal hematoma.

Source: The Heidelberg Bleeding Classification: Classification of Bleeding Events After Ischemic Stroke and Reperfusion Therapy. von Kummer R, Broderick JP, Campbell BC, Demchuk A, et al. *Stroke*. 2015 Oct;46(10):2981–2986.

was shown to alter the clinical course of ischemic stroke and found to be a significant predictor of neurological deterioration with higher mortality and poor 3-month outcome (8,10).

The advent of MT dictated an expansion in the classification of hemorrhage after reperfusion therapy with or without the use of r-tPA. The IV r-tPA trials were focused on parenchymal hemorrhage because ICH is a predominant complication after thrombolytic therapy (24,28). However, subarachnoid hemorrhage (SAH) can also be observed after MT due to perforating or dissecting injury during device deployment, as well as stretch injury on perforating vessels from traction on the large arteries of the circle of Willis when retrieving the thrombectomy devices (24,28). The Heidelberg Bleeding Classification (HBC) for ICH was created by a consensus of stroke experts in 2015 and is now commonly employed in ongoing trials. The HBC amplifies the ECASS classification for ICHs after reperfusion therapy by including previously nonclassifiable hemorrhages, providing a formal approach for more precise anatomical descriptions, and better assessing for ICH symptomatology (Table 5.1 and Figure 5.2) (24,28). When comparing the rate of sICH in different trials, it remains important to take into consideration the differences between these classifications (24,28).

In multiple meta-analyses of randomized clinical trials for IV r-tPA (NINDS, ATLANTIS, ECASS I, II, III, EPITHET, and IST-3) and most community-based studies, the rate of sICH was 5% to 7% with an associated mortality close to 50% (8,23,29–33). An additional meta-analysis showed the risk of fatal intracranial hemorrhage from alteplase was 2.7% (compared to 0.4% with placebo) within 7 days; this risk was similar regardless of age, stroke severity, or time to treatment (6). Alteplase treatment had no significant effect on other early or late causes of death, including death at 90 days. These studies suggest that IV r-tPA leads to a good outcome in 33% to 35% of cases and can be used safely to treat AIS in regular clinical practice regardless of patient age, stroke severity, or the associated increased risk of symptomatic or fatal ICH in the first days after treatment (6,8,23,29–33). The benefit of IV r-tPA decreases continuously over time ("time is brain") as shown in a registry that analyzed data from over 58,000 patients treated with alteplase within 4.5 hours of AIS symptom onset (2,4–6). In this registry, each 15-minute delay in time to r-tPA treatment was associated with a 4% increase in the odds of sICH but importantly, did not mitigate the treatment benefit regardless of time strata (4).

RISK FACTORS

There are multiple risk factors associated with the development of sICH and poor neurologic outcomes after treatment with r-tPA and include age, weight and gender, stroke severity, early ischemic changes (EICs) in neuroimaging, cerebral microbleeds (CMBs), hyperglycemia and diabetes, hypertension, antiplatelet therapy, thrombocytopenia, atrial fibrillation (AF), and embolic stroke.

Age

Advanced age is associated with multiple comorbidities and worse outcomes regardless of r-tPA-related complications. Nevertheless, patients aged 80 years or older who are eligible for thrombolysis within 3 hours seem to benefit from treatment despite a higher mortality rate compared with younger patients. Of note, thrombolysis in patients older than 80 years old is a relative contraindication in the 3- to 4.5-hour time window (6,34–37).

Weight and Gender

In the SITS-MOST trial, body weight greater than 210 pounds (95 kg) has been associated with higher incidence of sICH despite the lower per-kilogram dose of alteplase. In the same study, male gender was associated with higher mortality rates and is concordant with other studies (33,37,38).

Stroke Severity and EICs on Neuroimaging

Larger areas of ischemia are generally associated with severe neurologic deficits and higher NIHSS scores. The larger the volume of damaged tissue, the greater the risk of HT. The SITS-MOST study has shown NIHSS score ≥10 to be associated with increased risk for sICH (2,6,33,37,39). However, strokes with high NIHSS scores without early neuroimaging evidence of large infarct changes will still benefit from thrombolysis within the therapeutic window according to a 2014 meta-analysis of individual patient data from 6,756 subjects (6).

In addition to ruling out hemorrhage, tumors, and prior infarcts, the baseline CT may provide useful information regarding the risk and benefit ratio related to r-tPA administration. Grading scales, such as the Alberta Stroke Program Early CT Score (ASPECTS), may also be helpful in assessing ischemic changes on CT in order to identify AIS patients unlikely to make an independent recovery despite thrombolytic treatment (38–40). A normal CT scan has an ASPECTS value of 10 points, while a score of 7 or less is associated with an odds ratio (OR) of 4.6 for sICH (33,37,39,41). EICs, either alone or with a hyperdense middle cerebral artery sign (HMCAS), are not a contraindication for thrombolysis and include subtle or small areas of hypodensity, loss of gray–white differentiation, cerebral edema, and obscuration of the lentiform nucleus (2,34,38,39,41). However, clearly defined, extensive regions of obvious hypodensity consistent with irreversible injury on baseline head CT should raise suspicion as to the true time of ischemic stroke onset, and thrombolytic treatment should be carefully considered. EIC with HMCAS involving more than one-third of the middle cerebral artery (MCA) territory is associated with sICH (OR of 9.38, vs. 3.17) and is an exclusion criterion for IV r-tPA in the 3- to 4.5-hour window (2,34,37,39,41). In these cases, MT is the treatment of choice regardless of whether patients receive IV r-tPA for the same ischemic stroke event (2,40). MT has not been associated with increased rates of sICH or mortality according to meta-analysis of multiple trials (7,40). The mechanisms for reperfusion hemorrhage after MT are similar to those described for IV thrombolysis. However, SAH is a complication more commonly seen after MT in comparison to IV r-tPA alone due to the mechanical nature of the procedure as previously described. In most cases, minor asymptomatic SAH occurs without functional impact at discharge. Only extensive SAH or those accompanied by severe PHs after MT may worsen clinical outcome at discharge (25,42).

Cerebral Microbleeds

Recent meta-analyses found that the presence of CMBs on brain MRI before treatment was associated with an increased risk of ICH in patients treated with IV thrombolysis for AIS (2,43,44). According to the guidelines, in otherwise eligible patients who have previously had a high burden of CMBs (>10) demonstrated on MRI, treatment with IV alteplase may be associated with an increased risk of sICH. Although the benefits are uncertain due to contradictory data, treatment is likely reasonable depending on the stroke severity (2,43–45).

Hyperglycemia and Diabetes

Evidence indicates that persistent in-hospital hyperglycemia (glucose >180 mg/dL) during the first 24 hours after reperfusion therapy predisposes to sICH and has been associated with diminished neurologic improvement, greater infarct size, and worse clinical outcome at 3 months after treatment (2,46–49). It is reasonable to treat hyperglycemia to achieve blood glucose levels in a range of 140 to 180 mg/dL (7.8-10 mmol/L) and to closely monitor to prevent hypoglycemia

(2,46–49). Some studies suggest that hyperglycemia may augment brain injury by several mechanisms including increased tissue acidosis from anaerobic metabolism, free radical generation, and increased BBB permeability increasing the risk of HT (3,13–23,46–49). Regarding diabetes treatment, several retrospective studies have reported that in diabetic patients with AIS, previous and continued use of sulfonylureas is associated with reduced sICH (48,49).

Hypertension

Approximately 75% of patients present with elevated blood pressure at the time of ischemic stroke (50). Several studies have confirmed significantly higher rates of sICH with elevated pretreatment and posttreatment blood pressure readings (systolic blood pressure [SBP] >185 and diastolic blood pressure [DBP] >110) (38,50). The rate of sICH with IV r-tPA administration and uncontrolled hypertension at presentation is 26% (37,51). The SITS-International Stroke Thrombolysis Register (ISTR) database was used in a retrospective analysis of the relationships between blood pressure and the development of PH 2, mortality, and independence at 3 months (32,52,53). The SITS-ISTR concluded that high blood pressure was associated with a worse outcome; however, as a categorical variable, blood pressure had a linear association with sICH and a U-shaped association with mortality and independence. In addition, SBP of 141 to150 mmHg was associated with the most favorable outcomes (32,52,53). The 2018 American Heart Association/American Stroke Association (AHA/ASA) guidelines have special considerations regarding blood pressure control in patients with AIS who are eligible for IV thrombolytic therapy. Before initiation of thrombolysis, the blood pressure must be at or below 185 mmHg systolic (SBP) and 110 mmHg diastolic (DBP). Once thrombolytic therapy has been administered, the blood pressure must be maintained below 180/105 mmHg within 24 hours following r-tPA (2). In patients treated with thrombolysis, lowering the systemic blood pressure has been associated with clinical deterioration and increased incidence of sICH in observational studies in the first 24 hours after stroke onset due to loss of CBF autoregulation (54–56). Under normal physiological conditions, CBF remains independent of mean arterial blood pressure across a wide range not withstanding extreme low and high values (3,15,57,58). However, the regional CBF in the ischemic penumbra is dependent upon the systemic blood pressure due to loss of CBF autoregulation, which results in vasodilatation and low perfusion pressure distal to the occluded vessel (3,23,57–59). The goal of permissive HTN is to optimize blood flow to the ischemic penumbra until IV r-tPA and intra-arterial recanalization therapies can be employed or optimization of the collateral vasculature can occur (2,34,52,59). Nevertheless, the optimal lower end range of desired blood pressure is unclear in patients requiring antihypertensive treatment for thrombolysis. The only evidence-based guideline recommendation is to keep SBP less than 180 and DBP less than 105, despite the risk of worsening blood flow and increasing HT within the ischemic penumbra if blood pressure is driven too low (7,52). The recommended values based on expert opinions are to keep SBP between 150 and 180 mmHg prior to reperfusion, and targeting SBP to less than140 mmHg once reperfusion is achieved with r-tPA or MT (2,52). For patients with ischemic stroke who are not treated with thrombolytic therapy, the 2018 AHA/ASA guidelines recommend withholding antihypertensive therapies unless SBP is greater than 220 mmHg or DBP is greater than 120 mmHg (2,52,60). When treatment is indicated, cautious lowering of blood pressure by 15% during the first 24 hours after stroke onset is recommended (2,52,60).

Antiplatelet Therapy

Approximately 30% of patients have taken aspirin prior to hospitalization and treatment with r-tPA (38,61). Small retrospective studies suggest that dual antiplatelet therapy (DAPT) with aspirin and clopidogrel has a higher risk of sICH than single antiplatelet therapy or no antiplatelet use (38,62). Despite the higher potential risk of sICH with DAPT, outcomes do not seem to be affected (38,61,62). Hence, the benefits of r-tPA outweigh any potential increased risk of sICH in patients taking antiplatelet therapy before stroke onset. On the other hand, the 2018 AHA/ASA guidelines recommend holding aspirin administration for 24 hours after thrombolysis (2). The development of secondary HT of an ischemic infarct does not preclude the early use of aspirin, particularly when the hemorrhage is petechial (2). It is not clear that stopping aspirin influences hematoma progression; however, aspirin administration is often withheld in patients who develop PH 1 or PH 2 (2). Aspirin should be given once the patient's neurologic condition becomes stable.

Thrombocytopenia

In patients without history of thrombocytopenia, treatment with IV alteplase can be initiated before platelet count is available but should be discontinued if it is less than 100,000/mm^3. A low platelet count has been associated with the development of early HT and sICH in patients with nonlacunar ischemic stroke (2,45,63). It has been hypothesized that the decreased overall number of platelets available for activation and aggregation directly increases the risk of HT (2,3,45,63).

AF and Embolic Stroke

AF is correlated with more severe ischemic strokes and longer transient ischemic attacks than emboli from carotid disease, presumably due to embolization of larger particles (64–68). Hence, embolic stroke due to AF results in more severe baseline hypoperfusion and leads to greater infarct area, higher incidence of severe HT, and worse stroke outcomes (45,68). In previous studies, the volume of infarction edema on the initial CT scan has been independently related to the risk of HT after cardioembolic stroke. In particular, the probability of HT resulting in asymptomatic ICH was about 95% if the volume of infarction edema did not exceed 10 cm^3 (45,68).

PREVENTION

Successful treatment of AIS with IV r-tPA is highly time dependent with efficacy quickly diminishing over time. Thrombolytic therapy should be administered to all AIS patients who have met the inclusion criteria within 3 hours of symptom onset and to a more selective group of eligible acute stroke patients (based on ECASS III exclusion criteria) within 4.5 hours of last known normal (2). Centers should attempt to achieve door-to-needle times of less than 60 minutes in ≥50% of stroke patients who are candidates for thrombolytic therapy (2). It has been demonstrated that thrombolytic treatment can be beneficial up to 4.5 hours. However, sICH rates appear to increase within the 5- to 6-hour time frame (60). The best way to prevent the development of sICH is adherence to 2018 AHA/ASA treatment guidelines. These guidelines detail standard thrombolytic inclusion and exclusion criteria, posttreatment protocols of blood pressure management, and proper use of antiplatelet/anticoagulant medications (2,38).

It is well known that sICH has a significant negative impact on the outcome of ischemic stroke, and hence, this small but real risk of sICH still discourages many clinicians from administering r-tPA. This is particularly true for patients with multiple comorbidities and risk factors for sICH (38,45,69,70). For this reason, several risk assessment methods and predictive tools for prognosis have been created to identify patients with AIS who are at increased risk for developing sICH after thrombolytic therapy. A clinical score that predicts the risk of sICH would be useful in addition to standard inclusion criteria for r-tPA administration and may increase the number of patients treated with thrombolysis (70). The challenge in designing clinical scores is to utilize a select few parameters that can accurately predict sICH while maintaining computational simplicity (70). At least seven clinical risk factor scores have been developed and include the Hemorrhage After Thrombolysis (HAT) score, SEDAN score, Stroke-Thrombolytic Predictive Instrument (Stroke-TPI), Stroke Prognostication using Age and NIHSS (SPAN)-100 index, Safe Implementation of Thrombolysis in Stroke–symptomatic IntraCerebral Hemorrhage (SITS- sICH) risk score, Glucose Race Age Sex Pressure Stroke Severity (GRASPS) score, and Multicenter Stroke Survey (MSS); see Table 5.2 (33,70–79). However, additional validation studies are needed to confirm the utility of these scores before they can be used in routine clinical practice (71,80,81).

The development of blood markers that may predict the risk of HT of AIS after IV r-tPA has been investigated in multiple studies. The principle behind the development of these blood markers is based on the understanding that HT is the result of the disruption of the microvasculature endothelial components leading to an increase in the permeability of the BBB (3,17–21). Serum levels of molecules considered to be biomarkers of endothelial damage, such as MMP-9/MMP-2, cellular fibronectin, and caveolin-1 have been reported as being able to predict HT in patients treated with r-tPA (3,17–21). However, before these biomarkers become applicable in routine clinical practice, faster tests to perform the analyses are required, and further studies must be undertaken to validate and generalize the results.

BBB disruption in AIS has been demonstrated as early parenchymal and vascular enhancement due to contrast extravasation on CT and MRI, which is also predictive of HT after r-tPA administration (3,82). Increasing evidence suggests that permeability imaging features might be good predictors of HT. One approach to identifying patients at risk of HT is to seek evidence of BBB damage before thrombolysis. In this respect, there are promising permeability imaging methods using both CT and MRI. One of these promising methods to determine BBB permeability consists of modeling the transfer constant (K^{trans}), a metric of BBB integrity, based on the measurement of the intravascular tracer leakage into the extravascular space (3,83,84). However, the best BBB-permeability volume threshold to predict HT by perfusion CT (PCT) has not been established yet, in large part due to differences in image acquisition and data modeling (3,83,84). Despite these differences, recent studies using high-permeability region size on PCT (HP_{rs}-PCT) and a threshold of 7 mL/100 g/min could reliably identify patients at low risk of

Table 5.2 Risk Assessment Methods and Predictive Tools for Patients With Increased Risk for Developing sICH After Thrombolytic Therapy

Score/Criteria for sICH	Components	Cutoff Values, Score Points (pts)	Total Score	Overall Risk Level	Percentages
SITS-MOST (SITS sICH)	ASA + clopidogrel ASA alone NIHSS BG, mg/dl Age, years SBP, mmHg Weight, kg Onset to treatment, min History of HTN	Yes, 3 pts Yes, 2 pts 7–12, 1 pt ≥13, 1 pt ≥180, 2 pts ≥72, 1 pt ≥146, 1 pt ≥95, 1 pt ≥180, 1 pt Yes, 1 pt	0–2 pts 3–5 pts 6–8 pts ≥9 pts	Risk of sICH Low Average Moderate High	Rate of sICH 0.4% 1.5% 3.6% 9.2%
HAT (NINDS sICH)	History of diabetes mellitus **or** BG ≥ 200 Pretreatment NIHSS Initial CT with hypodense MCA	Yes, 1 pt 15–19, 1 pt ≥20, 2 pts ≥1/3, 2 pts <1/3, 1 pt	0 pts 1 pt 2 pts 3 pts ≥4 pts	Risk of sICH 2% 5% 10% 15% 44%	Risk of fatal hemorrhage 0% 3% 7% 6% 33%

(continued)

Table 5.2 Risk Assessment Methods and Predictive Tools for Patients With Increased Risk for Developing sICH After Thrombolytic Therapy (*continued*)

Score/Criteria for sICH	Components	Cutoff Values, Score Points (pts)	Total Score	Overall Risk Level	Percentages
SPAN (NINDS sICH) Determines favorable outcome (within 3 months) and ICH risk after r-tPA	Age NIHSS on admission	SPAN positive SPAN negative	If age + NIHSS is ≥100 If age + NIHSS is <100	Outcome Nonfavorable 5.6% of cases Favorable 55.4% of cases	ICH risk 42% 12%
SEDAN (ECASS sICH)	Blood **S**ugar **E**arly infarct signs on CT Hyper**D**ense cerebral artery sign on CT **A**ge **N**IHSS	145–216, 1 pt >216, 2 pts Yes, 1 pt Yes, 1 pt >75, 1 pt ≥10, 1 pt	 0 1 2 3 4 5	Risk of sICH 1.6% 3.3% 5.4% 8.8% 12.3% 16.9%	
MSS (NINDS sICH) MSS Score	Age NIHSS admission BG Platelets, 103 mm^3	>60, 1 pt >10, 1 pt >149, 1 pt <150, 1 pt	 0 pts 1 pt 2 pts ≥3 pts	ICH risk after IV r-tPA 2.6% 9.7% 15.1% 37.9%	A similar pattern was seen with symptomatic and asymptomatic ICH separately, and with radiographically defined parenchymal hemorrhage

(*continued*)

Table 5.2 Risk Assessment Methods and Predictive Tools for Patients With Increased Risk for Developing sICH After Thrombolytic Therapy (*continued*)

Score/Criteria for sICH	Components	Cutoff Values, Score Points (pts)	Total Score	Overall Risk Level	Percentages
GRASPS (NINDS sICH)	B**G** **R**ace **A**ge **S**ex **P**ressure: SBP **S**troke Severity: NIHSS admission	<100, 2 pts 100–149, 6 pts ≥150, 8 pts Asian, 9 pts No Asian, 0 pt <60, 8 pts 61–70, 11 pts 71–80, 15 pts >80, 17 pts Male, 4 pts Female, 0 pt <120, 10 pts 120–149, 14 pts 150–179, 18 pts ≥180, 21 pts 0–5, 25 pts 6–10, 27 pts 11–15, 34 pts 16–20, 40 pts >20, 42 pts	45–57 pts 58–63 pts 64–68 pts 69–71 pts 78–79 pts 82 pts 85 pts	Risk of sICH within 36 hours after IV r-tPA 1% 2% 3% 4% 8% 10% 13%	

BG, blood glucose; ECASS, European Cooperative Acute Stroke Study; GRASPS, Glucose Race Age Sex Pressure Stroke Severity; HAT, Hemorrhage After Thrombolysis; HTN, hypertension; ICH, intracerebral hemorrhage; IV, intravenous; MCA, middle cerebral artery; MSS, Multicenter Stroke Survey; NIHSS, National Institutes of Health Stroke Scale; NINDS, National Institute of Neurological Disorders and Stroke; r-tPA, recombinant tissue plasminogen activator; SBP, systolic blood pressure; SITS-MOST, Safe Implementation of Thrombolysis in Stroke-Monitoring Study; sICH, symptomatic intracerebral hemorrhage; SPAN, Stroke Prognostication using Age and NIHSS.

developing HT and PH 2 after r-tPA administration (82–86). By using this approach, patients with low risk of bleeding beyond the current therapeutic window for r-tPA administration could potentially be identified and safely treated. Regarding MRI studies, there are two modalities, HARM and ASL (arterial spin labeling), that are able to identify BBB-permeability changes (21,87–90). HARM is defined as delayed enhancement of the subarachnoid or subpial space on post-contrast fluid-attenuated inversion recovery (FLAIR) images due to contrast material leakage from ischemic tissue to the subarachnoid space (21,86–88). HARM is associated with upregulation of MMP-9 and increased monocyte count during BBB disruption in AIS (91). The presence of HARM has been correlated with specific stroke etiologies including large artery atherosclerosis and cardioembolic stroke. In contrast, small vessel occlusion has been associated with the absence of HARM. MCA and cortical infarction have more pronounced HARM compared to infarctions at other vascular territories and anatomic compartments (87–89). ASL techniques enable CBF measurements without the use of a contrast agent and are sensitive in detecting hyperemic lesions (HLs) in several conditions such as ischemic stroke, tumor, seizures, and Moyamoya disease. HLs (defined as a region where relative CBF ≥1.4 normal) detected on pretreatment ASL maps are associated with subsequent BBB disruption and HT in AIS (90). The identification of HLs may allow for the prediction and localization of BBB disruption and HT in AIS patients eligible for endovascular therapy (90). However, further studies will need to be done to determine how HP_{rs}-PCT, MRI-HARM, and MRI-ASL might refine clinical decision making in AIS patients treated within and beyond the current r-tPA therapeutic window (84–90).

IDENTIFICATION AND MANAGEMENT

After administration of IV r-tPA, all patients should be admitted to a neurocritical care or stroke unit for close monitoring generally for a period of 24 hours (2). These measures are based on AHA guidelines with both protocolized serial neurologic monitoring and also vital sign assessment that is designed to maximize early recognition of complications and facilitates their management to improve outcomes (2).

sICH should be suspected in any patient who develops sudden deterioration in level of consciousness, new headache, nausea and vomiting, or a sudden rise in blood pressure after thrombolytic therapy, especially within the first 24 hours of treatment. The first steps in the management are to stop the infusion of r-tPA until sICH is ruled out by obtaining a STAT noncontrast head CT or MRI.

Laboratory studies must include typing and crossmatching, PT, PTT, platelet count, and fibrinogen (2,22,23).

The recommended management of sICH in the 2018 AHA/ASA guidelines for management of AIS is based on small case series and expert opinions with the guidelines acknowledging limited evidence to support the details of care (2,22,23). The treatment goal is the replacement of coagulation factors and platelets to rapidly correct the fibrinolytic state produced by r-tPA and prevent both ICH expansion and concomitant worsening of neurological outcome (2,22,23). According to the guidelines, the administration of the following agents to treat sICH and reverse the effects of thrombolytic therapy includes: (a) cryoprecipitate (including factor VIII), 10 units immediately infused over 10 to 30 minutes (onset in 1 hour, peaks in 12 hours) and more as needed to achieve a serum fibrinogen level of ≥200 mg/dL; (b) tranexamic acid (10–15 mg/kg) 1,000 mg IV infused over 10 to 20 minutes; or aminocaproic acid 4 to 5 g IV during the first hour, followed by 1 g IV until bleeding is controlled (peak onset in 3 hours) (2,22,23). In some circumstances, the use of complementary therapy agents includes the following: (a) prothrombin complex concentrate as adjuvant to cryoprecipitate for patients on warfarin prior to alteplase treatment, or fresh frozen plasma as adjuvant to cryoprecipitate if prothrombin complex concentrate is not available; (b) vitamin K (10 mg IV) as adjuvant for patients on warfarin prior to alteplase treatment; (c) platelets (6–8 units) for patients with thrombocytopenia of less than 100,000/microliter; (d) protamine sulfate 1 mg for every 100 units of unfractionated heparin given in the preceding 4 hours, or administration of recombinant factor VIIa (2,22,23).

Supportive therapy includes management of blood pressure, intracranial pressure, cerebral perfusion pressure, and glucose control (2,22,23). Regarding blood pressure management, the only guideline recommendation based on consensus of expert opinion and clinical experience is blood pressure reduction by 15% (2). In patients with sICH, blood pressure targets are unclear due to conflicting data, but the goal is to achieve a balance between providing adequate blood flow to the ischemic territory and lowering the blood pressure to reduce the risk of hematoma expansion (91). Among patients with H1 or H2 and incomplete recanalization, higher blood pressure targets may be necessary to maintain adequate collateral blood flow to the ischemic penumbra and to reduce risk of infarct growth. On the other hand, in patients with full recanalization, strict blood pressure control with a target of normal blood pressure may be reasonable (91).

Finally, urgent neurosurgery and hematology consultations are indicated when sICH is diagnosed (2,22,23). Surgical intervention to reverse or prevent herniation may be lifesaving. Neither hemicraniectomy and/or craniotomy and hematoma evacuation has proven efficacy in sICH post r-tPA (92,93). Neurosurgeons may be reluctant to perform a ventriculostomy or craniotomy in the acute setting while the patient is coagulopathic owing to the difficulty with achieving hemostasis (2,23,24). However, both of these interventions may be necessary and should be considered on a case-by-case basis. In a retrospective analysis of data from the GUSTO-I trial of thrombolysis for myocardial infarction, 30-day survival was significantly higher with surgical hematoma evacuation than without (65% vs. 35%) (94). Additionally in the same trial, there was a trend favoring improved functional outcome with a higher incidence of nondisabling stroke in those with evacuation compared with those without (20% vs. 12%) (94).

CONCLUSIONS

HT is a frequent, spontaneous, and natural consequence of infarction and reperfusion characterized by a range of ischemia-related blood extravasation. It results from a robust inflammatory response that results in disruption of the BBB and increased paracellular permeability. In contrast, sICH is a rare complication after IV alteplase treatment with an incidence of 5% to 7% (95). Although it remains an important clinical event that requires early recognition and treatment, the small risk for sICH should not discourage treatment with IV r-TPA or MT for patients who meet treatment criteria. The best ways to prevent the development of sICH is adherence to treatment guidelines. Several risk assessment methods and predictive tools for prognosis have been created to identify patients with AIS who are at an increased risk for developing sICH after thrombolytic therapy. However, additional validation studies are needed to confirm the utility of these methods before they should be used in clinical practice.

REFERENCES

1. Benjamin EJ, Blaha MJ, Chiuve SE, et al. Heart disease and stroke statistics—2017 update: a report from the American Heart Association. *Circulation*. 2017;135:e229–e445. doi:10.1161/CIR.0000000000000485
2. Powers WJ, Rabinstein AA, Ackerson T, et al. American Heart Association Stroke Council. 2018 Guidelines for the early management of patients with acute ischemic stroke: a guideline for healthcare professionals from the American Heart Association/American Stroke Association. *Stroke*. 2018;49(3):e46–e110. doi:10.1161/str.0000000000000163

3. Khatri R, McKinney AM, Swenson B, et al. Blood-brain barrier, reperfusion injury, and hemorrhagic transformation in acute ischemic stroke. *Neurol.* 2012;79 (13 Suppl 1):S52–S57. doi:10.1212/wnl.0b013e3182697e70
4. Saver JL, Fonarow GC, Smith EE, et al. Time to treatment with intravenous tissue plasminogen activator and outcome from acute ischemic stroke. *JAMA.* 2013;309:2480. doi:10.1001/jama.2013.6959
5. Wardlaw JM, Murray V, Berge E, et al. Recombinant tissue plasminogen activator for acute ischaemic stroke: an updated systematic review and meta-analysis. *Lancet.* 2012;379:2364. doi:10.1016/s0140-6736(12)60738-7
6. Emberson J, Lees KR, Lyden P, et al. Effect of treatment delay, age, and stroke severity on the effects of intravenous thrombolysis with alteplase for acute ischemic stroke: a meta-analysis of individual patient data from randomized trials. *Lancet.* 2014;384:1929. doi:10.1016/s0140-6736(14)60584-5
7. Prabhakaran S, Ruff I, Bernstein RA. Acute stroke intervention: a systematic review. *JAMA.* 2015;313:1451. doi:10.1001/jama.2015.3058
8. Whiteley WN, Emberson J, Lees KR, et al. Risk of intracerebral haemorrhage with alteplase after acute ischaemic stroke: a secondary analysis of an individual patient data meta-analysis. *Lancet Neurol.* 2016;15:925. doi:10.1016/s1474-4422(16)30076-x
9. Lees KR, Emberson J, Blackwell L, et al. Effects of alteplase for acute stroke on the distribution of functional outcomes: a pooled analysis of 9 trials. *Stroke.* 2016;47:2373. doi:10.1161/strokeaha.116.013644
10. Sussman ES, Connolly ES Jr. Hemorrhagic transformation: a review of the rate of hemorrhage in the major clinical trials of acute ischemic stroke. *Front Neurol.* 2013;4:69. doi:10.3389/fneur.2013.00069
11. Jaillard A, Cornu C, Durieux A, et al. Hemorrhagic transformation in acute ischemic stroke. The MAST-E study. MAST-E Group. *Stroke.* 1999;30:1326–1332. doi:10.1161/01.str.30.7.1326
12. Bang OY, Saver JL, Kim SJ, et al. Collateral flow averts hemorrhagic transformation after endovascular therapy for acute ischemic stroke. *Stroke.* 2011;42:2235–2239. doi:10.1161/strokeaha.110.604603
13. Wang X, Lo EH. Triggers and mediators of hemorrhagic transformation in cerebral ischemia. *Mol Neurobiol.* 2003;28:229–244. doi:10.1385/mn:28:3:229
14. Hamann GF, Okada Y, del Zoppo GJ. Hemorrhagic transformation and microvascular integrity during focal cerebral ischemia/reperfusion. *J Cereb Blood Flow Metab.* 1996;16(6):1373–1378. doi:10.1097/00004647-199611000-00036
15. Reggie Lee HC, Goyanes-Vasquez JJ, Couto e Silva A, et al. Fatty acid methyl esters as a potential therapy against cerebral ischemia. *OCL.* 2016;23(1):D108. doi:10.1051/ocl/2015040

16. Castellanos M, Serena J. Applicability of biomarkers in ischemic stroke. *Cerebrovasc Dis.* 2007;24(suppl 1):7–15. doi:10.1159/000107374
17. Castellanos M, Sobrino T, Millán M, et al. Serum cellular bronectin and matrix metalloproteinase-9 as screening biomarkers for the prediction of parenchymal hematoma after thrombolytic therapy in acute ischemic stroke: a multicenter confirmatory study. *Stroke.* 2007;38:1855–1859. doi:10.1161/strokeaha.106.481556
18. Xu L, Guo R, Xie Y, et al. Caveolae: molecular insights and therapeutic targets for stroke. *Expert Opin Ther Targets.* 2015;19:633–650. doi:10.1517/14728222.2015.1009446
19. Castellanos M, Van Eendenburg C, Gubern C, et al. Low levels of caveolin-1 predict symptomatic bleeding after thrombolytic therapy in patients with acute ischemic stroke. *Stroke.* 2018;49(6):1525–1527. doi:10.1161/strokeaha.118.020683
20. Suofu Y, Clark JF, Broderick JP, et al. Matrix metalloproteinase-2 or -9 deletions protect against hemorrhagic transformation during early stage of cerebral ischemia and reperfusion. *Neuroscience.* 2012;212:180–189. doi:10.1016/j.neuroscience.2012.03.036
21. Warach S, Latour LL. Evidence of reperfusion injury, exacerbated by thrombolytic therapy, in human focal brain ischemia using a novel imaging marker of early blood-brain barrier disruption. *Stroke.* 2004;35:2659–2661. doi:10.1161/01.str.0000144051.32131.09
22. National Institute of Neurological Disorders and Stroke rt-PA Stroke Study Group. Tissue plasminogen activator for acute ischemic stroke. *N Engl J Med.* 1995;14;333(24):1581–1587. doi:10.1056/nejm199512143332401
23. Yaghi S, Eisenberger A, Willey JZ. Symptomatic intracerebral hemorrhage in acute ischemic stroke after thrombolysis with intravenous recombinant tissue plasminogen activator: a review of natural history and treatment. *JAMA Neurol.* 2014;71(9):1181–1185. doi:10.1001/jamaneurol.2014.1210
24. von Kummer R, Broderick JP, Campbell BC, et al. The Heidelberg Bleeding Classification: classification of bleeding events after ischemic stroke and reperfusion therapy. *Stroke.* 2015;46(10):2981–2986. doi:10.1161/strokeaha.115.010049
25. Gumbinger C, Gruschka P, Böttinger M, et al. Improved prediction of poor outcome after thrombolysis using conservative definitions of symptomatic hemorrhage. *Stroke.* 2012;43(1):240–242. doi:10.1161/strokeaha.111.623033
26. Demaerschalk BM, Kleindorfer DO, Adeoye OM, et al. Scientific rationale for the inclusion and exclusion criteria for intravenous alteplase in acute ischemic stroke: a statement for healthcare professionals from the American Heart Association/American Stroke Association. *Stroke.* 47(2):581–641. doi:10.1161/str.0000000000000086

27. Neuberger U, Möhlenbruch MA, Herweh C, et al. Classification of bleeding events: comparison of ECASS III (European Cooperative Acute Stroke Study) and the New Heidelberg Bleeding Classification. *Stroke*. 2017;48(7):1983–1985. doi:10.1161/strokeaha.117.016735s
28. Rao NM, Levine SR, Gornbein JA, et al. Defining clinically relevant cerebral hemorrhage after thrombolytic therapy for stroke: analysis of the National Institute of Neurological Disorders and Stroke tissue-type plasminogen activator trials. *Stroke*. 2014;45(9):2728–2733. doi:10.1161/strokeaha.114.005135
29. Albers GW, Bates VE, Clark WM, et al. Intravenous tissue-type plasminogen activator for treatment of acute stroke: the Standard Treatment with Alteplase to Reverse Stroke (STARS) study. *JAMA*. 2000;283:1145. doi:10.1001/jama.283.9.1145
30. LaMonte MP, Bahouth MN, Magder LS, et al. A regional system of stroke care provides thrombolytic outcomes comparable with the NINDS stroke trial. *Ann Emerg Med*. 2009;54:319. doi:10.1016/j.annemergmed.2008.09.022
31. Hill MD, Buchan AM. Canadian alteplase for stroke effectiveness study (CASES) investigators. Thrombolysis for acute ischemic stroke: results of the Canadian Alteplase for stroke effectiveness study. *Can Med Assoc J*. 2005;172:1307. doi:10.1503/cmaj.1041561
32. Wahlgren N, Ahmed N, Dávalos A, et al. Thrombolysis with alteplase for acute ischaemic stroke in the Safe Implementation of Thrombolysis in Stroke-Monitoring Study (SITS-MOST): an observational study. *Lancet*. 2007;369:275. doi:10.1016/s0140-6736(07)60149-4
33. Mazya M, Egido JA, Ford GA, et al. Predicting the risk of symptomatic intracerebral hemorrhage in ischemic stroke treated with intravenous alteplase: safe Implementation of Treatments in Stroke (SITS) symptomatic intracerebral hemorrhage risk score. *Stroke*. 2012;43:1524. doi:10.1161/strokeaha.111.644815
34. Cronin CA, Shah N, Morovati T, et al. No increased risk of symptomatic intracerebral hemorrhage after thrombolysis in patients with European Cooperative Acute Stroke Study (ECASS) exclusion criteria. *Stroke*. 2012;43:1684. doi:10.1161/strokeaha.112.656587
35. Hill MD, Coutts SB. Alteplase in acute ischaemic stroke: the need for speed. *Lancet*. 2014;384:1904. doi:10.1016/s0140-6736(14)60662-0
36. Miller D, Simpson J, Silver B. Safety of thrombolysis in acute ischemic stroke: a review of complications, risk factors, and newer technologies. *Neurohospitalist*. 2011;1(3):138–147. doi:10.1177/1941875211408731
37. Tanne D, Kasner SE, Demchuk AM, et al. Markers of increased risk of intracerebral hemorrhage after intravenous recombinant tissue plasminogen activator therapy for acute ischemic stroke in clinical practice: the Multicenter rt-PA Stroke Survey. *Circ*. 2002;105(14):1679–1685. doi:10.1161/01.cir.0000012747.53592.6a

38. Wahlgren N, Ahmed N, Eriksson N, et al. Multivariable analysis of outcome predictors and adjustment of main outcome results to baseline data profile in randomized controlled trials: safe implementation of thrombolysis in Stroke-Monitoring Study (SITS-MOST). *Stroke.* 2008;39(12):3316–3322. doi:10.1161/strokeaha.107.510768
39. Barber PA, Demchuk AM, Zhang J, et al. Validity and reliability of a quantitative computed tomography score in predicting outcome of hyperacute stroke before thrombolytic therapy. ASPECTS Study Group. Alberta stroke programme early CT Score. *Lancet.* 2000;355:1670. doi:10.1016/s0140-6736(00)02237-6
40. Goyal M, Menon BK, van Zwam WH, et al. Endovascular thrombectomy after large-vessel ischaemic stroke: a meta-analysis of individual patient data from five randomised trials. *Lancet.* 2016;387:1723. doi:10.1016/s0140-6736(16)00163-x
41. Pexman JH, Barber PA, Hill MD, et al. Use of the Alberta stroke program early CT Score (ASPECTS) for assessing CT scans in patients with acute stroke. *AJNR Am J Neuroradiol.* 2001;22:1534. doi:10.3174/ajnr.a0975
42. Shi ZS1, Liebeskind DS, Loh Y, et al. Predictors of subarachnoid hemorrhage in acute ischemic stroke with endovascular therapy. *Stroke.* 2010;41(12):2775–2781. doi:10.1161/strokeaha.110.587063
43. Charidimou A, Shoamanesh A, Wilson D, et al. Cerebral microbleeds and postthrombolysis intracerebral hemorrhage risk updated meta-analysis. *Neurol.* 2015;85:927. doi:10.1212/wnl.0000000000001923
44. Tsivgoulis G, Zand R, Katsanos AH, et al. Risk of symptomatic intracerebral hemorrhage after intravenous thrombolysis in patients with acute ischemic stroke and high cerebral microbleed burden: a meta-analysis. *JAMA Neurol.* 2016;73:675. doi:10.1001/jamaneurol.2016.0292
45. Zhang J, Yang Y, Sun H, et al. Hemorrhagic transformation after cerebral infarction: current concepts and challenges. *Ann Transl Med.* 2014;2(8):81. doi:10.5535/arm.2014.38.5.698
46. Alvarez-Sabín J, Molina CA, Montaner J, et al. Effects of admission hyperglycemia on stroke outcome in reperfused tissue plasminogen activator—treated patients. *Stroke.* 2003;34:1235. doi:10.1161/01.str.0000068406.30514.31
47. Ahmed N, Dávalos A, Eriksson N, et al. Association of admission blood glucose and outcome in patients treated with intravenous thrombolysis: results from the Safe Implementation of Treatments in Stroke International Stroke Thrombolysis Register (SITS-ISTR). *Arch Neurol.* 2010;67:1123. doi:10.1001/archneurol.2010.210
48. Masrur S, Cox M, Bhatt DL, et al. Association of acute and chronic hyperglycemia with acute ischemic stroke outcomes post-thrombolysis: findings from get with the guidelines-stroke. *J Am Heart Assoc.* 2015;4:e002193. doi:10.1161/jaha.115.002193
49. Kunte H, Busch MA, Trostdorf K, et al. Hemorrhagic transformation of ischemic stroke in diabetics on sulfonylureas. *Ann Neurol.* 2012;72:799–806. doi:10.1002/ana.23680

50. Rodriguez-Garcia JL, Botia E, de La Sierra A, et al. Significance of elevated blood pressure and its management on the short-term outcome of patients with acute ischemic stroke. *Am J Hypertens.* 2005;18(3):379–384. doi:10.1016/j.amjhyper.2004.10.004
51. Tsivgoulis G, Frey JL, Flaster M, et al. Pre-tissue plasminogen activator blood pressure levels and risk of symptomatic intracerebral hemorrhage. *Stroke.* 2009;40(11):3631–3634. doi:10.1161/strokeaha.109.564096
52. McManus M, Liebeskind DS. Blood pressure in acute ischemic stroke. *J Clin Neurol.* 2016;12(2):137–146. doi:10.3988/jcn.2016.12.2.137
53. Ahmed N, Wahlgren N, Brainin M, et al. Relationship of blood pressure, antihypertensive therapy, and outcome in ischemic stroke treated with intravenous thrombolysis: retrospective analysis from Safe Implementation of Thrombolysis in Stroke-International Stroke Thrombolysis Register (SITS-ISTR). *Stroke.* 2009;40:2442–2449. doi:10.1161/strokeaha.109.548602
54. Oliveira-Filho J, Silva SC, Trabuco CC, et al. Detrimental effect of blood pressure reduction in the first 24 hours of acute stroke onset. *Neurol.* 2003;61:1047. doi:10.1212/01.wnl.0000092498.75010.57
55. Vlcek M, Schillinger M, Lang W, et al. Association between course of blood pressure within the first 24 hours and functional recovery after acute ischemic stroke. *Ann Emerg Med.* 2003;42:619. doi:10.1016/s0196-0644(03)00609-7
56. Castillo J, Leira R, García MM, et al. Blood pressure decrease during the acute phase of ischemic stroke is associated with brain injury and poor stroke outcome. *Stroke.* 2004;35:520. doi:10.1161/01.str.0000109769.22917.b0
57. Aiyagari V, Gorelick PB. Management of blood pressure for acute and recurrent stroke. *Stroke.* 2009;40:2251. doi:10.1161/strokeaha.108.531574
58. National Institute for Health and Clinical Excellence. *Stroke: The diagnosis and acute management of stroke and transient ischaemic attacks.* London, UK: Royal College of Physicians; 2008. http://www.nice.org.uk/CG068
59. Qureshi AI. Acute hypertensive response in patients with stroke: pathophysiology and management. *Circulation.* 2008;118:176. doi:10.1161/circulationaha.107.723874
60. Clark WM, Albers GW, Madden KP, et al. The rtPA (alteplase) 0- to 6-hour acute stroke trial, part A (A0276g): results of a double-blind, placebo-controlled, multicenter study. Thrombolytic therapy in acute ischemic stroke study investigators. *Stroke.* 2000;31(4):811–816. doi:10.1161/01.str.31.4.811
61. Dowlatshahi D, Hakim A, Fang J, et al. Pre admission antithrombotics are associated with improved outcomes following ischaemic stroke: a cohort from the Registry of the Canadian Stroke Network. *Int J Stroke.* 2009;4(5):328–334. doi:10.1111/j.1747-4949.2009.00331.x

62. Hermann A, Dzialowski I, Koch R, et al. Combined anti-platelet therapy with aspirin and clopidogrel: risk factor for thrombolysis-related intracerebral hemorrhage in acute ischemic stroke? *J Neurol Sci.* 2009;284(1–2):155–157. doi:10.1016/j.jns.2009.05.003
63. Prodan CI, Stoner JA, Cowan LD, et al. Lower coated platelet levels are associated with early hemorrhagic transformation in patients with non-lacunar brain infarction. *J Thromb Haemost.* 2010;8:1185–1190. doi:10.1111/j.1538-7836.2010.03851.x
64. Anderson DC, Kappelle LJ, Eliasziw M, et al. Occurrence of hemispheric and retinal ischemia in atrial fibrillation compared with carotid stenosis. *Stroke.* 2002;33:1963. doi:10.1161/01.str.0000023445.20454.a8
65. Harrison MJ, Marshall J. Atrial fibrillation, TIAs and completed strokes. *Stroke.* 1984;15:441. doi:10.1161/01.str.15.3.441
66. Lin HJ, Wolf PA, Kelly-Hayes M, et al. Stroke severity in atrial fibrillation. The Framingham Study. *Stroke.* 1996;27:1760. doi:10.1161/01.str.27.10.1760
67. Tu HT, Campbell BC, Christensen S, et al. Worse stroke outcome in atrial fibrillation is explained by more severe hypoperfusion, infarct growth, and hemorrhagic transformation. *Int J Stroke.* 2013;10(4):534–540. doi:10.1111/ijs.12007
68. Hornig CR, Bauer T, Simon C, et al. Hemorrhagic transformation in cardioembolic cerebral infarction. *Stroke.* 1993;24:465–468. doi:10.1161/01.str.24.3.465
69. Brown DL, Barsan WG, Lisabeth LD, et al. Survey of emergency physicians about recombinant tissue plasminogen activator for acute ischemic stroke. *Ann Emerg Med.* 2005;46(1):56–60. doi:10.1016/j.annemergmed.2004.12.025
70. Asuzu D, Nystrom K, Amin H, et al. Comparison of 8 scores for predicting symptomatic intracerebral hemorrhage after IV thrombolysis. *Neurocrit Care.* 2015;22(2):229–233. doi:10.1007/s12028-014-0060-2
71. Lou M, Safdar A, Mehdiratta M, et al. The HAT Score: a simple grading scale for predicting hemorrhage after thrombolysis. *Neurology.* 2008;71(18):1417–1423. doi:10.1212/01.wnl.0000330297.58334.dd
72. Strbian D, Meretoja A, Ahlhelm FJ, et al. Predicting outcome of IV thrombolysis-treated ischemic stroke patients: the DRAGON score. *Neurology.* 2012;78(6):427–432. doi:10.1212/wnl.0b013e318245d2a9
73. Kent DM, Selker HP, Ruthazer R, et al. The stroke-thrombolytic predictive instrument: a predictive instrument for intravenous thrombolysis in acute ischemic stroke. *Stroke.* 2006;37(12):2957–2962. doi:10.1161/01.str.0000249054.96644.c6
74. McMeekin P, Flynn D, Ford GA, et al. Validating the stroke-thrombolytic predictive instrument in a population in the United Kingdom. *Stroke.* 2012;43(12):3378–3381. doi:10.1161/strokeaha.112.671073

75. Saposnik G, Guzik AK, Reeves M, et al. Stroke prognostication using age and NIH stroke scale: SPAN-100. *Neurology*. 2013;80(1):21–28. doi:10.1212/wnl.0b013e31827b1ace

76. Cucchiara B, Tanne D, Levine SR, et al. A risk score to predict intracranial hemorrhage after recombinant tissue plasminogen activator for acute ischemic stroke. *J Stroke Cerebrovasc Dis*. 2008;17(6):331–333. doi:10.1016/j.jstrokecerebrovasdis.2008.03.012

77. Sung SF, Chen SC, Lin HJ, et al. Comparison of risk-scoring systems in predicting symptomatic intracerebral hemorrhage after intravenous thrombolysis. *Stroke*. 2013;44(6):1561–1566. doi:10.1161/strokeaha.111.000651

78. Strbian D, Engelter S, Michel P, et al. Symptomatic intracranial hemorrhage after stroke thrombolysis: the SEDAN score. *Ann Neurol*. 2012;71(5):634–641. doi:10.1002/ana.23546

79. Kent DM, Ruthazer R, Decker C, et al. Development and validation of a simplified Stroke-Thrombolytic Predictive Instrument. *Neurology*. 2015;85(11):942–949. doi:10.1212/wnl.0000000000001925

80. Strbian D, Michel P, Seiffge DJ, et al. Symptomatic intracranial hemorrhage after stroke thrombolysis: comparison of prediction scores. *Stroke*. 2014;45(3):752–758. doi:10.1161/strokeaha.113.003806

81. Li M, Wang-Qin RQ, Wang YL, et al. Symptomatic intracerebral hemorrhage after intravenous thrombolysis in Chinese patients: comparison of prediction models. *J Stroke Cerebrovasc Dis*. 2015;24(6):1235–1243. doi:10.1016/j.jstrokecerebrovasdis.2015.01.026

82. Puig J, Blasco G, Daunis-i-Estadella P, et al. High-permeability region size on perfusion CT predicts hemorrhagic transformation after intravenous thrombolysis in stroke. *PLoS ONE*. 2017;12(11):e0188238. doi:10.1371/journal.pone.0188238

83. Patlak CS, Blasberg RG, Fenstermacher JD. Graphical evaluation of blood-to-brain transfer constants from multiple-time uptake data. *J Cereb Blood Flow Metab*. 1983;3:1–7. doi:10.1038/jcbfm.1983.1

84. Tofts PS, Brix G, Buckley DL, et al. Estimating kinetic parameters from dynamic contrast-enhanced T(1)-weighted MRI of a diffusable tracer: standardized quantities and symbols. *J Magn Reson Imaging*. 1999;10:223–232. doi:10.1002/(sici)1522-2586(199909)10:3<223::aid-jmri2>3.0.co;2-s

85. Paciaroni M, Agnelli G, Corea F, et al. Early hemorrhagic transformation of brain infarction: rate, predictive factors, and influence on clinical outcome: results of a prospective multicenter study. *Stroke*. 2008;39:2249–2256. doi:10.1161/strokeaha.107.510321

86. Ozkul-Wermester O, Guegan-Massardier E, Triquenot A, et al. Increased blood-brain barrier permeability on perfusion computed tomography predicts hemorrhagic transformation in acute ischemic stroke. *Eur Neurol*. 2014;72:45–53. doi:10.1159/000358297

87. Lee KM, Kim JH, Kim E, et al. Early stage of hyperintense acute reperfusion marker on contrast-enhanced FLAIR images in patients with acute stroke. *AJR Am J Roentgenol.* 2016;206(6):1272–1275. doi:10.2214/ajr.15.14857
88. Choi HY, Lee KM, Kim HG, et al. Role of hyperintense acute reperfusion marker for Classifying the Stroke Etiology. *Front Neurol.* 2017;8:630. doi:10.3389/fneur.2017.00630
89. Nadareishvili Z, Luby M, Leigh R, et al. An MRI Hyperintense Acute Reperfusion Marker is related to Elevated Peripheral Monocyte Count in acute ischemic stroke. *J Neuroimaging.* 2018;28(1):57–60. doi:10.1111/jon.12462
90. Niibo T, Ohta H, Miyata S, et al. Prediction of blood brain barrier disruption and intracerebral hemorrhagic infarction using arterial spin-labeling magnetic resonance imaging. *Stroke.* 2017;48(1):117–122. doi:10.1161/strokeaha.116.013923
91. Yaghi S, Willey J, Cucchiara B, et al. Treatment and outcome of hemorrhagic transformation after intravenous alteplase in acute ischemic stroke. A scientific statement for healthcare professionals from the American Heart Association/American Stroke Association. *Stroke.* 2017;48:e343–e361. doi:10.1161/str.0000000000000152
92. Vahedi K, Hofmeijer J, Juettler E, et al. Early decompressive surgery in malignant infarction of the middle cerebral artery: a pooled analysis of three randomised controlled trials. *Lancet Neurol.* 2007;6:215. doi:10.1016/s1474-4422(07)70036-4
93. Hofmeijer J, Kappelle LJ, Algra A, et al. Surgical decompression for space-occupying cerebral infarction (the Hemicraniectomy After Middle Cerebral Artery infarction with Life-threatening Edema Trial [HAMLET]): a multicentre, open, randomised trial. *Lancet Neurol.* 2009;8:326–333. doi:10.1016/S1474-4422(09)70047-X
94. Mahaffey KW, Granger CB, Sloan MA, et al. Neurosurgical evacuation of intracranial hemorrhage after thrombolytic therapy for acute myocardial infarction: experience from the GUSTO-I trial. Global Utilization of Streptokinase and tissue-plasminogen activator (tPA) for Occluded Coronary Arteries. *Am Heart J.* 1999;138:493. doi:10.1016/s0002-8703(99)70152-3
95. Cucchiara B, Kasner SE, Tanne D, et al. Factors associated with intracerebral hemorrhage after thrombolytic therapy for ischemic stroke: pooled analysis of placebo data from the Stroke-Acute Ischemic NXY Treatment (SAINT) I and SAINT II Trials. *Stroke.* 2009;40(9):3067–3072. doi:10.1161/strokeaha.109.554386

6 Endovascular and Postprocedural Complications

Lee A. Birnbaum, Justin Mascitelli, and Cameron McDougall

KEY POINTS

- Endovascular mechanical thrombectomy (MT) has an overall low complication rate.
- Patient selection with advanced neuroimaging not only improves clinical outcomes, but likely minimizes complications, specifically symptomatic intracerebral hemorrhage (sICH).
- A variety of direct clot and proximal aspiration techniques are often used in conjunction with a stentriever to maximize recanalization rates and minimize emboli to new vascular territories.
- The use of either conscious sedation or general anesthesia is not associated with increased procedural complications and should be selected on a case-by-case basis that optimizes safety and outcome.

INTRODUCTION

The endovascular treatment of acute ischemic stroke has evolved significantly over the past 20 years. The initial randomized trials of endovascular therapies for acute large vessel occlusion (LVO) utilized intra-arterial (IA) chemical thrombolysis with recombinant pro-urokinase (rpro-UK) for proximal middle cerebral artery (MCA) strokes. The PROACT (1) and PROACT II (2) trials demonstrated both improved recanalization and clinical outcomes despite increased early symptomatic intracranial hemorrhage. These favorable results were further supported several years later in the MERCI trial (3), which utilized a novel endovascular thrombectomy device, the Merci Retriever, rather than chemical thrombolysis alone. The overall clinical benefit of MT in the MERCI trial provided the catalyst for endovascular device development that included a variety of direct aspiration catheters and stentrievers.

 DOI: 10.1891/9780826124791.0006

This newer generation of thrombectomy devices has been shown to result in better recanalization rates, better clinical outcomes, and in 2015, overwhelming benefit in multiple randomized clinical trials. As a result, the American Heart Association/American Stroke Association (AHA/ASA) published a 2015 Focused Update, which recommended the use of stentrievers in selected acute stroke LVO patients within 6 hours from last known well (LKW) (Class I, Level of Evidence A) (4). More recent randomized trials of MT examined extended time windows up to 24 hours and utilized advanced neuroimaging with cerebral perfusion. These trials were recently published and also demonstrated overwhelming efficacy in the MT groups. Subsequently, the 2018 AHA/ASA guidelines recommended MT in selected acute stroke LVO patients within 16 hours of LKW (Class I, Level of Evidence A) (5). The recommendation for 16 to 24 hours of LKW is based solely on a single randomized trial and therefore, does not meet criteria for 1A evidence.

Procedure-related complications from MT that are reported in the literature include sICH, emboli to new vascular territories, vessel dissection or rupture, vasospasm of the access vessel, stent detachment, and groin hematoma. Compared to MT alone, the combination of intravenous (IV) tissue plasminogen activator (tPA) with MT for LVO does not significantly increase the rate of procedural complication and may signal a trend toward better recanalization rates and clinical outcomes (6). The effect of combination IA tPA and MT on clinical outcomes, however, is less clear and may increase the rate of sICH compared to MT alone. Despite a small risk of procedure-related complications, MT for eligible LVO patients within 24 hours significantly improves clinical outcomes and has become the standard of care.

PATIENT SELECTION

Avoidance of procedural complications begins with appropriate patient selection that can be challenging in an emergent situation. Additionally, who should undergo MT is something of a moving target as the time windows and inclusion criteria continue to expand. It has long been recognized that revascularization in the setting of infarction is a significant risk factor for sICH (7). However, avoiding MT in patients with large completed infarctions is not always straightforward, and several variables should be considered. First, even patients with large infarctions may still benefit from MT despite the risk for reperfusion hemorrhage (8). Hemorrhagic transformation (HT) in the setting of infarction may or may not have a negative clinical impact (9). Intracerebral hemorrhage (ICH) is generally only considered relevant when accompanied by a significant change in a validated outcome metric, often an increase of 4 or more points on the National Institutes of Health Stroke Scale (NIHSS) (10). While patient inclusion for MT is expanding, technological imaging advances, such as the widespread availability of perfusion software, are filtering this larger patient pool to exclude patients with nonsalvageable infarction (11).

Another consideration in case selection includes the patient's overall premorbid level of function. Much of the randomized controlled trial (RCT) evidence demonstrating benefit from MT excluded patients with poor premorbid condition. Certainly, individualized decision making based on patient or family wishes, expectations, and overall goals of care is paramount and can help direct the informed consent discussion. For example, an elderly patient with dementia and a baseline modified Rankin Scale (mRS) of 4 (unable to attend to own bodily needs without assistance, unable to walk unassisted) is unlikely to benefit from MT. Even when successful, it is unlikely to improve the patient's quality of life in a meaningful way. Furthermore, significant arterial atherosclerosis, calcification, and tortuosity, as well as other medical comorbidities of advanced age often increase the inherent risk of the procedure.

ARTERIAL ACCESS

While a full discussion about minimizing the risks of endovascular access is beyond the scope of this chapter, some points do warrant at least a brief examination. Access during MT may carry increased risk due to the acuity of the situation as well as the prior administration of thrombolytic agents. If patients have received IV tPA or are known to take blood thinners, then a micropuncture kit should be used to obtain access. Because accurate common femoral artery access is pivotal, utilizing ultrasound guidance is often time well spent to ensure that access trauma is minimized and the height of the entry point is within acceptable range. Consideration may be made to leave the sheath in situ following the procedure while the thrombolytic agent is allowed to wear off. While this is probably a safer option, it has the distinct disadvantage of often necessitating a long period of manual compression at the bedside for what is typically a 6- to 9-French access sheath. Transradial access eliminates the risks associated with retroperitoneal hematoma. However, it is less desirable, and frequently not possible, with larger balloon guide catheters.

Because timely revascularization is critical, the operator should weigh anatomical considerations that may limit both transradial and common femoral access. In that situation, direct common carotid access with ultrasound guidance may be considered. The technique involves placement of a low-profile sheath that enters the artery obliquely, minimizes the puncture caliber, and avoids the jugular vein. In the setting of thrombolytic administration, strong consideration should be given to leaving the sheath in place until the effects have dissipated and manual pressure can be used to achieve hemostasis (12). Closure devices for common carotid access must be considered carefully, if at all, with passive devices probably being the safest. It should be mentioned that devices such as Exoseal (Cordis, Baar Switzerland) or Angio-Seal (Terumo, Somerset, New Jersey), which rely on pulsatile retrograde blood flow to indicate when to deploy the device, do not function well as blood flow is orthograde to the sheath in the carotid. Alternatively, when there is extreme concern regarding neck hematoma, direct surgical carotid exposure with the sheath in place and primary carotid repair is also an option.

SYMPTOMATIC INTRACEREBRAL HEMORRHAGE

sICH is the most common complication of MT for acute LVO. Fortunately, HT from reperfusion of an ischemic infarct is often incidental and generally requires an increase of 4 or more points on the NIHSS to be considered symptomatic. HT has been classified into hemorrhagic infarction (HI), a heterogeneous pattern without mass effect, and parenchymal hematoma (PH), a more homogeneous hematoma with mass effect. HI and PH have been further stratified into types 1 and 2 (Table 6.1), of which PH 2 has been associated with a significantly increased risk of early neurological deterioration and death (13). The rate of sICH has declined in recent

Table 6.1 Classification of Hemorrhagic Transformation

Hemorrhage Classification	Radiographic Appearance
Hemorrhagic infarction type 1	Small hyperdense petechiae within infarct area
Hemorrhagic infarction type 2	More confluent hyperdensity throughout infarct area without mass effect
Parenchymal hematoma type 1	Homogeneous hyperdensity of <30% infarct area with some mass effect
Parenchymal hematoma type 2	Homogeneous hyperdensity of >30% infarct area with significant mass effect and/or homogeneous hyperdensity outside infarct area

years due to advancements in thrombectomy devices that minimize the need for IA chemical thrombolysis and utilization of advanced neuroimaging to exclude malignant LVOs that are at greatest risk for HT. In the initial thrombectomy PROACT trials, IA rpro-UK was directly delivered to the MCA clot with adjunctive IV heparin bolus and infusion for 4 hours. The rates of sICH were 15.4% (4/26) and 10% (11/108) in PROACT I and II, respectively.

Although the recent LVO trials in 2015 included subjects who received IV thrombolysis, the majority underwent MT alone, rarely had IA thrombolysis, and almost never had IV heparin infusion. Following these parameters, the rates of sICH in the recent MT trials are significantly less than the 10% to 15% reported in the PROACT trials (Table 6.2). The recent randomized trials of SWIFT PRIME (14) and EXTEND IA (15) utilized brain perfusion imaging for screening, excluded malignant stroke profiles, and reported sICH rates of zero. Thus, the utilization of perfusion imaging likely improves final outcomes by excluding those with the greatest risk of sICH (large core infarct and small penumbra) and including those with the greatest potential for good clinical outcome (small core infarct and large penumbra). These perfusion ratios of core and penumbra have been termed "nontarget mismatch" and "target mismatch," respectively.

The recently published DAWN (16) and DEFUSE 3 (17) thrombectomy trials utilized perfusion imaging to include LKW 6 to 24 hours and reported sICH rates of 6% and 7%, respectively. Compared to the 2015 trials that mostly enrolled LKW up to 6 hours, these sICH rates are greater than those reported in SWIFT PRIME and EXTEND IA (that utilized perfusion imaging) but consistent with MR CLEAN (18), ESCAPE (19), and REVASCAT (20) (that relied on CT angiography only). Thus, the DAWN and DEFUSE 3 sICH rates are not unreasonable when considering the extended time window up to 24 hours and liberal inclusion thresholds for infarct core. The DAWN trial included subjects with core infarct on perfusion imaging up to 20 to 50 mL depending on age and NIHSS, albeit the qualifying median volume of ischemic core was relatively small, approximately 8 mL (16). The DEFUSE 3 trial included subjects with an ischemic core up to 70 mL depending on absolute volume of penumbra, albeit the qualifying median volume of ischemic core was also relatively small, approximately 10 mL (17).

sICH remains a potential complication of MT and in recent clinical trials occurs in less than 10% of cases. The rate of sICH should continue to decline as devices become even more effective and advanced neuroimaging including perfusion becomes standardized in patient selection.

Table 6.2 Procedure-Related Complication Rates by Trial

	PROACT I (1)	PROACT II (2)	SWIFT PRIME (14)	MR CLEAN (18)	ESCAPE (19)	EXTEND IA (15)	REVASCAT (20)	DAWN (16)	DEFUSE 3 (17)
sICH	15.4%	10%	0%	7.7%	3.6%	0%	1.9%	6%	7%
ENT	n/a	n/a	n/a	8.6%	4.9%	5.7%	4.9%	4%	n/a
AP	n/a	n/a	n/a	0.9%	0.6	2.9%	4.9%	0%	n/a
AD	n/a	n/a	n/a	1.7%	0.6	n/a	3.9%	2%	n/a

AD, arterial dissection; AP, arterial perforation; ENT, embolization to new territory; n/a, not available; sICH, symptomatic intracerebral hemorrhage.

EMBOLI TO NEW VASCULAR TERRITORIES

Emboli to new vascular territories occurred in up to 10% of MT cases in the recent MT trials (Table 6.2). This complication is particularly troublesome when an MCA thrombectomy results in an anterior cerebral artery (ACA) embolic event due to incomplete clot retrieval. The outcome from this scenario can be devastating as the ipsilateral collateral flow becomes attenuated and hemispheric infarction progresses rapidly. When an embolism traverses to the ipsilateral ACA, a second thrombectomy is often performed in the new vascular territory to restore collaterals and reperfusion.

Thrombectomy is more likely to result in emboli to new vascular territories when aspiration is not employed. The ADAPT study showed that direct aspiration alone or in combination with a stentriever, the Solumbra technique, minimizes this risk. Of the 100 treated lesions within ADAPT, no instances of embolization to a new territory were reported (21). In addition, proximal aspiration via a balloon guide catheter in the cervical segment of the internal carotid artery (ICA) may be used independently or in conjunction with the ADAPT technique. With the balloon inflated in the cervical ICA, flow arrest ensues and aspiration is performed through the guide catheter. The PROTECT trial combined both direct and proximal aspiration techniques and reported embolization into a previously unaffected territory in only 1 of 40 subjects (2.5%) (22). In summary, a variety of aspiration techniques have been shown to be safe and minimize emboli to new vascular territories.

IATROGENIC ARTERIAL INJURY

The rate of arterial dissection (AD) or arterial perforation (AP) ranged from 0.5% to 5% in the recent clinical trials of LVO (Table 6.2). Arterial injuries may occur in the extracranial or intracranial circulation and result from wires, catheters, thrombectomy devices, or balloon angioplasty. MT procedures require the placement of a large bore guide catheter high in the cervical ICA or vertebral artery (VA). Typically, the guide catheter is advanced rapidly (due to the urgency of the procedure), using stiff guidewires (for greater support in this particular population of patients), with poor visualization of the cervical arteries (due to patient movement). Additionally, balloon guide catheters are typically inflated in the cervical ICA or VA. Intracranially, microwires are advanced "blindly" beyond the occlusion, large bore aspiration catheters are advanced into the distal circulation (i.e., M2 segment), and stent retrievers cause endothelial trauma with clot retraction. These necessary techniques enable vessel recanalization but increase the risk of intracranial arterial injury.

Prior to MT devices, IA thrombolysis was often performed with the aid of smaller microwires and microcatheters that minimized the likelihood of intracranial vessel injury but also limited interventions to IA thrombolysis and balloon angioplasty. Currently, MT devices are widely used as primary reperfusion therapies due to their safety and efficacy but require more supportive microcatheters for intracranial delivery. These larger microcatheters often provide less flexibility to manage tortuous, distal intracranial anatomy, such as the MCA M2 and M3 segments. Even more so, aspiration catheters are most difficult to advance intracranial due to their inherent large diameter that enables optimal suction. The larger aspiration catheters often require both a supportive guide sheath in the cervical ICA and a microcatheter in a distal artery to facilitate safe intracranial advancement. Additionally, larger microwires are sometimes used to add support when advancing aspiration catheters.

To minimize the risk of vessel injury, a variety of angiographic techniques are employed. Operators often place a J-shaped curve on the microwire that permits safer navigation beyond an intracranial thrombus and into distal branches that cannot be visualized on angiography due to flow arrest. Additionally, the microwire size should be selected based on the perceived difficulty with intracranial anatomy, as well as the degree of distal microcatheter positioning needed to adequately deliver a device. In a similar fashion, the microcatheter size should be selected to optimize performance based on perceived anatomical challenges. When balloon angioplasty is performed, a precision syringe or insufflator is recommended to ensure accurate inflation volumes and minimize the risk of vessel rupture from balloon overinflation.

If a vessel perforation occurs, immediate attention to halt extravasation is required to avoid death. A small vessel perforation from a microwire may resolve spontaneously; however, in the setting of IV or IA thrombolysis, extravasation may continue and require an occlusive intervention. When required, vessel embolization is most readily achieved with coils and/or liquid embolic agents depending on the microcatheter and degree of perforation. Vessel rupture from a herniated catheter or an overinflated balloon angioplasty results in a large tear that invariably requires vessel takedown. The sequela of vessel occlusion is ischemic stroke to varying degrees but avoids certain death from uncontrolled extravasation.

Although vessel rupture is often life-threatening, AD may be asymptomatic or safely managed with antithrombotics. Only occasionally do ADs lead to occlusive or thromboembolic complications with neurological deficits. An AD usually appears angiographically as a pocket of contrast along the vessel wall that does not clear over time or as a double lumen with an intimal flap. AD may result in occlusion, stenosis, string sign, aneurysm, or pseudoaneurysm (23). The risk of iatrogenic AD ranges from 0.6% to 3.9% in RCTs and 1% to 6.7% in non-RCTs (24). Extracranial ADs are more common than intracranial ADs.

The treatment of iatrogenic AD is usually medical in nature. The majority of ADs can be treated with antiplatelet medication alone, typically aspirin. Anticoagulation may also be considered, but there is no evidence that it is superior to antiplatelet therapy (25). If there is associated thrombus formation at the site of the dissection, local IA administration of a glycoprotein (GP) IIb/IIIa inhibitor may be considered to directly lyse the thrombus. In the event of symptomatic decreased cerebral perfusion, permanent stenting of the AD is an option. The patient is often given aspirin and an IV bolus of GP IIb/IIIa inhibitor immediately prior to stent placement. Then, a continuous infusion of the GP IIb/IIIa inhibitor should be maintained until the patient is started on a second oral antiplatelet agent, often clopidogrel.

TANDEM LESIONS

Approximately 15% of LVO strokes involve a tandem lesion of the carotid bifurcation (26). These lesions tend to respond poorly to thrombolytic therapy and thus, represent an important group of cases from thrombectomy series (27). Much has been written regarding the optimal management of such lesions without overall consensus (28). One approach is to focus on cerebral revascularization first and then, attempt to manage the carotid lesion, ideally without a stent. Balloon angioplasty alone may allow the carotid lesion to be dealt with at a later time and avoid commitment to antiplatelet agents in the setting of acute stroke with or without thrombolytics.

When carotid stenting is necessary, the patient should be loaded with an antiplatelet agent, preferably IV GP IIB/IIIA inhibitors because of their fast onset. The balance between avoiding stent-related thromboembolic phenomena and minimizing the risk of intracranial hemorrhage is often complicated and without consensus on the optimal approach (29). A frequent approach is to initiate a IIB/IIIA inhibitor (tirofiban or eptifibatide, Merck, West Point, Pennsylvania) during the case, followed by a continuous infusion. Follow-up neuroimaging is often obtained within 24 hours postprocedure to ensure a hemorrhagic complication has not occurred. In the absence of complication, the patient is loaded with standard oral dual antiplatelet agents, and then, the IIB/IIIA inhibitor is stopped, which allows for treatment overlap.

COMPLICATIONS OF ANESTHESIA

The effect of anesthesia type on outcome following MT is a controversial topic. There is evidence from a number of retrospective studies that suggests a higher risk of poor outcomes with general anesthesia in comparison to conscious sedation (30–32). On the other hand, two randomized trials, SIESTA (33) and ANSTROKE (34), found no significant difference in outcomes based on anesthesia. The discrepancy may be explained by confounding factors such as stroke severity, delays to treatment, and medical comorbidities. The presumed mechanism for worse outcomes associated with general anesthesia is associated with changes in vital signs at the time of induction, namely hypotension and hypocapnia, which result in cerebral vasoconstriction and decreased blood flow to the ischemic penumbra via leptomeningeal collaterals (35). There are no particular anesthetic agents that are more or less associated with poor outcome. Conscious sedation, however, may result in worse outcomes due to patient movement that often results in worse imaging quality and likely increases the risk for arterial injury. Overall, the use of conscious sedation or general anesthesia should be determined on a case-by-case basis that optimizes safety and outcome.

CONCLUSION

The overwhelming clinical benefits of MT for acute LVO strokes are a result of advanced neuroimaging, modern devices, and improved techniques that optimize recanalization rates and minimize procedural complications. Furthermore, cerebral perfusion imaging enables therapies to be safely and effectively delivered in time windows up to 24 hours from LKW. Some MT topics remain controversial due to equivocal results in randomized trials and include conscious sedation versus general anesthesia or clot aspiration versus stentriever. Therefore, operators should individualize their approach to MT, including advanced neuroimaging, angiographic techniques, and anesthesia, to best optimize good clinical outcomes.

REFERENCES

1. del Zoppo GJ, Higashida RT, Furlan AJ, et al. PROACT: a phase II randomized trial of recombinant pro-urokinase by direct arterial delivery in acute middle cerebral artery stroke. PROACT Investigators. Prolyse in acute cerebral thromboembolism. *Stroke*. 1998;29(1):4–11. doi:10.1161/01.str.29.1.4.

2. Furlan A, Higashida R, Wechsler L, et al. Intra-arterial prourokinase for acute ischemic stroke. The PROACT II study: a randomized controlled trial. Prolyse in acute cerebral thromboembolism. *JAMA*. 1999;282(21):2003–2011. doi:10.1001/jama.282.21.2003.
3. Smith WS, Sung G, Starkman S, et al. Safety and efficacy of mechanical embolectomy in acute ischemic stroke: results of the MERCI trial. *Stroke*. 2005;36(7):1432–1438. doi:10.1161/01.str.0000171066.25248.1d. Epub 2005 Jun 16.
4. Powers WJ, Derdeyn CP, Biller J, et al. 2015 American Heart Association/American Stroke Association focused update of the 2013 guidelines for the early management of patients with acute ischemic stroke regarding endovascular treatment: a guideline for healthcare professionals from the American Heart Association/American Stroke Association. *Stroke*. 2015;46(10):3020–3035. doi:10.1161/STR.0000000000000074. Epub 2015 Jun 29.
5. Powers WJ, Rabinstein AA, Ackerson T, et al. 2018 Guidelines for the early management of patients with acute ischemic stroke: a guideline for healthcare professionals from the American Heart Association/American Stroke Association. *Stroke*. 2018;49(3):e46–e110. doi:10.1161/STR.0000000000000158. Epub 2018 Jan 24. Review. Erratum in: *Stroke*. 2018;49(3):e138.
6. Mistry EA, Mistry AM, Nakawah MO, et al. Mechanical thrombectomy outcomes with and without intravenous thrombolysis in stroke patients: a meta-analysis. *Stroke*. 2017;48(9):2450–2456. doi:10.1161/STROKEAHA.117.017320. Epub 2017 Jul 26.
7. Khatri R, McKinney AM, Swenson B, et al. Blood-brain barrier, reperfusion injury, and hemorrhagic transformation in acute ischemic stroke. *Neurol*. 2012;79:S52–S57. doi:10.1212/wnl.0b013e3182697e70
8. Bhatt N, Atchaneeyasakul K, Marulanda-Londono E, et al. Mechanical thrombectomy in large vessel occlusion stroke patients with low CT ASPECT score (P5.258). *Neurol*. 2017;88(16 Supplement):P5.258.
9. Molina CA, Alvarez-Sabín J, Montaner J, et al. Thrombolysis-related hemorrhagic infarction: a marker of early reperfusion, reduced infarct size, and improved outcome in patients with proximal middle cerebral artery occlusion. *Stroke*. 2002;33:1551–1556. doi:10.1161/01.str.0000016323.13456.e5
10. Rao NM, Levine SR, Gornbein JA, et al. Defining clinically relevant cerebral hemorrhage after thrombolytic therapy for stroke: analysis of the National Institute of Neurological Disorders and Stroke tissue-type plasminogen activator trials. *Stroke*. 2014;45:2728–2733. doi:10.1161/strokeaha.114.005135
11. Protto S, Pienimaki JP, Seppanen J, et al. Low cerebral blood volume identifies poor outcome in stent retriever thrombectomy. *Cardiovasc Intervent Radiol*. 2017;40:502–509. doi:10.1007/s00270-016-1532-x

12. Mokin M, Snyder KV, Levy EI, et al. Direct carotid artery puncture access for endovascular treatment of acute ischemic stroke: technical aspects, advantages, and limitations. *J Neurointerv Surg*. 2015;7:108–113. doi:10.1136/neurintsurg-2013-011007
13. Fiorelli M, Bastianello S, von Kummer R, et al. Hemorrhagic transformation within 36 hours of a cerebral infarct: relationships with early clinical deterioration and 3-month outcome in the European Cooperative Acute Stroke Study I (ECASS I) cohort. *Stroke*. 1999;30(11):2280–2284. doi:10.1161/01.str.30.11.2280
14. Saver JL, Goyal M, Bonafe A, et al. Stent-retriever thrombectomy after intravenous t-PA vs. t-PA alone in stroke. *N Engl J Med*. 2015;372(24):2285–2295. doi:10.1056/NEJMoa1415061
15. Campbell BC, Mitchell PJ, Kleinig TJ, et al. Endovascular therapy for ischemic stroke with perfusion-imaging selection. *N Engl J Med*. 2015;372(11):1009–1018. doi:10.1056/NEJMoa1414792
16. Nogueira RG, Jadhav AP, Haussen DC, et al. Thrombectomy 6 to 24 hours after stroke with a mismatch between deficit and infarct. *N Engl J Med*. 2018;378(1):11–21. doi:10.1056/NEJMoa1706442
17. Albers GW, Marks MP, Kemp S, et al. Thrombectomy for stroke at 6 to 16 hours with selection by perfusion imaging. *N Engl J Med*. 2018;378(8):708–718. doi:10.1056/NEJMoa1713973
18. Berkhemer OA, Fransen PS, Beumer D, et al. A randomized trial of intraarterial treatment for acute ischemic stroke. *N Engl J Med*. 2015;372(1):11–20. doi:10.1056/NEJMoa1411587. Epub 2014 Dec 17. Erratum in: *N Engl J Med*. 2015 Jan 22;372(4):394.
19. Goyal M, Demchuk AM, Menon BK, et al. Randomized assessment of rapid endovascular treatment of ischemic stroke. *N Engl J Med*. 2015;372(11):1019–30. doi:10.1056/NEJMoa1414905
20. Jovin TG, Chamorro A, Cobo E, et al. Thrombectomy within 8 hours after symptom onset in ischemic stroke. *N Engl J Med*. 2015;372(24):2296–306. doi:10.1056/NEJMoa1503780
21. Turk AS, Frei D, Fiorella D, et al. ADAPT FAST study: a direct aspiration first pass technique for acute stroke thrombectomy. *J Neurointerv Surg*. 2014;6:260–264. doi:10.1136/neurintsurg-2014-011125
22. Maegerlein C, Moench S, Boeckh-Behrens T, et al. PROTECT: PRoximal balloon Occlusion TogEther with direCt Thrombus aspiration during stent retriever thrombectomy—evaluation of a double embolic protection approach in endovascular stroke treatment *J Neurointerv Surg*. 2017;10(8):751–755. doi:10.1136/neurintsurg-2017-013558
23. Davis MC, Deveikis JP, Harrigan MR. Clinical presentation, imaging, and management of complications due to neurointerventional procedures. *Semin Intervent Radiol*. 2015;32(2):98–107. doi:10.1055/s-0035-1549374.
24. Balami JS, White PM, McMeekin PJ, et al. Complications of endovascular treatment for acute ischemic stroke: prevention and management. *Int J Stroke*. 2018;13(4):348–361. doi:10.1177/1747493017743051

25. CADISS trial investigators, Markus HS, Hayter E, et al. Antiplatelet treatment compared with anticoagulation treatment for cervical artery dissection (CADISS): a randomised trial. *Lancet Neurol.* 2015;14(4):361–367. doi:10.1016/S1474-4422(15)70018-9. Epub 2015 Feb 12. Erratum in: *Lancet Neurol.* 2015;14(6):566.
26. Widimský P, Koznar B, Abelson M, et al. Stent or balloon: how to treat proximal internal carotid artery occlusion in the acute phase of ischemic stroke? Results of a short survey. *Cor et Vasa.* 2016;58:e204–e206. doi:10.1016/j.crvasa.2016.02.006
27. Christou I, Felberg RA, Demchuk AM, et al. Intravenous tissue plasminogen activator and flow improvement in acute ischemic stroke patients with internal carotid artery occlusion. *J Neuroimaging.* 2002;12:119–123. doi:10.1111/j.1552-6569.2002.tb00107.x
28. Wilson MP, Murad MH, Krings T, et al. Management of tandem occlusions in acute ischemic stroke—intracranial versus extracranial first and extracranial stenting versus angioplasty alone: a systematic review and meta-analysis. *J Neurointerv Surg.* 2018;10:721–728. doi:10.1136/neurintsurg-2017-013707
29. Malik AM, Vora NA, Lin R, et al. Endovascular treatment of tandem extracranial/intracranial anterior circulation occlusions: preliminary single-center experience. *Stroke.* 2011;42:1653–1657. doi:10.1161/strokeaha.110.595520
30. Jagani M, Brinjikji W, Rabinstein AA, et al. Hemodynamics during anesthesia for intra-arterial therapy of acute ischemic stroke. *J Neurointerv Surg.* 2016;8(9):883–888. doi:10.1136/neurintsurg-2015-011867
31. Bekelis K, Missios S, MacKenzie TA, et al. Anesthesia technique and outcomes of mechanical thrombectomy in patients with acute ischemic stroke. *Stroke.* 2017;48(2):361–366. doi:10.1161/STROKEAHA.116.015343
32. Ouyang F, Chen Y, Zhao Y, et al. Selection of patients and anesthetic types for endovascular treatment in acute ischemic stroke: a meta-analysis of randomized controlled trials. *PLoS One.* 2016;11(3):e0151210. doi:10.1371/journal.pone.0151210
33. Schönenberger S, Uhlmann L, Hacke W, et al. Effect of conscious sedation vs general anesthesia on early neurological improvement among patients with ischemic stroke undergoing endovascular thrombectomy: a randomized clinical trial. *JAMA.* 2016;316(19):1986–1996. doi:10.1001/jama.2016.16623. Erratum in: *JAMA.* 2017 Feb 7;317(5):538.
34. Löwhagen Hendén P, Rentzos A, Karlsson JE, et al. General anesthesia versus conscious sedation for endovascular treatment of acute ischemic stroke: the Anstroke trial (anesthesia during stroke). *Stroke.* 2017;48(6):1601–1607. doi:10.1161/STROKEAHA.117.016554.
35. Wang A, Abramowicz AE. Role of anesthesia in endovascular stroke therapy. *Curr Opin Anaesthesiol.* 2017;30(5):563–569. doi:10.1097/ACO.0000000000000507.

7 Reperfusion Injury in Ischemic Stroke

Pablo Coss and Shaheryar Hafeez

KEY POINTS

- Cerebral ischemic reperfusion injury (CIRI) refers to the biochemical cascade that occurs as a result of recanalizing an occluded artery.
- Reperfusion injury initiates a complex biological cascade that causes significant neurotoxicity.
- Free radicals, excitatory neurotransmitters, and disruption of blood–brain barrier (BBB) are some of the proposed mechanisms contributing to reperfusion injury.
- To prevent reperfusion injury, significant elevations in blood pressure (BP) should be prevented and promptly treated.
- Hypoglycemia and hyperglycemia should be avoided.
- Management of reperfusion injury is largely supportive.

INTRODUCTION

The treatment for ischemic stroke rests upon early revascularization of occluded arteries to restore blood flow and oxygen to ischemic but salvageable cerebral tissue and prevent impending neuronal cell death. The intravenous (IV) thrombolytic agent tissue plasminogen activator (tPA) and mechanical thrombectomy are the most effective techniques for reperfusion of ischemic brain tissue during acute ischemic strokes (AISs) that are due to thromboembolism (1). These techniques have been shown to reduce the final volume of infarcted tissue and decrease functional disability due to stroke when performed soon after the onset of stroke symptoms. But while recent advances in patient selection in the DAWN and DEFUSE trials have expanded the potential benefit of mechanical thrombectomy to some patients with longer duration of symptoms, the ultimate goal of improving patient functional outcome remains limited by two main factors: the speed at which irreversible cell

 DOI: 10.1891/9780826124791.0007

death occurs due to ischemia and the risk of augmented injury to the tissue as a result of restoring blood flow (2,3). The interplay of these two phenomena is a complex process, which is known as cerebral ischemic reperfusion injury. Here we examine the currently postulated pathophysiologic mechanisms that lead to CIRI, its clinical manifestations, and potential therapeutic targets that may one day improve outcomes of reperfusion further.

PATHOPHYSIOLOGY

CIRI refers to the biochemical cascade that occurs as a result of recanalizing an occluded artery, causing further tissue damage that parallels and antagonizes the benefits of restoring blood flow to the ischemic tissue (4,5). Here, we use CIRI and reperfusion injury interchangeably. The result of CIRI is either poor neurologic improvement or even worsening after recanalization of a large artery. To date, the bulk of our understanding of the pathophysiology underlying this phenomenon is derived from animal studies of middle cerebral artery (MCA) occlusion and reperfusion and inferences made from large clinical trials.

In patients with AIS, the primary pathologic insult to the cerebral tissues is energy failure that leads to a cycle of decreased metabolic substrates and oxygen. The widespread damage in ischemic stroke inhibits oxidative phosphorylation, not only in neurons, but also in glial cells, endothelial cells, microglia, and pericytes. Depletion of adenosine triphosphate (ATP) leads to dysfunction of various energy-dependent processes; among them the most vital is the Na^+–K^+-ATPase pump (6). This causes dysregulation of sodium and potassium gradients, which in turn leads to cell swelling, as well as failure of the Na^+/Ca^{2+} exchanger and buildup of intracellular calcium.

High intracellular calcium concentrations activate apoptotic cascades and also lead to the release of glutamate. Glutamate's role in excitotoxicity has been well established in various neurologic disease processes and is not reviewed in full. However, it predominantly acts through activation of N-methyl-D-aspartate (NMDA) and α-amino-3-hydroxy-5-methyl-4-isoxazolepropionic acid (AMPA) receptors and causes further increases in intracellular calcium concentrations, thereby propagating its deleterious effects to other cells (7).

Another important aspect of neurotoxicity during ischemia is oxidative and nitrative stress. Glutamate mediated excitotoxicity and anaerobic respiration leads to the generation of reactive oxygen species (ROS) such as superoxide anion, hydrogen peroxide, nitric oxide, and peroxynitrite (8). These molecules react with and alter the structure of various macromolecules within cells, such as

DNA, proteins, and lipids, thereby causing structural instability and dysfunction of various cellular processes.

ROS plays a role in another major aspect of ischemic neurotoxicity: inflammation. ROS induces the expression of proinflammatory genes in ischemic tissues and activates microglia. Microglia in turn release cytokines, including interleukin 1, interleukin 6, and tumor necrosis factor alpha. The massive cytokine release in the brain attracts and activates other elements of the immune system such as neutrophils, monocytes, lymphocytes, and natural killer cells. Proinflammatory cytokines also promote adhesion molecules on the leukocyte membranes and endothelial surface allowing for extravasation into the ischemic tissues. Leukocytes then contribute to the elaboration of ROS and proinflammatory cytokines (9,10). They also produce matrix metalloproteinases (MMPs), a family of proteins important in remodeling of the extracellular matrix. These complex biochemical processes not only lead to direct neuronal injury as a result of ischemia, but they also each set the stage for reperfusion injury and recent therapeutic targets.

Observations from clinical trials of IV tPA, such as the Echoplanar Imaging Thrombolytic Evaluation Trial (EPITHET) in 2008 (11), shed light on one aspect of reperfusion injury: a significant proportion of patients do not exhibit reperfusion of the ischemic tissue despite evidence of recanalization, leading to infarction of seemingly salvageable penumbra (12). This is referred to as the "no-reflow" phenomenon and was originally described following coronary recanalization during myocardial infarction (13). The mechanism of the no-reflow phenomenon is not currently well established in humans, but it is postulated from animal studies that ischemia results in damage and obstruction of the downstream microcirculation such that blood is not able to perfuse the ischemic tissue beds despite recanalization. Several events are thought to contribute to this. First, tissue edema and swelling of endothelial cells, pericytes, and astrocyte foot processes is thought to compress capillary lumens, which leads to a restriction of blood flow. Second, high levels of intracellular calcium within pericytes leads to vasoconstriction. Third, proinflammatory cascade produced by damaged endothelium leads to more perivascular inflammation, which can obstruct the vessel lumen. Endothelial damage also exposes local tissue factor causing fibrin accumulation leading to microthrombosis.

A second and perhaps more clinically relevant aspect of reperfusion injury is disruption of the BBB. All of the processes previously described play a role in BBB disruption. A lack of oxidative phosphorylation and increase in ROS can directly cause endothelial cell swelling and weakening of tight junctions between cells. Direct damage to the astrocytes that provide the necessary foot processes of the BBB can cause its disruption. Proinflammatory cytokines disrupt the BBB in an attempt to invade the brain tissue to clean up any inflammation or necrotic tissue that has developed from a stroke (14). As alluded to previously, metalloproteinases such as MMP-9, degrade the extracellular matrix of the basal lamina, which provides the framework of the BBB. These complex processes work in conjunction to break down the BBB allowing increased vascular permeability, edema, extravasation of cells, blood products, and metabolites, and loss of vasoregulatory mechanisms. This highly disruptive cascade of cellular mechanisms and breakdown of the BBB is thought to be the main pathologic event underlying the clinical manifestations of reperfusion injury, which can range from asymptomatic hemorrhagic transformation (HT) to life-threatening cerebral edema and intracranial hemorrhage.

IDENTIFICATION

Evidence of CIRI and its clinical manifestations following revascularization comes from animal studies and observations in clinical trials of poor neurologic improvement or paradoxical worsening of neurologic function due to ischemia, edema, and hemorrhage following reperfusion. But while HT and cerebral edema are readily observable and recognized as severe obstacles in stroke management, the case for worsening ischemic damage to penumbral tissue as a result of reperfusion injury is more elusive.

Restoration of blood flow to ischemic tissue but becomes ischemic again and later infarcts—despite a patent blood vessel and adequate flow—is evidence of secondary ischemic injury due to reperfusion. Olah et al. demonstrated this concept in rats with deliberate occlusion followed by reperfusion of the MCA vessel. MRI scans showed apparent diffuse coefficient (ADC) values initially decreased in ischemic brain tissue, improved after a few hours following reperfusion, only to decrease again hours later despite adequate perfusion (15). This finding was demonstrated in at least two other animal studies (16). One study that addressed this phenomenon in humans was performed by Kidwell who studied serial diffusion and perfusion-weighted MRI scans on a small cohort of patients who received intra-arterial tPA and achieved recanalization of the occluded artery (17). They found that areas that exhibited hyperperfusion were more likely to result in infarction than areas that did not exhibit hyperperfusion. This finding indicates that reperfusion injury or CIRI can occur.

Contrary to the aforementioned concerns in animal models and small cohort studies, the most recent thrombectomy trials, DAWN and DEFUSE 3, have not shown secondary ischemic injury to be a significant clinical problem if imaging and clinical profiles are favorable. In DEFUSE 3, infarct volumes and infarct growth at 24 hours were both similar between thrombectomy and medical arms. DAWN showed a significant reduction in the infarct volumes in the thrombectomy arm, and no difference in infarct growth at 24 hours. Both trials demonstrated significantly improved functional outcomes in the thrombectomy arms as their primary end points. Therefore, previous concerns regarding worsening an AIS with reperfusion therapy become less of a concern if there are favorable imaging and clinical characteristics. Nonetheless, it is possible that innovations in neuroprotective therapies, discussed later in this chapter, could reduce infarct size and growth or extend treatment times even further after successful reperfusion.

Hemorrhagic Transformation

HT is the most clinically evident manifestation of CIRI. The best evidence to discuss the natural history of rates of HT in AIS comes from the original National Institute of Neurological Disorders and Stroke (NINDS) and European Cooperative Acute Stroke Study (ECASS) III trials (18,19). The rate of *any* HT for ischemic strokes *not treated* with tPA or thrombectomy at 90 days was 7% in the seminal NINDS trial and 18% in ECASS III. The use of tPA significantly increased the incidence of HT to 13% in NINDS and 27% in ECASS III. *Symptomatic HT* occurred in 7% of patients given tPA in NINDS and 33% in ECASS III. The increase in symptomatic and asymptomatic hemorrhages after tPA has traditionally been thought of as being related to the tPA itself, but it can also be related to reperfusion of ischemic tissue. Both NINDS and ECASS III demonstrated a significant increase in symptomatic HT compared to placebo, more so in ECASS III likely due to the extended time window. Sixty-one percent of patients with symptomatic HT in the NINDS trial died, compared to an 11% overall mortality. In ECASS III, about 10% of the patients with symptomatic HT died, and all of them had received tPA, compared to 8% overall mortality. It became clear from this data that IV tPA increased the rate of asymptomatic and symptomatic HT, and that symptomatic HT was associated with worse outcomes. However, because early thrombolysis studies did not track rates of recanalization or reperfusion, it was difficult to establish a definitive causal link between the postulated mechanisms of reperfusion injury to HT. Some argue this is also because one needs to consider the degree of collateral flow that helps keep ischemic tissue from infarction before full revascularization can occur (20).

In the years since reperfusion has become the main goal of AIS therapy, several risk factors for intracerebral hemorrhage following reperfusion have been identified. They include time from symptom onset, age, coagulopathy, uncontrolled hyperglycemia, hypertension, severity of neurologic deficit, collateral flow status, and area of infarction as evident on cerebral imaging (21). As expected, these markers are reflections of the underlying mechanisms of reperfusion injury: dysfunction of large areas of BBB as well as extravasation of blood and fluid into the damaged parenchyma.

Categories have also been developed to stratify the severity of HT based on its radiographic appearance. The four major categories are hemorrhagic infarction (parenchymal hematoma [PH]) 1 and 2 and intraparenchymal hematoma (IH) 1 and 2. PH 1 refers to small hyperdense petechiae seen on neuroimaging. PH 2 refers to more confluent hyperdensities in the infarct zone without mass effect. IH 1 is a homogeneous hyperdensity that occupies less than 30% of the infarct zone and has some mass effect. IH 2 occupies more than 30% of the infarct zone with significant mass effect or extends beyond the infarct zone. These categories make it possible to draw finer correlations between risk factors, extent of HT, and functional outcomes. For example, it is now known that PH 1 is not a marker of poor outcome. On the contrary, PH 1 indicates successful recanalization. It is only PH 2 and IH that portend neurologic deterioration (21).

Radiographic Findings of Reperfusion Injury

The past two decades have also seen an abundance of radiographic evidence linking reperfusion and hyperperfusion to HT. Several imaging modalities and different characteristic findings on certain sequences have been postulated to help clinicals predict whether a stroke will have HT. Selim et al. demonstrated areas with low ADC values were an independent predictor of HT in ischemic stroke patients who received IV tPA (22). Kimura et al. suggested that recanalization as demonstrated on magnetic resonance angiography after tPA was an independent predictor of HT (23). Similarly, Seidel et al. showed reperfusion occurring more than 6 hours after symptom onset on bedside transcranial Doppler was associated with worse subtypes of HT than earlier reperfusion (24). A more direct link between reperfusion injury and poor outcomes was established by Warach et al. in 2004. In a prospective trial using gadolinium enhanced MRI, they described an imaging marker they termed "HARM," or "Hyperintense Acute Reperfusion Marker." HARM was defined as a delayed gadolinium enhancement of sulcal cerebrospinal fluid (CSF) spaces on fluid-attenuated inversion recovery (FLAIR) images. They surmised that HARM was a marker of early BBB disruption and could potentially be used to predict those patients who would have reperfusion injury. They were able to demonstrate using perfusion imaging that reperfusion was the strongest predictor of HARM, and that HARM in turn was associated with tPA use, subsequent HT, and poor clinical outcome at 90 days (25). Figure 7.1 demonstrates a case of reperfusion injury wherein perfusion imaging was used.

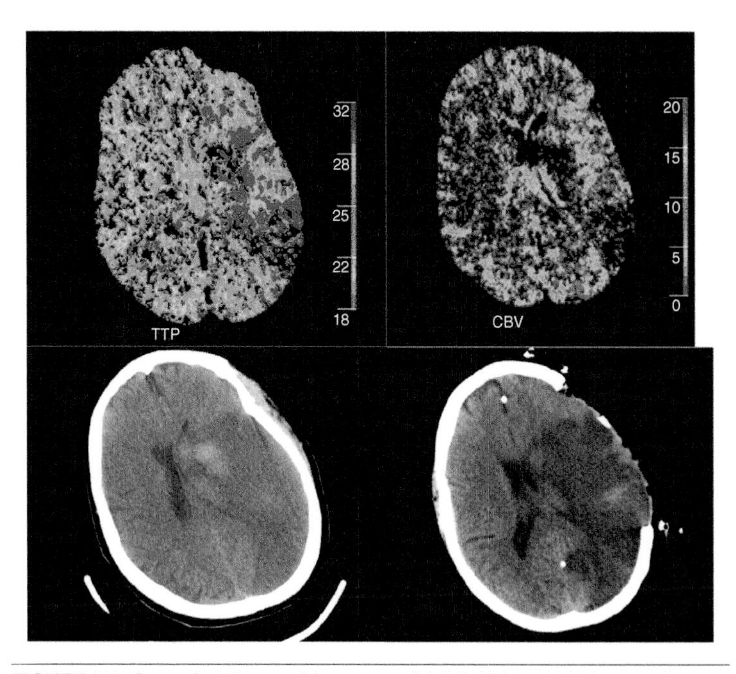

FIGURE 7.1 Case of a 37-year-old woman with left ICA and MCA occlusion with subsequent reperfusion injury. Top left: TTP perfusion CT scan showing decreased flow in the MCA territory. Top right: CBV perfusion CT showing relatively small core infarct volume with hyperperfusion in the MCA superior division territory. Bottom left: CT head showing unexpected large full territory MCA stroke with hemorrhagic transformation, edema, and midline shift despite successful TICI 2b recanalization. The patient did not receive tPA. Bottom right: CT head depicting large left MCA stroke with cerebral edema and hemorrhagic transformation necessitating left hemicraniectomy.

CBV, cerebral blood volume; ICA, internal carotid artery; MCA, middle cerebral artery; TICI, thrombolysis in cerebral infarction; tPA, tissue plasminogen activator; TTP, time to peak.

In 2014, Cho et al. also described HARM following carotid revascularization for severe carotid stenosis. While the study was small, HARM was not associated with new infarcts in this study (26). More recently, focal hyperperfusion seen on arterial spin labeling MRI and single-photon emission CT (SPECT) following thrombolysis or thrombectomy has also been associated with risk of HT (27).

The summation of the aforementioned evidence suggests early hyperperfusion, BBB disruption, and recanalization in some patients can cause CIRI. As imaging modalities continue to evolve, clinicians must be aware that reperfusion injury can be seen on different MRI sequences with or without contrast and SPECT imaging. These imaging findings may be helpful to identify areas of BBB disruption and may be used to target future therapy and help limit reperfusion injury. However, the success of the most recent stroke trials—due to improved patient selection—paints a different picture when it comes to reperfusion injury when recanalization is achieved. They give us some guidance and clues on how ischemic or penumbral tissue can affect normal brain and parenchyma that is at highest risk of infarction. The cumulative evidence showed a low rate of HT compared to control. However, the DAWN trial demonstrated a 6% risk of symptomatic HT, which represented a twofold increase compared to medical management, though it did not reach statistical significance. Similarly, DEFUSE 3 demonstrated a 7% risk of symptomatic HT, which was 3% higher than the control group, but not statistically significant. The ESCAPE trial was the lone outlier at an HT rate of 36.9% with a symptomatic intracranial hemorrhage rate of only 3.6% (28). The other trials showed HT occurred between 5.8% and 11.4% and a symptomatic intracranial hemorrhage rate between 1.9% and 7.7% (5) (Table 7.1). Thus, these trials suggest acute reperfusion therapy can have deleterious consequences of reperfusion injury and the risk of HT must be evaluated and considered carefully.

PREVENTION

The main strategy for prevention of reperfusion injury is optimal patient selection for reperfusion therapy, optimal glucose management, and targeted BP management. In multiple studies, hyperglycemia has been associated with worsening the ischemic penumbra and infarct size (29). During a stroke, glucose transporters decrease cellular uptake of available glucose to the infarcted tissue and upregulate in the penumbral tissue to increase glucose uptake. In acute stroke patients with MRI scans showing perfusion–diffusion mismatch, higher blood glucose concentration was associated with

Table 7.1 Rates of Hemorrhagic Transformation in Stroke After Endovascular Therapy in Selected Trials

Trial	MR CLEAN	ESCAPE	EXTEND-IA	SWIFT-PRIME	DAWN	RESVASCAT	DEFUSE3
Any Hemorrhagic Transformation	I: 6.9% C: 6.4%	I: 36.9% C:17.3%	I: 11.4% C: 8.6%	I: 5.1% C: 7.1%	I: 1.9% C: 1.0%	I: 5.8% C: 5.8%	I: 9% C: 3%
Symptomatic Hemorrhagic Transformation	I: 7.7% C: 6.4%	I: 3.6% C: 2.7%	I: 0% C: 5.7%	I: 0% C: 3.1%	I: 6% C: 3%	I: 1.9% C: 1.9%	I: 7% C: 4%

Source: Adapted from Al-Mufti F, Amuluru K, Roth W, et al. Cerebral ischemic reperfusion injury following recanalization of large vessel occlusions. *Neurosurgery.* 2018;82(6):781–789. doi:10.1093/neuros/nyx341
*I = Interventional or endovascular therapy group.
**C = control group.

a smaller percentage of mismatch indicating poor collateral flow from long-standing hyperglycemia or peri-ischemic cortical depolarization from hyperglycemia and further local ischemia (21).

The goal of BP management in patients with acute stroke is to optimize cerebral perfusion pressure and flow and limit hypotension, but also to prevent HT. This represents a balancing act clinicians must perform on a daily basis and occurs with wide practice variability. The best evidence for guidance on optimal BP management following large vessel occlusion (LVO) is a single center prospective examination of 217 consecutive AIS patients with LVO who had a mechanical thrombectomy with thrombolysis in cerebral infarction (TICI) 2b or TICI 3 revascularization. The patients were divided into three groups: BP less than 140/90 mmHg (intensive group), less than 160/90 mmHg (moderate group), and a permissive hypertension group. The three groups did not differ in rates of symptomatic intracranial hemorrhage, but 3-month mortality was higher in the permissive hypertension group compared to the moderate and intensive therapy groups. Additionally, the permissive hypertension group had less functional independence as well (30). This study suggests allowing luxury perfusion after thrombectomy has deleterious effects and may be due to impaired autoregulation or reperfusion injury of infarcted tissue. Optimal BP management post-thrombectomy has yet to be determined but permissive hypertension is likely to be harmful. There is no specific recommendation or guideline for BP management after revascularization.

Other strategies that clinicians can employ to reduce HT without sacrificing efficacy include using a lower dose of IV tPA. In the ENCHANTED trial, a lower tPA dosage of 0.6 mg/kg compared to the original 0.9 mg/kg was shown to be noninferior in the ordinal analysis of modified Rankin Scale scores while significantly lowering the risk of symptomatic intracerebral hemorrhage (31). Novel therapeutics are also showing promise. A 2016 Chinese study showed that early initiation of tirofiban, a glycoprotein IIb/IIIa inhibitor, reduced the risk of reocclusion after IV tPA and avoided higher risk of hemorrhagic complications. The most impressive results were that this therapy also significantly improved 3-month outcomes in AIS patients receiving alteplase (32).

MANAGEMENT

Trials such as the recent DEFUSE 3 and DAWN have harnessed the power of neuroimaging to better identify patients who stand to benefit from acute thrombectomy and are at lower risk of HT. This has allowed us to extend the window for intervention for select patients, but is not in and of itself intervening in the underlying disease process. Just as in reperfusion injury following myocardial infarction, a host of novel therapies, collectively termed "neuroprotective," have been trialed since the 1990s in efforts to mitigate cerebral ischemic and reperfusion injury. The promise of this line of thought lies in extending therapeutic windows and improving functional outcomes in conjunction with existing reperfusion therapies. These include a diverse assortment of agents such as metalloprotease inhibitors, neurotransmitter receptor antagonists, statins, free radical scavengers, immunosuppressive agents, hypothermia, and ischemic conditioning. Although most of these therapeutic agents and strategies have shown efficacy in preclinical trials, none have shown efficacy in phase 3 clinical trials and none are currently recommended for clinical practice. A few examples follow (33).

In 2014, the URICO-ICTUS trial, a randomized double-blind phase 2b/3 trial compared IV tPA alone to IV tPA in combination with uric acid for patients within 4.5 hours of stroke symptoms' onset (34). Uric acid is known to be a potent free radical scavenger and was hypothesized to reduce ischemic reperfusion injury and improve outcomes in conjunction with tPA. However, the trial failed to show a difference in functional outcomes at 90 days. In 2016, the Glyburide Advantage in Malignant Edema and Stroke (GAMES) trial attempted to reduce MMP-9 activation via an IV sulfonylurea receptor inhibitor in order to decrease malignant cerebral edema and the need for decompressive hemicraniectomy. The trial did reduce MMP-9 levels but failed to show a reduction in cerebral edema or a reduction in the need for decompressive surgery as compared to placebo (35).

In the face of many disappointments, attention has turned to factors other than the pharmacologic target. For example, in 2015, the Field Administration of Stroke Therapy-Magnesium (FAST-MAG) trial examined the use of IV magnesium initiated by emergency responders within 2 hours of symptom onset, hypothesizing that it was a delay in initiation of the drug that had resulted in previous negative trials (36). However, FAST too failed to show benefit in modified Rankin Scale at 90 days compared to placebo.The authors postulated that this was due to delayed penetrance of magnesium into the central nervous system, underscoring the need for therapeutics that are feasibly deployed, are themselves able to penetrate into the ischemic tissue, and exert their effect in time to intercede in the progression of ischemia and reperfusion injury.

Despite the lack of progress so far, neuroprotection continues to be an active field of inquiry. Recently a pilot trial of fingolimod, an immunomodulatory agent used to prevent lymphocyte migration into the central nervous system, has shown success when used with tPA at reducing NIH stroke scale scores, lesion volumes, and rates of hemorrhage (37). A larger study examining the role of fingolimod in addition to IV tPA and thrombectomy, called the FAMTAIS trial, is currently planned (38). Also ongoing is the CHemical Optimization of Intra-arterial Cerebral Embolectomy (CHOICE) trial, which is expected to terminate in 2019, and aims to evaluate whether *intra-arterial* tPA in addition to mechanical thrombectomy can prevent the no-reflow phenomenon by lysing microemboli that form due to recanalization.

CONCLUSION

CIRI is the biochemical cascade that occurs as a result of recanalizing an occluded artery, causing further tissue damage that parallels and antagonizes the benefits of restoring blood flow to the ischemic tissue. CIRI can worsen brain ischemia, cause HT, BBB disruption with subsequent cerebral edema, and is associated with worse outcomes. Clinical management of CIRI continues to hinge on prevention, early recognition, BP reduction, and optimal glucose management. As recanalization becomes more common, understanding what happens to the parenchyma, CSF, microglia, BBB, and vasculature after mechanical thrombectomy and pharmacologic clot lysis is vital. CIRI will become more common and mitigating its response will become a top priority.

REFERENCES

1. Powers W, Rabinstein AA, Ackerson T, et al. 2018 Guidelines for the Early Management of Patients with Acute Ischemic Stroke. *Stroke.* 2018;49:e46-e99.
2. Nogueira RG, Jadhav AP, Haussen DC, et al. Thrombectomy 6 to 24 hours after stroke with a mismatch between deficit and infarct. *N Engl J Med.* 2018;378(1):11–21. doi:10.1056/NEJMoa1706442
3. Albers GW, Marks MP, Kemp S, et al. Thrombectomy for stroke at 6 to 16 hours with selection by perfusion imaging. *N Engl J Med.* 2018;378(8):708–718. doi:10.1056/nejmoa1713973
4. Bai J, Lyden P. Revisiting cerebral post ischemic reperfusion injury: new insights in understanding reperfusion failure, hemorrhage, and edema. *Int J Stroke.* 2015;10(2):143–152. doi:10.1111/ijs.12434
5. Al-Mufti F, Amuluru K, Roth W, et al. Cerebral ischemic reperfusion injury following recanalization of large vessel occlusions. *Neurosurgery.* 2018;82(6):781–789. doi:10.1093/neuros/nyx341
6. Wang W, Li M, Chen Q, et al. Hemorrhagic transformation after tissue plasminogen activator reperfusion therapy for ischemic stroke: mechanisms, models, and biomarkers. *Mol Neurobiol.* 2015;52(3):1572–1579. doi:10.1007/s12035-014-8952-x
7. Zheng H, Chen C, Zhang J, et al. Mechanism and therapy of brain edema after intracerebral hemorrhage. *Cerebrovasc Dis.* 2016;42:155–169. doi:10.1159/000445170
8. Khan M, Dhammu TS, Matsuda F, et al. Blocking a vicious cycle nNOS/peroxynitrite/AMPK by S-nitroglutathione: implication for stroke therapy. *BMC Neurosci.* 2015;16:42. doi:10.1186/s12868-015-0179-x
9. Khoshnam SE, Winlow W, Farzaneh M, et al. Pathogenic mechanisms following ischemic stroke. *Neurol Sci.* 2017;38:1167–1186. doi:10.1007/s10072-017-2938-1
10. Jung JE. Reperfusion and neurovascular dysfunction in stroke: from basic mechanisms to potential strategies for neuroprotection. *Mol Neurobiol.* 2010;41(2–3):172–179. doi:10.1007/s12035-010-8102-z
11. Davis S. Effects of alteplase beyond 3 h after stroke in the Echoplanar Imaging Thrombolytic Evaluation Trial (EPITHET): a placebo-controlled randomised trial. *Lancet Neurol.* 2008;7:299–309. doi:10.1016/s1474-4422(08)70044-9
12. De Silva DA, Fink JN, Christensen S, et al. Assessing reperfusion and recanalization as markers of clinical outcomes after intravenous thrombolysis in the Echoplanar Imaging Thrombolytic Evaluation Trial (EPITHET). *Stroke.* 2009;40:2872–2874. doi:10.1161/strokeaha.108.543595
13. Braunwald E, Kloner RA. Myocardial reperfusion: a double-edged sword? *J Clin Invest.* 1985;76(5):1713–1719. doi:10.1172/jci112160

14. Nour M, Scalzo F, Liebeskind DS. Ischemia-reperfusion injury in stroke. *Intervent Neurol.* 2012;1:185–199. doi:10.1159/000353125
15. Olah L, Wecker S, Hoehn M. Secondary deterioration of apparent diffusion coefficient after 1-hour transient focal cerebral ischemia in rats. *J Cereb Blood Flow Metab.* 20:1474–1482. doi:10.1097/00004647-200010000-00009
16. Pan J, Konstas A-A, Bateman B, et al. Reperfusion injury following cerebral ischemia: pathophysiology, MR imaging, and potential therapies. *Neuroradiol.* 2007;49:93–102. doi:10.1007/s00234-006-0183-z
17. Kidwell CS, Saver JL, Mattiello J, et al. Diffusion-perfusion MRI characterization of post-recanalization hyperperfusion in humans. *Neurology.* 2001;57:2015–2021. doi:10.1212/wnl.57.11.2015
18. Hacke W, Kaste M, Bluhmki E, et al. Thrombolysis with alteplase 3 to 4.5 hours after acute ischemic stroke. *N Engl J Med.* 2008;359:1317–1329. doi:10.1056/nejmoa0804656
19. National Institute of Neurological Disorders and Stroke rt-PA Stroke Study Group. Tissue plasminogen activator for acute ischemic stroke. *N Engl J Med.* 1995;333(24):1581–1587. doi:10.1056/nejm199512143332401
20. Bang OY, Saver JL, Kim SJ, et al. Collateral flow averts hemorrhagic transformation after endovacular therapy for acute ischemic stroke. *Stroke.* 2011;42:2235–2239. doi:10.1161/strokeaha.110.604603
21. Zhang J, Yang Y, Sun H, Xing Y. Hemorrhagic transformation after cerebral infarction: current concepts and challenges. *Ann Transl Med.* 2014;2(8):81. doi:10.3978/j.issn.2305-5839.2014.08.08
22. Selim M, Fink JN, Kumar S, et al. Predictors of hemorrhagic transformation after intravenous recombinant tissue plasminogen activator: prognostic value of the initial apparent diffusion coefficient and diffusion-weighted lesion volume. *Stroke.* 2002;33:2047–2052. doi:10.1161/01.str.0000023577.65990.4e
23. Kimura K., Iguchi Y, Shibazaki K, et al. Recanalization between 1 and 24 hours after t-PA therapy is a strong predictor of cerebral hemorrhage in acute ischemic stroke patients. *J Neurol Sci.* 2008;270(1–2):48–52. doi:10.1016/j.jns.2008.01.013
24. Seidel G, Cangür H, Albers T, et al. Sonographic Evaluation of Hemorrhagic Transformation and Arterial Recanalization in Acute Hemispheric Ischemic Stroke. *Stroke.* 2009;40:119–123. doi:10.1161/strokeaha.108.516799
25. Warach S, Latour LL. Evidence of reperfusion injury, exacerbated by thrombolytic therapy, in human focal brain ischemia using a novel imaging marker of early blood-brain barrier disruption. *Stroke.* 2004;35:2659–2661. doi:10.1161/01.str.0000144051.32131.09
26. Cho A-H, Cho Y-P, Lee DH, et al. Reperfusion Injury on Magnetic Resonance Imaging After Carotid Revascularization. *Stroke.* 2014;45:602–604. doi:10.1161/strokeaha.113.003792

27. Okazaki S, Yamagami H, Yoshimoto T, et al. Cerebral Hyperperfusion on arterial spin labeling MRI after reperfusion therapy is related to hemorrhagic transformation. *J Cereb Blood Flow Metab.* 2017;37(9):3087–3090. doi:10.1177/0271678x17718099
28. Goyal M, Demchuk AM, Menon BK, et al. Randomized assessment of rapid endovascular treatment of ischemic stroke. *N Engl J Med.* 2015;372;1019–1030. doi:10.1056/NEJMoa1414905
29. Fuentes B, Castillo J, San José B, et al. The prognostic value of capillary glucose levels in acute stroke: the Glycemia in Acute Stroke (GLIAS) study. *Stroke.* 2009;40(2):562–568. doi:10.1161/strokeaha.108.519926
30. Goyal N, Tsivgoulis G, Pandhi A, et al. Blood pressure levels post mechanical thrombectomy and outcomes in large vessel occlusion strokes. *Neurology.* 2017;89:540–547. doi:10.1212/wnl.0000000000004184
31. Anderson CS, Robinson T, Lindley RI, et al. Low-Dose versus Standard-Dose Intravenous Alteplase in Acute Ischemic Stroke. *N Engl J Med.* 2016;374:2313–2323. doi:10.1056/NEJMoa1515510.
32. Li W, Lin L, Zhang M, et al. Safety and preliminary efficacy of early tirofiban treatment after alteplase in acute ischemic stroke patients. *Stroke.* 2016;47:2649–2651. doi:10.1161/strokeaha.116.014413
33. Chamorro A. Neuroprotectants in the Era of Reperfusion Therapy. *J Stroke.* 2018;20(2):197–207. doi:10.5853/jos.2017.02901
34. Chamorro A, Amaro S, Castellanos M, et al. Safety and efficacy of uric acid in patients with acute stroke (URICO-ICTUS): a randomised, double-blind phase 2b/3 trial. *Lancet Neurol.* 2014;13:453–460. doi: 10.1016/s1474-4422(14)70054-7
35. Sheth KN., Elm JJ, Molyneaux BJ, et al. Safety and efficacy of intravenous glyburide on brain swelling after large hemispheric infarction (GAMES-RP): a randomised, double-blind, placebo-controlled phase 2 trial. *Lancet Neurol.* 2016;15(11):1160–1169. doi:10.1016/S1474-4422(16)30196-X
36. Saver JL, Starkman S, Eckstein M, et al. Prehospital Use of Magnesium Sulfate as Neuroprotection in Acute Stroke. *N Engl J Med.*2015;372:528–536. doi:10.1056/NEJMoa1408827
37. Zhu Z, Fu Y, Tian D, et al. Combination of the immune modulator fingolimod with alteplase in acute ischemic stroke: a pilot trial. *Circulation.* 2015;132:1104–1112. doi:10.1161/circulationaha.115.016371
38. Zhang S, Zhou Y, Zhang R, et al. Rationale and design of combination of an immune modulator Fingolimod with Alteplase with Mechanical Thrombectomy in Acute Ischemic Stroke (FAMTAIS) trial. *Int J Stroke.* 2017;12(8):906–909. dosi:10.1177/1747493017710340

8 Stroke-Related Seizures

Bilal Butt, Stefania Maraka, and Christos Lazaridis

KEY POINTS

- Cerebrovascular disease is a major cause of epilepsy after middle age (1).
- Poststroke seizures can manifest either as an early sequel or as a late complication (2).
- Intracerebral hemorrhage (ICH) and hemorrhagic transformation are predictors of early seizures (ESs) after stroke (3).
- Stroke severity and cortical involvement are significant predictors of late seizures (LSs) (3).
- Prophylactic treatment is not routinely recommended (4).

INTRODUCTION

Stroke is the fourth leading cause of death in the United States with a combined direct and indirect cost exceeding 68 billion dollars per year (5). The relationship between seizures and stroke has been reported as early as 1864 by John Hughlings Jackson (6). Ischemic and hemorrhagic strokes amount to approximately 11% of all adult epilepsy cases (5,7) and represent the main etiology of symptomatic seizures in older adults, especially in patients over 60 years old (5,8).

EPIDEMIOLOGY, MORBIDITY, AND MORTALITY

Conventionally, stroke-related seizures are classified as ESs or LSs. The most frequently reported time landmark to differentiate ESs versus LSs is 7 to 14 days after an ischemic stroke (9). However, there is wide variation in the literature with ES being defined anywhere between 24 hours and 4 weeks poststroke. For that reason, the reported incidence of ESs varies from 2% to 33% with 50% to 78% of the seizures occurring within the first 24 hours (10,11).

Factors associated with an increased likelihood of seizures are: cortical infarct location, central nervous system infection,

 DOI: 10.1891/9780826124791.0008

or concurrent traumatic brain injury (TBI) (4). Risk factors for the development of ES are hemorrhagic subtype, stroke severity, age younger than 65 years old, and alcohol use (11). Diabetes mellitus, smoking, hyperlipidemia, ischemic heart disease, atrial fibrillation, and previous transient ischemic attacks (TIAs) were not associated with ESs (3). ESs are twice as frequent in hemorrhagic compared to ischemic subtypes with 6.3% incidence in ICH, 7.9% in subarachnoid hemorrhage (SAH), and 2.4% in ischemic stroke (11). The most important risk factor for post-ICH ESs is cortical involvement (12,13). Although ischemic stroke is associated with a lower incidence of ESs as compared to ICH, it nevertheless results in a higher overall burden of poststroke epilepsy (PSE) due to higher incidence and prevalence (3,14). The cumulative incidence of LSs is approximately 3%. Similarly with ESs, the risk of having LSs is increased with cortical involvement and young age (15). LSs peak within 6 to 12 months after stroke (4); a summary of features of ESs versus LSs is provided in Table 8.1.

The risk of seizure recurrence and PSE differs between ESs and LSs. The 10-year risk of seizure recurrence is reported as 20% and 60% for ESs and LSs respectively (2,16). In 2014, the definition of

Table 8.1 Summary of Features Distinguishing ESs Versus LSs

	ES	LS
Incidence (varies based on definition)	2%–33%	3%
Timeline (varies in the literature)	7–14 days with most occurring within 24 hours	Beyond 14 days and peak at 6–12 months
Common risk factors	ICH, hemorrhagic transformation of ischemic stroke, stroke severity, age younger than 65 years old, and alcohol use	Stroke severity and cortical involvement
Pathophysiology	Cellular biochemical dysfunction leading to electrically irritable tissue	Gliosis
Management	No routine use of prophylactic AEDs. Treatment of seizures as per guidelines for epilepsy	

AED, antiepileptic drug; ES, early seizure; ICH, intracerebral hemorrhage; LS, late seizure.

epilepsy was modified to include the event of one unprovoked seizure provided that the chance of recurrence (over the next 10 years) is sufficiently high (17). Therefore, even with one episode of LSs, diagnosis of epilepsy can be established. A meta-analysis has found gender and family history not to be significant risk factors for the development of PSE (3). There is a recent effort to create a predictive scoring system for PSE; the CAVE score has been developed to predict LS and PSE after ICH. The "C" refers to cortical involvement, "A" for age less than 65 years old, "V" for volume greater than 10 mL, and "E" for ES within 7 days after hemorrhage. Each item denotes a score of 1 and the higher the score the greater the risk of PSE. However, further studies are needed to validate the CAVE score before routine use (4,18).

The reported combined incidence of subcortical strokes and seizures has been from 0% to 23%. Causality remains uncertain; some consider seizures to be impossible in the case of isolated lacunar infarctions (11,19). As mentioned later in this chapter, subcortical strokes could conceivably influence neuronal networks leading to epileptiform activity. Brainstem strokes, particularly in the pons, can cause convulsive movements of the extremities giving the appearance of seizures; however, they are more plausibly related to ischemia of corticospinal fibers (20).

Last, other studies investigating different risk factors for post-stroke seizures have shown no association between seizures and presence of hydrocephalus, intracranial shift, Glasgow Coma Scale, or degree of neurological deficit (11,21). The association between a cardioembolic mechanism and acute symptomatic seizures is controversial (13,15,22). Further prospective studies to assess stroke subtypes based on the TOAST criteria and seizures are needed.

A recent systematic review and meta-analysis reported an association between ES and LS with a greater risk of poststroke disability. This risk was higher at the time of discharge and then decreased 3 months after the stroke event (3,11). For the group of patients on treatment with antiepileptic drugs (AEDs), the drug–drug interactions with medications used for secondary prevention of stroke including antithrombotics, statins, and blood pressure medications could lead to increased risk of stroke recurrence (9). Finally, when patients with poststroke seizure develop epilepsy this may lead to further anxiety, worsen recovery and overall quality of life (4).

Occurrence of seizures within 24 hours of stroke is associated with higher 30-day mortality, which might be a reflection of the extent of neuronal damage (5). Interestingly, Serafini et al. did not find an association between ESs and increased mortality at 1 month or association between LSs and increased mortality at 24 months (15). Nevertheless, in other investigations the occurrence of PSE has been shown to lead to poor prognosis and increased mortality (4,11).

PATHOPHYSIOLOGY

The pathophysiology of seizures after stroke is currently not fully elucidated, but several mechanisms have been hypothesized. Cellular biochemical dysfunction with membrane instability of injured cells, glutamate neurotransmitter release secondary to hypoxia, free radical damage, or transient depolarizations of the ischemic penumbra with a resulting electrically irritable tissue are some of the proposed mechanisms (23). The disruption of the blood–brain barrier (BBB) has been the most researched hypothesis for poststroke seizures. Following disruption of the BBB, albumin enters the brain parenchyma whereby it binds to astrocytes and activates them. Activated astrocytes reduce uptake of potassium and glutamate, which in turn induces neuronal hyperexcitability. In addition, disrupted BBB can result in extravasated thrombin, which can increase neuronal electrical activity and can induce a seizure (4). Early and late poststroke seizures have different pathophysiological mechanisms. ESs are thought to be a result of cellular biochemical dysfunction leading to electrically irritable tissue. Acute ischemia leads to increased extracellular concentrations of the excitatory neurotransmitter glutamate, which causes secondary neuronal injury (24). However, LSs are believed to be caused by gliosis and the development of a meningocerebral cicatrix. The gliotic scar has been recognized as a nidus for LSs. Changes in membrane properties, selective neuronal loss, and collateral sprouting can result in hyperexcitability and neuronal synchrony sufficient to cause seizures (9,24).

As already stated, ICH is more likely to result in ESs as compared to ischemic strokes (15). The pathophysiological mechanism of seizures from ICH is not well defined but there are different hypotheses in the literature. One possible mechanism is the sudden development of a space-occupying lesion with mass effect. Furthermore, blood products might be responsible for increased epileptogenicity, and in particular the presence of hemosiderin (11,15). The impact of ICH volume on development of seizures has been controversial (25). De Herdt et al. did not report a correlation between the volume of ICH and ES, while Yang et al. showed ES to be associated with younger age and larger ICH volume (25,26). Hemorrhagic transformation of cerebral infarction also led to a greater risk of PSE. Hemorrhagic transformation, especially in cortical regions, could increase the excitability of the affected cortical ischemic penumbra (3). Zhang et al. reported more excitability in the presence of hemorrhagic transformation and also suggested that it could act as an independent predictor of status epilepticus in patients with acute ischemic stroke (3,27).

Even though poststroke seizures have been typically associated with cortical localization, subcortical strokes could also be related to seizures. The pathophysiology of seizures after subcortical strokes has not been defined. It might be due to coexistence of cortical microinfarcts, which have been detected with 1.5 to 3 Tesla MRI. Another possible explanation is the disruption of subcortical connecting fibers leading to secondary cortical degeneration.

The frequency of seizures associated with TIA is low at 1.8% to 3.7%. Limb shaking TIAs can look like a focal seizure and are believed to be caused by focal cerebral hypoperfusion due to carotid artery occlusive disease. Unfortunately, phenomenologically distinguishing limb shaking TIAs from a focal seizure can be hard, and hence the true frequency of such seizures is uncertain (24).

Although not directly related to epileptic seizures recorded by surface EEG, another pathological electro-ischemic phenomenon is worth mentioning. These phenomena are cortical spreading depolarization(s) (CSD) and associated cortical spreading depression and ischemia. Spreading depolarizations are propagating (2–5 mm/min) waves of mass depolarization of gray matter. In injured cortex (from diverse types of brain pathologies), depolarizations can be prolonged leading to unfavorable supply–demand relationships, and energy failure. This process is part of a vicious circle including propagating microvascular constriction, termed spreading ischemia. These processes are now considered potentially significant contributors in the development and/or exacerbation of secondary injury in the settings of ischemic stroke, ICH, and SAH, as well as in TBI. The clinical gold-standard method to record CSDs is by electrocorticography (ECoG) from subdural electrode strips that are placed operatively through craniotomies or burr holes. The use of linear strips allows continuous monitoring of a 5 cm extent of cerebral cortex for up to 2 weeks in the ICU (28). A potential etiology for CSD is the opening of the BBB that has also been implicated in pathophysiology of seizures poststroke. Following malignant stroke, the incidence of CSDs ranges from 35% to 88%, and their presence has been implicated in penumbral cell death and infarct extension (29).

PREVENTION

The American Heart Association (AHA) does not recommend routine prophylactic administration of AEDs poststroke (30). Statin use in the acute phase of stroke may reduce the risk of ESs, and may prevent the progression of initial poststroke seizure into chronic epilepsy (4,31). This may be related to direct anticonvulsant or anti-inflammatory effects of statins, and in the prevention of BBB breakdown (4). Perampanel is a novel, highly selective noncompetitive postsynaptic α-amino-3-hydroxy-5-methyl-4-isoxazolepropionic acid (AMPA) glutamate receptor antagonist (4). Although no clinical evidence exists for its use in PSE, it is believed to have some potential in preventing epileptogenesis by blocking glutamate excitotoxicity (known to play an important role in PSE pathogenesis) (4). The need for prophylaxis for PSE with newer generation AEDs is still unclear and hence randomized controlled trials are needed to answer this.

IDENTIFICATION

Seizures with tonic–clonic semiology or focal motor jerking can be readily picked up on clinical examination. However, some seizures can have subtle clinical findings and therefore can be missed. Such subtle clinical presentation can involve behavioral arrest, alteration of awareness, nystagmus, focal sensory, facial twitching, autonomic fluctuations, and intermittent speech impairment. Electrophysiological studies are required for detection of those subclinical events (5). Additionally, stroke patients are at risk for nonconvulsive status epilepticus (NCSE), particularly in the setting of ESs; 9% of patients with acute cerebral ischemia are reported to have nonconvulsive seizures with a 7% incidence of NCSE (32,33). The subtle nature or lack of clinical manifestations of NCSE can be hard to detect in the acute phase of stroke and hence continuous electroencephalography (cEEG) is required for detection (4). Furthermore, cEEG recording is prudent to obtain in stroke patients with depressed mental status disproportionate to the extent of structural brain injury (12).

MANAGEMENT

Appropriate timing for anticonvulsant initiation remains unclear for poststroke seizures. There is no data to suggest that early use will prevent lesion-related epilepsy or that treatment of ESs will prevent the occurrence of LSs (12). According to the AHA, prophylactic antiseizure medication for ICH is not recommended (Class III, Level of Evidence B) (12). In fact, studies suggest that the use of prophylactic seizure medication (primarily phenytoin) was associated with increased death and disability in ICH (12). Prophylactic treatment with valproic acid showed no reduction in seizure incidence over 1 year in patients with ICH (12,34).

The 2018 AHA guidelines do not include specific recommendations for the treatment of postischemic stroke seizures (35). Due to lack of high-level evidence, there is large variation in treatment practices after an isolated poststroke seizure; especially after ES that carries less risk for development of PSE. Many clinicians would start AED treatment on repeated unprovoked poststroke seizures; however, there is no good evidence to inform the appropriate duration of treatment. Clinical seizures post-ICH should be treated with standard AEDs (Class I, Level of Evidence A) (12). Traditional first-line AEDs, in the acute setting of seizures, include lorazepam, phenytoin, valproic acid, levetiracetam, and phenobarbital. In the setting of more intractable seizures, and status epilepticus, it may be necessary to use continuous infusion of second-line agents such as midazolam, propofol, pentobarbital, or ketamine. A more recent option includes intravenous lacosamide that has been widely used due to limited drug interactions and systemic toxicity. In terms of efficacy, there is minimal data comparing AEDs in this setting. Therefore, specific AED choice for poststroke seizures depends on potential side effects and impact on stroke recovery (5). Treatment of EEG abnormalities should be considered based on the morphology and type of abnormality. For instance, rhythmic epileptiform discharges such as periodic lateralized epileptiform discharges (PLEDs) and bilateral independent periodic epileptiform discharges (BiPEDs) can evolve to electrographic seizures. The presence of PLEDs on EEG might suggest the need for treatment since up to 75% of these patients have been found to develop ESs (24). On the contrary, intermittent rhythmic discharges and periodic diffuse discharges rarely evolve to seizures and no treatment is warranted (5).

CONCLUSION

Stroke is a major cause of seizures, and detection may not always be straightforward. Recognition, prevention, and management of seizures, and epilepsy, are of critical importance in order to maximize poststroke recovery. Seizures are more common in hemorrhagic stroke than ischemic, and those with late-occurring episodes are at a greater risk for epilepsy (11). Primary ICH, hemorrhagic transformation, and alcohol use are associated with ESs, while cortical lesions and stroke severity may predict LSs (3). Current evidence on pharmacologic management of stroke-related seizures does not support the use of AEDs for primary prevention (14). Our current understanding of the pathophysiology, epidemiology, risk factors, and treatment of PSE remains incomplete; enhanced identification of factors placing patients at high risk could result in targeted, preventive AED administration (24).

REFERENCES

1. Forsgren L, Beghi E, Oun A, et al. The epidemiology of epilepsy in Europe—a systematic review. *Eur J Neurol.* 2005;12(4):245–253. doi:10.1111/j.1468-1331.2004.00992.x
2. Zelano J. Poststroke epilepsy: update and future directions. *Ther Adv Neurol Disord.* 2016;9(5):424–435. doi:10.1177/1756285616654423
3. Zhang C, Wang X, Wang Y, et al. Risk factors for post-stroke seizures: a systematic review and meta-analysis. *Epilepsy Res.* 2014;108(10):1806–1816. doi:10.1016/j.eplepsyres.2014.09.030
4. Tanaka T, Ihara M. Post-stroke epilepsy. *Neurochem Int.* 2017;107:219–228. doi:10.1016/j.neuint.2017.02.002
5. Chung JM. Seizures in the acute stroke setting. *Neurol Res.* 2014;36(5):403–406. doi:10.1179/1743132814y.0000000352
6. Chadehumbe MA, Khatri P, Khoury JC, et al. Seizures are common in the acute setting of childhood stroke: a population-based study. *J Child Neurol.* 2009;24(1):9–12. doi:10.1177/0883073808320756
7. Hauser WA, Annegers JF, Kurland LT. Incidence of epilepsy and unprovoked seizures in Rochester, Minnesota: 1935–1984. *Epilepsia.* 1993;34(3):453–468. doi:10.1111/j.1528-1157.1993.tb02586.x
8. Forsgren L, Bucht G, Eriksson S, et al. Incidence and clinical characterization of unprovoked seizures in adults: a prospective population-based study. *Epilepsia.* 1996;37(3):224–249. doi:10.1111/j.1528-1157.1996.tb00017.x
9. Chan L, Hu C-J, Fan Y-C, et al., Incidence of poststroke seizures: a meta-analysis. *J Clin Neurosci.* 2017; 47:347–351. doi:10.1016/j.jocn.2017.10.088
10. Hamidou B, Aboa-Eboulé C, Durier J, et al. Prognostic value of early epileptic seizures on mortality and functional disability in acute stroke: the Dijon Stroke Registry (1985–2010). *J Neurol.* 2013;260(4):1043–1051. doi:10.1007/s00415-012-6756-3
11. Bladin CF, Alexandrov AV, Bellavance A, et al. Seizures after stroke: a prospective multicenter study. *Arch Neurol.* 2000;57(11):1617–1622. doi:10.1001/archneur.57.11.1617
12. Hemphill JC 3rd, Greenberg SM, Anderson CS, et al. Guidelines for the management of spontaneous intracerebral emorrhage: a guideline for healthcare professionals from the American Heart Association/American Stroke Association. *Stroke.* 2015;46(7):2032–2060. doi:10.1161/str.0000000000000069

13. Beghi E, D'Alessandro R, Beretta S, et al. Incidence and predictors of acute symptomatic seizures after stroke. *Neurology*. 2011;77(20):1785–1793. doi:10.1212/wnl.0b013e3182364878
14. Wang JZ, Vyas MV, Saposnik G, et al. Incidence and management of seizures after ischemic stroke: systematic review and meta-analysis. *Neurol*. 2017;89(12):1220–1228. doi:10.1212/wnl.0000000000004407
15. Serafini A, Gigli GL, Gregoraci G, et al. Are early seizures predictive of epilepsy after a stroke? Results of a Population-Based Study. *Neuroepidemiology*. 2015;45(1):50–58. doi:10.1159/000382078
16. Hesdorffer DC, Benn EKT, Cascino GD, et al. Is a first acute symptomatic seizure epilepsy? Mortality and risk for recurrent seizure. *Epilepsia*. 2009;50(5):1102–1108. doi:10.1111/j.1528-1167.2008.01945.x
17. Fisher RS. Redefining epilepsy. *Curr Opin Neurol*. 2015;28(2):130–135. doi:10.1097/wco.0000000000000174
18. Haapaniemi E, Strbian D, Rossi C, et al. The CAVE score for predicting late seizures after intracerebral hemorrhage. *Stroke*. 2014;45(7):1971–1976. doi:10.1161/strokeaha.114.004686
19. Fisher CM. Lacunar strokes and infarcts: a review. *Neurology*. 1982; 32(8):871–876. doi:10.1212/wnl.32.8.871
20. Saposnik G, Caplan LR. Convulsive-like movements in brainstem stroke. *Arch Neurol*. 2001;58(4):654–657. doi:10.1001/archneur.58.4.654
21. Berger AR, Lipton RB, Lesser ML, et al. Early seizures following intracerebral hemorrhage: implications for therapy. *Neurology*. 1988;38(9):1363–1365. doi:10.1212/wnl.38.9.1363
22. Giroud M, Gras P, Fayolle H, et al. Early seizures after acute stroke: a study of 1,640 cases. *Epilepsia*. 1994;35(5):959–964. doi:10.1111/j.1528-1157.1994.tb02540.x
23. Mohamed C, Kissani N. Early seizures in acute stroke. *Pan Afr Med J*. 2015;20:136. doi:10.11604/pamj.2015.20.136.5925
24. Camilo O, Goldstein LB. Seizures and epilepsy after ischemic stroke. *Stroke*. 2004;35(7):1769–1775. doi:10.1161/01.str.0000130989.17100.96
25. De Herdt V, Dumont F, Henon H, et al. Early seizures in intracerebral hemorrhage: incidence, associated factors, and outcome. *Neurology*. 2011;77(20):1794–1800. doi:10.1212/wnl.0b013e31823648a6
26. Yang TM, Lin W-C, Chang W-N, et al. Predictors and outcome of seizures after spontaneous intracerebral hemorrhage. Clinical article. *J Neurosurg*. 2009;111(1):87–93. doi:10.3171/2009.2.jns081622
27. Bateman BT, Claassen J, Willey JZ, et al. Convulsive status epilepticus after ischemic stroke and intracerebral hemorrhage: frequency, predictors, and impact on outcome in a large administrative dataset. *Neurocrit Care*. 2007;7(3):187–1893.doi:10.1007/s12028-007-0056-2
28. Hartings JA. Spreading depolarization monitoring in neurocritical care of acute brain injury. *Curr Opin Crit Care*. 2017;23(2):94–102. doi:10.1097/mcc.0000000000000395

29. Kramer DR, Fujii T, Ohiorhenuan I, et al. Cortical spreading depolarization: pathophysiology, implications, and future directions. *J Clin Neurosci.* 2016;24:22–27. doi:10.1016/j.jocn.2015.08.004
30. Winstein CJ, Stein J, Arena R, et al. Guidelines for adult stroke rehabilitation and recovery: a guideline for healthcare professionals from the American Heart Association/American Stroke Association. *Stroke.* 2016;47(6):e98–e169. doi:10.1161/str.0000000000000098
31. Guo J, Guo J, Li J, et al. Statin treatment reduces the risk of post-stroke seizures. *Neurology.* 2015. 85(8):701–707. doi:10.1212/wnl.0000000000001814
32. Claassen J, Mayer SA, Kowalski RG, et al. Detection of electrographic seizures with continuous EEG monitoring in critically ill patients. *Neurology.* 2004;62(10):1743–1748. doi:10.1212/01.wnl.0000125184.88797.62
33. Bentes C, Martins H, Peralta AR, et al. Post-stroke seizures are clinically underestimated. *J Neurol.* 2017;264(9):1978–1985. doi:10.1007/s00415-017-8586-9
34. Gilad R, Boaz M, Dabby R, et al. Are post intracerebral hemorrhage seizures prevented by anti-epileptic treatment? *Epilepsy Res.* 2011;95(3):227–231. doi:10.1016/j.eplepsyres.2011.04.002
35. Jauch EC, Saver JL, Adams HP, et al. Guidelines for the early management of patients with acute ischemic stroke: a guideline for healthcare professionals from the American Heart Association/American Stroke Association. *Stroke.* 2013;44(3):870–947.

9 Rebleeding, Vasospasm, and Hydrocephalus After Subarachnoid Hemorrhage

Mohammed H. Aref and A. Samy Youssef

KEY POINTS

- Spontaneous subarachnoid hemorrhage (SAH) accounts for 5% to 10% all strokes in the United States, with 30% to 40%, 30-day risk of mortality.
- Intracranial aneurysmal rupture accounts for 80% of spontaneous SAH.
- Ninety percent of rebleeding from a ruptured aneurysm occurs within the first 6 hours after the initial rupture and it increases the mortality rate to 70% to 90%.
- Angiographic vasospasm can affect 50% to 90% of patients with SAH.
- Delayed ischemic neurological deficit (DIND) refers to the development of clinical vasospasm, and this can affect half of the patients with angiographic vasospasm.
- Once a patient is suspected to have vasospasm, other metabolic and pathological conditions need to be ruled out.
- Fifteen to fifty-eight percent with SAH may develop acute hydrocephalus and up to 37% can develop chronic hydrocephalus.

INTRODUCTION

Spontaneous SAH is a devastating illness as it accounts for 5% to 10% of all strokes in the United States (1) with a 30% to 40%, 30-day risk of mortality (2). Ruptured intracerebral aneurysm(s) causes 80% of spontaneous SAH. The prevalence of aneurysms in the general population is about 1% to 2% and can be as high as 9% in some populations (3). It is important to distinguish between spontaneous and traumatic SAH as the differences in morbidity between them are significant. This chapter focuses on spontaneous aneurysmal SAH.

© Springer Publishing Company DOI: 10.1891/9780826124791.0009

Identifying, diagnosing, and prompt management of spontaneous SAH are paramount, not only due to its high initial mortality rate, but also the high morbidity as 50% of the survivors suffer permanent severe neurological sequelae (2).

Several factors are associated with the high risk of morbidity and mortality including time to identification of initial hemorrhage, rehemorrhage, surgical complications, vasospasm leading to delayed cerebral ischemia, hydrocephalus, and associated cardiac and pulmonary complications. In analyzing only mortality, Lantigua et al. found that up to 55% of the patients die due to initial hemorrhage, 17% due to rebleeding, and 15% from directly related medical complications. Eighteen percent of these deaths were in hospital, which further illustrates the gravity of the illness (4).

Since there is a limited window of opportunity in attempting to control and manage initial hemorrhage, much of the focus in aneurysmal SAH management is directed at managing subsequent complications, such as rebleeding, vasospasm, DIND, hydrocephalus, and medical complications. The rate of angiographic vasospasm ranges between 50% and 90%; two-thirds of these patients would suffer moderate-to-severe vasospasm.

Early recognition of vasospasm has become a cornerstone in aneurysmal SAH management as 50% of those patients will become symptomatic, of whom 50% will develop a cerebral infarct (5).

Rebleeding is strongly associated with increased mortality as high as 70% to 90%. The highest risk of rehemorrhage is during the first 24 hours with a range of 4% to 13.6% and peak time being at 2 hours. It remains statistically high up to 8 hours; then it declines to about 1% to 2% daily for the first two weeks (6,7).

Hydrocephalus is a commonly encountered complication following aneurysmal SAH with an incidence rate of 25% to 30% (8). Hydrocephalus occurs both acutely and in a delayed fashion. Acute hydrocephalus is associated with higher grade SAH, and thick or intraventricular blood clot.

Despite the advancement in diagnosis and treatment protocols of SAH, aneurysmal SAH remains a challenging disease to neurosurgeons and neurocritical care providers.

PATHOPHYSIOLOGY

Rebleeding

Rebleeding from a cerebral aneurysm is a major contributor to increased mortality, with a mortality rate reaching up to 70% to 90% of patients. In a review by Larsen et al., it was found that 8%

to 23% of patients rebled within the first 72 hours (9), with 90% of rehemorrhages occurring in the first 6 hours.

The rate of rebleeding is 4% in the first 24 hours, and 1.5% per day afterward with a cumulative risk of 19% in the first 2 weeks as per the International Cooperative Study of Timing of Aneurysm Surgery (7). A later study from Japan found that the rate of hemorrhage in the first 24 hours was up to 17% (6). Risk factors of rebleeding include poor clinical condition, hypertension, large aneurysm size, and large intracerebral or intraventricular hemorrhage (Box 9.1).

Earlier evidence suggests that ventriculostomy and cerebrospinal fluid (CSF) drainage might increase risk of rebleeding (10,11). This is attributed to draining CSF and rapidly reducing intracranial pressure (ICP) thereby increasing the transmural pressure and releasing the tamponade effect created by the high ICP. Later studies (12,13) suggest that the overall risk is not significant, and no ventriculostomy should be withheld if there a clinical indication for it. However, in the study by McIver et al. they do recommend moderate CSF drainage in order to minimize the risk of rebleeding (13).

Vasospasm

Vasospasm is a sustained contraction of the arterial vascular smooth muscles causing narrowing of the vessel. Hemoglobin released from the clot causes calcium influx and activation of calcium/calmodulin dependent myosin light chain, which leads to a chain of events that result in smooth muscle contraction.

Up to 50% to 90% of aneurysmal SAH patients can develop angiographic vasospasm, half of whom will develop clinical vasospasm, which is also referred to as delayed ischemic neurological deficit. Ultimately if untreated, vasospasm can lead to cerebral infarction.

Box 9.1 Risk Factors of Rebleeding

Poor clinical condition
Hypertension
Large aneurysm size
Large intracerebral hemorrhage
Intraventricular hemorrhage

Table 9.1 The Fisher and Modified Fisher Scale

Grade	Modified Fisher	% With Vasospasm	Fisher	% With Vasospasm
0	No SAH	-	-	
1	Thin SAH, no IVH	24	Focal thin	21
2	Thin SAH with IVH	33	Diffuse thin SAH	25
3	Thick SAH, no IVH	33	Thick SAH	37
4	Thick SAH with IVH	40	Focal or diffuse thin SAH with significant ICH or IVH	31

ICH, intracerebral hemorrhage; IVH, intraventricular hemorrhage; SAH, subarachnoid hemorrhage.

The peak time for vasospasm is at 7 days following the ictus of SAH, with a range of 3 to 21 days. However, vasospasm can occur early within the first 48 hours in 10% to 15% of patients (14).

Several factors can predict the likelihood of vasospasm following a ruptured cerebral aneurysm. The most important of these is the amount and the distribution of the subarachnoid blood. This was the rationale behind developing the Fisher scale (15) followed by the Modified Fisher scale later (Table 9.1) (16). The modified scale looked at the degree of cisternal and ventricular hemorrhage and was found to have a greater correlation and higher predictive value of vasospasm (17).

Other factors that have been considered as risk factors for vasospasm are intraventricular hematoma, persistent subarachnoid blood, poor neurological status, history of smoking, hypertension, diabetes, and cocaine use (Box 9.2) (18–20).

In a review by Findlay et al. (5), they suggested that endothelin-1 overproduction, nitric oxide underproduction, and arterial vessel wall narrowing because of an inflammatory process are three main factors in the pathogenesis of vasospasm.

Nitric oxide is a vital key vasodilator naturally produced by vascular endothelial cells, whereas endothelin-1 is a potent vasoconstrictor. Following SAH, the blood clot undergoes auto-oxidation thereby releasing superoxide anion radicals, which lead to lipid peroxidation (21,22). These free radicals along with the lipid

Box 9.2 Risk Factors for Vasospasm

Intraventricular hematoma
Persistent subarachnoid blood
Poor neurological status
History of smoking
Hypertension
Cocaine use
Diabetes

peroxides injure endothelial cells and smooth muscles of the vessel wall. Subsequently, this leads to decreased secretion of nitric oxide (vasodilator) and overproduction of endothelin-1 (vasoconstrictor) leading to vasospasm (23).

Following SAH, other inflammatory mediators such as complement C3a and adhesion molecule-1 are elevated, and these are associated with worse outcomes and vasospasm (24,25).

Hydrocephalus

Hydrocephalus is a common complication following aneurysmal SAH. The incidence ranges from 15% to 58% in the acute stage, and 4% to 37% in the chronic stage (26), which is defined as at 2 weeks or longer. It is important to keep in mind that there exists a subset of patients who can develop delayed hydrocephalus up to 1 year following SAH. The incidence is 0.9% for those who did not need a ventriculostomy when they were hospitalized versus 5.7% for those who received a ventriculostomy (27).

The exact mechanism of hydrocephalus remains unclear, but it is widely conceived to be a result of obstruction caused by blood in the ventricles and/or arachnoid cisterns. Chronic hydrocephalus following SAH is thought to be a result of scarring at the level of arachnoid granulations leading to impaired CSF absorption (8,28,29).

Several predictive features to the development of chronic hydrocephalus include: old age, high Hunt and Hess (H&H) grade, high Fisher grade, low Glasgow Coma Scale (GCS), intraventricular hemorrhage on admission, and acute hydrocephalus. Aneurysmal hemorrhage from either the anterior communicating artery or posterior circulation had a higher probability of causing hydrocephalus (26,30).

Other factors that were found to increase the risk of hydrocephalus are hyperglycemia on admission, bicaudate index of ≥0.20

(distance between the two heads of caudate over the distance of the outer table of the skull at the same level), and the development of nosocomial meningitis (31); see Box 9.3.

Inflammatory processes affecting arachnoid granulations' absorption capacity has been found to be linked to the development of hydrocephalus. In a study by Wostrack et al., it was found that the presence of interleukin-6 (IL-6), an inflammatory mediator, of ≥10,000 pg/ml was significantly associated with future shunt dependency (32). This finding is supported by other studies, which showed that patients who underwent microsurgical clipping are at higher risk of developing vasospasm.

PREVENTION

Rebleeding

The most effective method of preventing rebleeding is immediate treatment of the ruptured aneurysm (33). Up until the actual treatment is performed, medical management should be optimized such as strict systolic blood pressure (SBP) below 160 mmHg (34).

CSF drainage was discussed earlier and was found to have no association with rehemorrhage with moderate amount of drainage (12,13).

A trial of using NovoSeven (recombinant activated factor VII)) to prevent rebleeding was suspended following increased complications related to thrombosis (35), and thromboembolic complications (36). Similarly, a study that looked at administering tranexamic acid to prevent rebleeding by Vermeulen et al. (37) found no benefit of such intervention given the subsequent ischemic complications in the intervention group.

Box 9.3 Risk Factors for Developing Hydrocephalus

Old age
High Hunt and Hess/Fisher grade
Low GCS
Intraventricular hemorrhage
ACOM or posterior circulation aneurysm
Hyperglycemia
Bicaudate index ≥0.20
Nosocomial meningitis

ACOM, anterior communicating; GCS, Glasgow Coma Scale.

Vasospasm

There is a great interest in studying methods or agents that would reduce the incidence of vasospasm. As the understanding of the pathophysiology deepens, more theories and agents are tested. So far, a definitive preventive method has not been described. Nevertheless, there are multiple clinical trials done with variable degrees of success, and as a result, some agents have fallen out of favor, while other agents/methods were shown to be promising.

Simvastatin has long been described as an agent that reduces the chance of vasospasm in earlier trials. The drug fell out of favor following the publication of a phase 3 international randomized clinical trial; simvastatin in aneurysmal subarachnoid hemorrhage (STASH) (38). The study showed that patients who were given 40 mg of simvastatin did not benefit from such intervention. Magnesium infusion also fell out of favor upon completion of the randomized trial of magnesium for aneurysmal subarachnoid hemorrhage (MASH-2) (39). Nimodipine is the only evidence-based agent used in vasospasm management, despite the fact that it was not found to reduce vasospasm; however, it did significantly improve outcomes (40).

Other agents that have been tested include cilostazol, clazosentan (endothelin receptor antagonist) (41), intracisternal recombinant tissue plasminogen activator (rtPa) for clot clearance (42,43), tirilazad mesylate, and nicardipine (44). A meta-analysis of randomized clinical trials about the efficacy of cilostazol (oral phosphodiesterase 3 inhibitor) showed a significant decrease in the risk of clinical vasospasm and possible decrease of angiographic vasospasm (45). In a systematic review and meta-analysis that looked at vasospasm treatment, cilostazol was found to be the only agent associated with significantly positive results when compared to clazosentan, rtPa, and nicardipine (46).

Tirilazad mesylate is a free radical scavenger and lipid peroxidation inhibitor. A randomized double-blind controlled trial by Kassell et al. showed some benefit in men over women; however, the results were not statistically significant (47).

Several interventional strategies such as lamina terminalis fenestration, continuous CSF drainage, and balloon angioplasty have been implemented in the management of vasospasm.

Microsurgical clipping with lamina terminalis fenestration was studied by Andaluz et al. (48) and was found to reduce risk of vasospasm from 54% to 30%. However, a later study found no difference between those who underwent lamina terminalis fenestration versus those who did not (49).

CSF drainage via a lumbar drain has been studied in several reports with variable results. Combined results did show statistically significant benefit in a meta-analysis (50,51).

Prophylactic transluminal balloon angioplasty was tested in a multicenter randomized clinical trial (52). The findings suggested that there was a statistically significant decrease in the need for therapeutic angioplasty; however, there was no change in the Glasgow Outcome Score at 3 months. The 3% risk of vessel perforation and 6% thromboembolic complication related to the procedure raise a safety concern regarding prophylactically utilizing it.

Hydrocephalus

Acute hydrocephalus following aneurysmal SAH is almost impossible to prevent as it is directly related to the amount, location, and distribution of hemorrhage within the cisterns and/or ventricles. One strategy in patients with aneurysmal SAH presenting initially without hydrocephalus is to rapidly treat the aneurysm to prevent rerupture, which might increase the odds of developing acute hydrocephalus.

Chronic hydrocephalus requiring CSF shunting following aneurysmal SAH affects one-third of the patients. Several methods have been described to reduce the incidence of chronic hydrocephalus such as lumbar drain, external ventricular drain (EVD), cisternal drainage and irrigation, ventricular irrigation, and thrombolysis and have had variable degrees of success. Also, intrathecal deferoxamine (53) has been studied in a rat model and was found to reduce chronic hydrocephalus by 20%, but this is yet to be translated to human trials. Cilostazol administration was also found to reduce the chance of chronic hydrocephalus (54).

There is conflicting evidence regarding the impact of microsurgical clipping on the incidence of hydrocephalus (55). Some studies showed that aneurysm clipping, with fenestration of the lamina terminalis and evacuation of cisternal blood, can reduce the risk of hydrocephalus up to 80% (56). However, there is contradictory evidence published by Yamada et al. (30) that patients who underwent microsurgical clipping were at higher risk of developing hydrocephalus. Their explanation was that microsurgical clipping could aggravate CSF inflammation and subsequently arachnoid granulation dysfunction. This is supported by a study by Wostrack et al., which found that the presence of IL-6 (an inflammatory mediator) of ≥10,000 pg/ml was significantly associated with future shunt dependency (32). Currently there is an ongoing randomized trial looking at the effect of lamina terminalis fenestration and development of hydrocephalus (57).

CSF drainage may accelerate the clearance of blood constituents and is believed to reduce the chance of obstruction of the arachnoid villi. A study in which CSF was drained for 6 days was found to reduce the risk of developing chronic hydrocephalus 4.86 times (58).

Intrathecal fibrinolysis use is feared in patients with aneurysmal SAH due to the potential risk of rehemorrhage. Several animal and human studies of the use of fibrinolytics in intraventricular hemorrhage showed promising results in reducing the chance of shunt dependency. These studies are yet to be translated to the SAH patient population (59–62).

Another approach to reducing hydrocephalus is endoscopic third ventriculostomy following SAH with intraventricular extension. It was found to reduce the duration of EVD placement and rate of permanent shunt placement (63).

IDENTIFICATION

Rebleeding

Rebleeding is usually accompanied by an acute exacerbation of symptoms and rapid decline in clinical status. The symptoms and clinical signs are proportional to the location and degree of hemorrhage and baseline clinical status. CT scan is the imaging modality of choice in such situations, due to its rapidity and because acute blood could be easily distinguishable.

Vasospasm

A patient with SAH should be in a high dependency unit (i.e., ICU) for at least the first 2 weeks, which corresponds to the peak incidence of vasospasm in most patients as discussed earlier. The key to diagnosing vasospasm is frequent and thorough neurological examination. Any subtle new deficit should be thoroughly investigated, as deficits from vasospasm manifest in a gradually progressive fashion. Once a change of neurological exam is detected, the next step would be to rule out other common causes such as cerebral edema, electrolyte imbalance, cerebral salt wasting, seizure, infection, rehemorrhage, and hydrocephalus (Box 9.4). This would include moving the patient to an ICU if not already there, complete laboratory blood investigations, and a brain CT scan. If a thorough investigation failed to explain the change in neurological status, then specific investigations for vasospasm should be initiated. The tests are divided into those that detect cerebral blood flow (CBF) reductions (CT perfusion, single-photon emission CT, thermal diffusion flowmetry), tests that detect cerebral ischemia

Box 9.4 Conditions That Should Be Investigated When Vasospasm Is Suspected

Cerebral edema
Electrolyte imbalance
Cerebral salt wasting
Seizure
Infection
Rebleeding
Hydrocephalus

(diffusion-weighted imaging [DWI] MRI, near-infrared spectroscopy, microdialysis, jugular venous oxygen saturation), and vascular studies (transcranial Doppler [TCD], CT angiography [CTA], and digital subtraction cerebral angiography [DSA]) (5).

Despite the high sensitivity of TCD in detecting vasospasm, it is not used uniformly across neurosurgical institutions due to lack of evidence suggesting improved outcomes (64). TCD is most useful when utilized for middle cerebral artery (MCA) velocities. The sensitivity of TCD increases with velocity values less than 120 cm/sec with negative predictive value (NPV) of vasospasm 90%, and greater than 200 cm/sec with positive predictive value (PPV) of vasospasm 90% (65,66). Lindegaard ratio, which is calculated by dividing the blood flow velocity of the MCA (Vmca) by the velocity of internal carotid artery (Vica)—Vmca/Vica—has been reported to help distinguish hyperemic and vasospastic states. A ratio of greater than 3 is consistent with vasospasm (67). The evidence for the diagnostic value of TCD is stronger for MCA and basilar artery, and weaker for other arteries of the circle of Willis (68). Tables 9.2 to 9.4 (69,70) show interpretation of TCD values in various intracranial arteries. The advantages of TCD are its ease of use at the bedside, and lack of harmful radiation.

The lack of adequate information by TCD either because of intermediate velocity or involvement of vessels other than MCA prompts additional testing. CTA has a sensitivity of 93% and specificity of 80% in detecting vasospasm (5). It is a quick test, which makes it one of the most valuable tests in investigating vasospasm, and has been recommended as the initial screening test (71). Cerebral angiography is useful in cases where the CTA was inconclusive, or in cases that failed to improve following medical treatment of vasospasm. It offers the additional benefit of treating vasospasm by intra-arterial agents or balloon angioplasty.

Table 9.2 Transcranial Doppler Criteria for MCA Vasospasm

Flow Velocity cm/s	MCA/Extracranial Internal Carotid	Interpretation
<120	3	Hyperemia
>80	3–4	Hyperemia + possible mild spasm
≥120	3–4	Mild spasm + hyperemia
≥120	4–5	Moderate spasm + hyperemia
>120	5–6	Moderate spasm
≥180	6	Moderate-to-severe spasm
≥200	≥6	Severe spasm
>200	4–6	Moderate spasm + hyperemia
>200	3–4	Hyperemia + mild/residual spasm
>200	<3	Hyperemia

MCA, middle cerebral artery.

Source: From Kumar G, Alexandrov AV. Vasospasm surveillance with transcranial Doppler sonography in subarachnoid hemorrhage. *J Ultrasound Med.* 2015;34(8):1345–1350. doi:10.7863/ultra.34.8.1345; Lindegaard K-F, Nornes H, Bakke SJ, et al. Cerebral vasospasm diagnosis by means of angiography and blood velocity measurements. *Acta Neurochir (Wien).* 1989;100(1):12–24. doi:10.1007/bf01405268

Diagnosing and recognizing vasospasm is multifaceted, and it is variable from one center to another. The optimum strategy when encountering a SAH patient with a neurological deficit is to

Table 9.3 Transcranial Doppler Grading for Basilar Artery Vasospasm

Flow Velocity (cm/s)	BA/EC VA (Soustiel's Ratio)	Interpretation
>70	>2	Vasospasm
>85	>2.5	Moderate-to-severe vasospasm
>85	>3	Severe vasospasm

BA, basilar artery; EC VA, extracranial vertebral artery.

Source: From Sviri GE, Ghodke B, Britz GW, et al. Transcranial Doppler grading criteria for basilar artery vasospasm. *Neurosurgery*. 2006;59(2):360–366. doi:10.1227/01.neu.0000223502.93013.6e

Table 9.4 Transcranial Doppler Grading for Internal Carotid, Anterior Cerebral Artery, Posterior Cerebral Artery, and Vertebral Artery Vasospasm

	Flow Velocity (cm/s)		
Artery	**Possible Vasospasm**	**Probable Vasospasm**	**Definite Vasospasm**
ICA	>80	>110	>130
ACA	>90	>110	>120
PCA	>60	>80	>90
VA	>60	>80	>90

ACA, anterior cerebral artery; ICA, internal carotid artery; PCA, posterior cerebral artery, VA, vertebral artery.

Source: From Kumar G, Alexandrov AV. Vasospasm surveillance with transcranial Doppler sonography in subarachnoid hemorrhage. *J Ultrasound Med*. 2015;34(8):1345–1350. doi:10.7863/ultra.34.8.1345

place the patient in a high dependency unit with frequent thorough neurological examination, raise systolic pressure if an aneurysm has been secured, blood work with EEG if necessary, followed by CTA. A DSA should follow if still in doubt, or if the deficit remains despite adequate medical treatment.

Hydrocephalus

Early identification of hydrocephalus is paramount to prevent further complications. Clinically, patients would present with an altered level of consciousness, and if left untreated it may evolve into papilledema, and upward gaze palsy. Radiographic parameters that suggest hydrocephalus include: Evans ratio greater than 0.3 (frontal horns/biparietal diameter), frontal horns/internal cranial diameter at the same level greater than 50% (Figure 9.1), ballooning of frontal horns and third ventricle, temporal horns greater than 2 mm in diameter, and periventricular edema.

Another way of diagnosing hydrocephalus is determining whether the ventricles are larger than the 95th percentile for age.

MANAGEMENT

Rebleeding

Once a patient exhibits symptoms or signs suggestive of rebleeding, an urgent CT is to be done to make the diagnosis. If diagnosed, the patient should undergo the same measures that he or

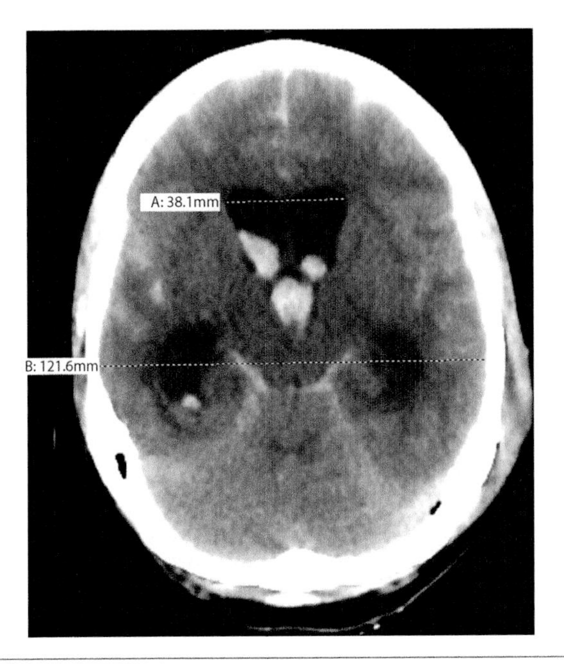

Figure 9.1 Patient with subarachnoid hemorrhage and intraventricular hemorrhage with acute hydrocephalus by Evans ratio criteria.

she initially had upon admission (ICU admission, controlling blood pressure, prompt diagnosis of the aneurysm). A rehemorrhage should be a trigger not to delay aneurysm treatment any further, except if clinically not fit for treatment.

Vasospasm

Vasospasm management starts upon admission by ensuring euvolemia, starting nimodipine, promptly treating the aneurysm, daily TCD, and being vigilant about any ensuing vasospasm. When vasospasm is established the goal is to maintain adequate CBF. Hypervolemia and hemodilution, which are part of the historic triple H therapy (hypertension, hypervolemia, and hemodilution), fell out of favor due to evidence suggesting possible harm. What remains unchanged is hypertension. Hypertension is induced using norepinephrine (max of 20 mcg/kg/min) or phenylephrine (max 180 mcg/kg/min) to raise the SBP to a target of up to 220 mmHg. These measures have not been found to increase the risk of rehemorrhage from an unsecured aneurysm (72). In addition to the aforementioned measures, milrinone (phosphodiesterase 3 inhibitor), which acts as a vasodilator may be infused as per the Montreal Neurological Institute protocol (0.1–0.2 mg/kg IV bolus followed by 0.75 mcg/kg/min infusion up to 1.25 mcg/kg/min) (73). If despite these procedures the patient fails to improve or cannot tolerate these measures, the patient should be immediately taken to the angiography suite for an endovascular intervention. Chemical angioplasty using agents such as, nimodipine, nicardipine, and milrinone is initially trialled and if adequate reperfusion fails then balloon angioplasty is utilized (Figures 9.2 and 9.3).

Complications associated with chemical angioplasty include hypotension and tachycardia, depending on the agent used. Balloon angioplasty is utilized in refractory vasospasm with improvement in vasospasm in up to 97% of the patients with 78.8% experiencing clinical improvement (74). Although balloon angioplasty may be perceived as a procedure that may carry higher complications than chemical angioplasty alone, several studies have shown balloon angioplasty to be as safe as chemical angioplasty alone (74). Arterial angioplasty should be promptly planned within 2 hours of development of clinical vasospasm for maximum benefit (75).

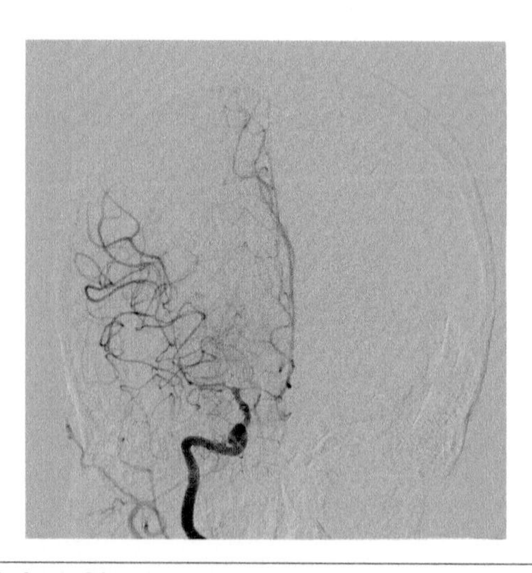

Figure 9.2 Patient with severe vasospasm in anterior cerebral artery and MCA vessels taken for chemical angioplasty.

MCA, middle cerebral artery.

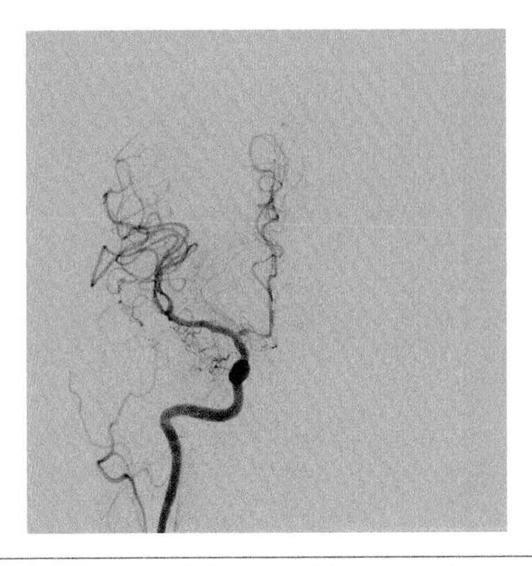

Figure 9.3 After treatment with intra-arterial verapamil. Improvement of MCA vasospasm, with persistent ACA vasospasm.

ACA, anterior cerebral artery; MCA, middle cerebral artery.

Hydrocephalus

Up to 20% of SAH patients develop acute hydrocephalus. Any patient with a decreased level of consciousness should promptly receive an EVD if presenting with a ventriculocranial ratio of 20% to 25% greater than the 95th percentile for age.

It should be noted that the complications associated with shunt insertion include rebleeding (0%–49%), infection (8%), and hematoma along the tract (8%). The risk of rebleeding due to drainage was discussed previously and was found not to be significant with a moderate amount of drainage (76,77).

CONCLUSION

Aneurysmal SAH remains a devastating condition despite our improved understanding of the etiology of aneurysm formation and improved population-wide surveillance strategies. SAH can be complicated by rebleeding, vasospasm, and hydrocephalus. Those patients have a high rate of morbidity and mortality, and many of the survivors would end up with severe lifelong deficits.

Prompt diagnosis and treatment of the ruptured aneurysm to prevent rehemorrhage and managing vasospasm remain the most important pillars in the treatment of SAH.

REFERENCES

1. Lawton MT, Vates GE. Subarachnoid hemorrhage. *N Engl J Med.* 2017;377(3):257–266. doi:10.1056/nejmcp1605827
2. Taufique Z, May T, Meyers E, et al. Predictors of poor quality of life 1 year after subarachnoid hemorrhage. *Neurosurgery.* 2016;78(2):256–264. doi:10.1227/neu.0000000000001042
3. Winn R. *Youmans and Winn Neurological Surgery.* Philadelphia, PA: Elsevier; 2017; vol 7.
4. Lantigua H, Ortega-Gutierrez S, Schmidt JM, et al. Subarachnoid hemorrhage: who dies, and why? *Crit Care.* 2015;19:309. doi:10.1186/s13054-015-1036-0
5. Findlay JM, Nisar J, Darsaut T. Cerebral vasospasm: a review. *Can J Neurol Sci.* 2016;43(1):15–32. doi:10.1017/cjn.2015.288
6. Fujii Y, Takeuchi S, Sasaki O, et al. Ultra-early rebleeding in spontaneous subarachnoid hemorrhage. *J Neurosurg.* 1996;84(1):35–42. doi:10.3171/jns.1996.84.1.0035
7. Haley EC, Kassell NF, Torner JC. The International Cooperative Study on the Timing of Aneurysm Surgery. The North American experience. *Stroke.* 1992;23(2):205–214. doi:10.1161/01.str.23.2.205
8. Germanwala AV, Huang J, Tamargo RJ. Hydrocephalus after aneurysmal subarachnoid hemorrhage. *Neurosurg Clin N Am.* 2010;21(2):263–270. doi:10.1016/j.nec.2009.10.013
9. Larsen CC, Astrup J. Rebleeding after aneurysmal subarachnoid hemorrhage: a literature review. *World Neurosurg.* 2013;79(2):307–312. doi:10.1016/j.wneu.2012.06.023
10. Paré L, Delfino R, Leblanc R, The relationship of ventricular drainage to aneurysmal rebleeding. *J Neurosurg.* 1992;76(3):422–427. doi:10.3171/jns.1992.76.3.0422
11. Voldby B, Enevoldsen EM. Intracranial pressure changes following aneurysm rupture: part 2: associated cerebrospinal fluid lactacidosis. *J Neurosurg.* 1982;56(2):197–204. doi:10.3171/jns.1982.56.2.0197
12. Hellingman CA, van den Bergh WM, Beijer IS, et al. Risk of rebleeding after treatment of acute hydrocephalus in patients with aneurysmal subarachnoid hemorrhage. *Stroke.* 2007;38(1):96–99. doi:10.1161/01.str.0000251841.51332.1d
13. McIver JI, Friedman JA, Wijdicks EFM, et al. Preoperative ventriculostomy and rebleeding after aneurysmal subarachnoid hemorrhage. *J Neurosurg.* 2002;97(5):1042–1044. doi:10.3171/jns.2002.97.5.1042
14. Qureshi AI, Sung GY, Suri MA, et al. Prognostic value and determinants of ultraearly angiographic vasospasm after aneurysmal subarachnoid hemorrhage. *Neurosurgey.* 1999;44(5):967-973.
15. Fisher C, Kistler J, Davis J. Relation of cerebral vasospasm to subarachnoid hemorrhage visualized by computerized tomographic scanning. *Neurosurgery.* 1980;6(1):1–9. doi:10.1097/00006123-198001000-00001

16. Frontera JA, Claassen J, Schmidt JM, et al. Prediction of symptomatic vasospasm after subarachnoid hemorrhage: the modified Fisher scale. *Neurosurgery*. 2006;59(1):21–27. doi:10.1227/01.neu.0000218821.34014.1b
17. Gross BA, Lai PMR, Frerichs KU, et al. Treatment modality and vasospasm after aneurysmal subarachnoid hemorrhage. *World Neurosurg*. 2014;82(6):e725–e730. doi:10.1016/j.wneu.2013.08.017
18. Otite F, Mink S, Tan CO, et al. Impaired cerebral autoregulation is associated with vasospasm and delayed cerebral ischemia in subarachnoid hemorrhage. *Stroke*. 2014;45(3):677–682. doi:10.1161/strokeaha.113.002630
19. Sheth SA, Hausrath D, Numis AL, et al. Intraoperative rerupture during surgical treatment of aneurysmal subarachnoid hemorrhage is not associated with an increased risk of vasospasm. *J Neurosurg*. 2014;120(2):409–414. doi:10.3171/2013.10.jns13934
20. Ibrahim GM, Morgan BR, Macdonald RL. Patient phenotypes associated with outcomes after aneurysmal subarachnoid hemorrhage. *Stroke*. 2014;45(3):670–676. doi:10.1161/strokeaha.113.003078
21. Sasaki T, Wakai S, Asano T, et al. The effect of a lipid hydroperoxide of arachidonic acid on the canine basilar artery: an experimental study on cerebral vasospasm. *J Neurosurg*. 1981;54(3):357–365. doi:10.3171/jns.1981.54.3.0357
22. Kamezaki T, Yanaka K, Nagase S, et al. Increased levels of lipid peroxides as predictive of symptomatic vasospasm and poor outcome after aneurysmal subarachnoid hemorrhage. *J Neurosurg*. 2002;97(6):1302–1305. doi:10.3171/jns.2002.97.6.1302
23. Iuliano BA, Pluta RM, Jung C, et al. Endothelial dysfunction in a primate model of cerebral vasospasm. *J Neurosurg*. 2004;100(2):287–294. doi:10.3171/jns.2004.100.2.0287
24. Mocco J, Mack WJ, Kim GH, et al. Rise in serum soluble intercellular adhesion molecule—1 levels with vasospasm following aneurysmal subarachnoid hemorrhage. *J Neurosurg*. 2002;97(3):537–541. doi:10.3171/jns.2002.97.3.0537
25. Mack WJ, Ducruet AF, Hickman ZL, et al. Early plasma complement C3a levels correlate with functional outcome after aneurysmal subarachnoid hemorrhage. *Neurosurgery*. 2007;61(2):255–261. doi:10.1227/01.neu.0000255518.96837.8e
26. Xie Z, Hu X, Zan X, et al. Predictors of shunt-dependent hydrocephalus after aneurysmal subarachnoid hemorrhage? a systematic review and meta-analysis. *World Neurosurg*. 2017;106:844–860 e6. doi:10.1016/j.wneu.2017.06.119
27. Walcott BP, Iorgulescu JB, Stapleton CJ, et al. Incidence, timing, and predictors of delayed shunting for hydrocephalus after aneurysmal subarachnoid hemorrhage. *Neurocrit Care*. 2015;23(1):54–58. doi:10.1007/s12028-014-0072-y

28. Dóczi T, Nemessányi Z, Szegváry Z, et al. Disturbances of cerebrospinal fluid circulation during the acute stage of subarachnoid hemorrhage. *Neurosurgery*. 1983;12(4):435–438. doi:10.1227/00006123-198304000-00011
29. Ellington E, Margolis G. Block of arachnoid villus by subarachnoid hemorrhage. *J Neurosurg*. 1969;30(6):651–657. doi:10.3171/jns.1969.30.6.0651
30. Yamada S, Ishikawa M, Yamamoto K, et al. Aneurysm location and clipping versus coiling for development of secondary normal-pressure hydrocephalus after aneurysmal subarachnoid hemorrhage: Japanese Stroke DataBank. *J Neurosurg*. 2015;123(6):1555–1561. doi:10.3171/2015.1.jns142761
31. Rincon F, Gordon E, Starke RM, et al. Predictors of long-term shunt-dependent hydrocephalus after aneurysmal subarachnoid hemorrhage. Clinical article. *J Neurosurg*. 2010;113(4):774–780. doi:10.3171/2010.2.jns09376
32. Wostrack M, Reeb T, Martin J, et al. Shunt-dependent hydrocephalus after aneurysmal subarachnoid hemorrhage: the role of intrathecal interleukin-6. *Neurocrit Care*. 2014;21(1):78–84. doi:10.1007/s12028-014-9991-x
33. Kassell NF, Drake CG. Timing of Aneurysm Surgery. *Neurosurgery*. 1982;10(4):514–519. doi:10.1227/00006123-198204000-00019
34. Ohkuma H, Tsurutani H, Suzuki S. Incidence and significance of early aneurysmal rebleeding before neurosurgical or neurological management. *Stroke*. 2001;32(5):1176–1180. doi:10.1161/01.str.32.5.1176
35. Pickard JD, Kirkpatrick PJ, Melsen T, et al. Potential role of NovoSeven® in the prevention of rebleeding following aneurysmal subarachnoid haemorrhage. *Blood Coagul Fibrinolysis*. 2000;11:S117–S120. doi:10.1097/00001721-200004001-00022
36. Simpson E, Lin Y, Stanworth S, et al. Recombinant factor VIIa for the prevention and treatment of bleeding in patients without haemophilia. *Cochrane Database Syst Rev*. 2012;(3):Cd005011. doi:10.1002/14651858.cd005011.pub4
37. Vermeulen M, Lindsay KW, Murray GD, et al. Antifibrinolytic Treatment in Subarachnoid Hemorrhage. *N Engl J Med*. 1984;311(7):432–437. doi:10.1056/nejm198408163110703
38. Kirkpatrick PJ, Turner CL, Smith C, et al. Simvastatin in aneurysmal subarachnoid haemorrhage (STASH): a multicentre randomised phase 3 trial. *Lancet Neurol*. 2014;13(7):666–675. doi:10.1016/s1474-4422(14)70084-5
39. Mees SMD, Algra A, Vandertop WP, et al. Magnesium for aneurysmal subarachnoid haemorrhage (MASH-2): a randomised placebo-controlled trial. *Lancet*. 2012;380(9836):44–49. doi:10.1016/s0140-6736(12)60724-7
40. Pickard JD, Murray GD, Illingworth R, et al. Effect of oral nimodipine on cerebral infarction and outcome after subarachnoid haemorrhage: British aneurysm nimodipine trial. *Br Med J*. 1989;298(6674):636–642. doi:10.1136/bmj.298.6674.636

41. Macdonald RL, Higashida RT, Keller E, et al. Clazosentan, an endothelin receptor antagonist, in patients with aneurysmal subarachnoid haemorrhage undergoing surgical clipping: a randomised, double-blind, placebo-controlled phase 3 trial (CONSCIOUS-2). *Lancet Neurol.* 2011;10(7):618–625. doi:10.1016/s1474-4422(11)70108-9
42. Findlay JM, Kassell NF, Weir BKA, et al. A Randomized trial of intraoperative, intracisternal tissue plasminogen activator for the prevention of vasospasm. *Neurosurgery.* 1995;37(1):168–178.
43. Amin-Hanjani S, Ogilvy CS, Barker FG. Does intracisternal thrombolysis prevent vasospasm after aneurysmal subarachnoid hemorrhage? A meta-analysis. *Neurosurgery.* 2004;54(2):326–335. doi:10.1227/01.neu.0000103488.94855.4f
44. Barth M, Capelle H-H, Weidauer S, et al. Effect of nicardipine prolonged-release implants on cerebral vasospasm and clinical outcome after severe aneurysmal subarachnoid hemorrhage. *Stroke.* 2007;38(2):330–336. doi:10.1161/01.str.0000254601.74596.0f
45. Saber, H, Serkin Z, Ibrahim M, et al. Efficacy of cilostazol in prevention of symptomatic vasospasm after aneurysmal subarachnoid hemorrhage: a meta-analysis of randomized clinical trials (P5. 066). *Neurology.* 2017;88(16 Supplement): P5. 066.
46. Boulouis G, Labeyrie MA, Raymond J, et al. Treatment of cerebral vasospasm following aneurysmal subarachnoid haemorrhage: a systematic review and meta-analysis. *Eur Radiol.* 2017;27(8):3333–3342. doi:10.1007/s00330-016-4702-y
47. Kassell NF, Haley C, Apperson-Hansen C, et al. Randomized, double-blind, vehicle-controlled trial of tirilazad mesylate in patients with aneurysmal subarachnoid hemorrhage: a cooperative study in Europe, Australia, and New Zealand. *J Neurosurg.* 1996;84(2):221–228. doi:10.3171/jns.1996.84.2.0221
48. Andaluz N, Zuccarello M. Fenestration of the lamina terminalis as a valuable adjunct in aneurysm surgery. *Neurosurgery.* 2004;55(5):1050–1059. doi:10.1227/01.neu.0000140837.63105.78
49. Komotar RJ, Hahn DK, Kim GH, et al. The impact of microsurgical fenestration of the lamina terminalis on shunt-dependent hydrocephalus and vasospasm after aneurysmal subarachnoid hemorrhage. *Neurosurgery.* 2008;62(1):123–134. doi:10.1227/01.neu.0000311069.48862.c8
50. Kasuya H, Shimizu T, Kagawa M. The effect of continuous drainage of cerebrospinal fluid in patients with subarachnoid hemorrhage: a retrospective analysis of 108 patients. *Neurosurgery.* 1991;28(1):56–59.
51. Klimo P Jr, Kestle JRW, MacDonald JD, Schmidt RH. Marked reduction of cerebral vasospasm with lumbar drainage of cerebrospinal fluid after subarachnoid hemorrhage. *J Neurosurg.* 2004;100(2):215–224. doi:10.3171/jns.2004.100.2.0215

52. Zwienenberg-Lee M, Hartman J, Rudisill N, et al. Effect of prophylactic transluminal balloon angioplasty on cerebral vasospasm and outcome in patients with Fisher grade III subarachnoid hemorrhage. *Stroke.* 2008;39(6):1759–1765. doi:10.1161/strokeaha.107.502666
53. Meng H, Li F, Hu R, et al. Deferoxamine alleviates chronic hydrocephalus after intraventricular hemorrhage through iron chelation and Wnt1/Wnt3a inhibition. *Brain Res.* 2015;1602:44–52. doi:10.1016/j.brainres.2014.08.039
54. Nakatsuka Y, Kawakita F, Yasuda R, et al. Preventive effects of cilostazol against the development of shunt-dependent hydrocephalus after subarachnoid hemorrhage. *J Neurosurg.* 2017;127(2):319–326. doi:10.3171/2016.5.jns152907
55. Komotar RJ, Hahn DK, Kim GH, et al. Efficacy of lamina terminalis fenestration in reducing shunt-dependent hydrocephalus following aneurysmal subarachnoid hemorrhage: a systematic review. *J Neurosurg.* 2009;111(1):147–154. doi:10.3171/2009.1.jns0821
56. Komotar RJ, Olivi A, Rigamonti D, et al. Microsurgical fenestration of the lamina terminalis reduces the incidence of shunt-dependent hydrocephalus after aneurysmal subarachnoid hemorrhage. *Neurosurgery.* 2002;51(6):1403–1413. doi:10.1097/00006123-200212000-00010
57. Tao C, Fan C, Hu X, et al. The effect of fenestration of the lamina terminalis on the incidence of shunt-dependent hydrocephalus after aneurysmal subarachnoid hemorrhage (FISH): study protocol for a randomized controlled trial. *Medicine.* 2016;95(52):e5727. doi:10.1097/md.0000000000005727
58. Hirashima Y, Kurimoto M, Hayashi N, et al. Duration of cerebrospinal fluid drainage in patients with aneurysmal subarachnoid hemorrhage for prevention of symptomatic vasospasm and late hydrocephalus. *Neurol Med Chir (Tokyo).* 2005;45(4):177–183. doi:10.2176/nmc.45.177
59. Findlay JM, Grace MG, Weir BK. Treatment of intraventricular hemorrhage with tissue plasminogen activator. *Neurosurgery.* 1993;32(6):941–947. doi:10.1097/00006123-199306000-00010
60. Staykov D, Kuramatsu JB, Bardutzky J, et al. Efficacy and safety of combined intraventricular fibrinolysis with lumbar drainage for prevention of permanent shunt dependency after intracerebral hemorrhage with severe ventricular involvement: a randomized trial and individual patient data meta-analysis. *Ann Neurol.* 2017;81(1):93–103. doi:10.1002/ana.24834
61. Brinker T, Seifert V, Dietz H. Subacute hydrocephalus after experimental subarachnoid hemorrhage: its prevention by intrathecal fibrinolysis with recombinant tissue plasminogen activator. *Neurosurgery.* 1992;31(2):306–312. doi:10.1097/00006123-199208000-00016
62. Hanley DF, Lane K, McBee N, et al. Thrombolytic removal of intraventricular haemorrhage in treatment of severe stroke: results of the randomised, multicentre, multiregion, placebo-controlled CLEAR III trial. *Lancet.* 2017;389(10069):603–611. doi:10.1016/s0140-6736(16)32410-2

63. Obaid S, Weil A, Rahme R, et al. Endoscopic third ventriculostomy for obstructive hydrocephalus due to intraventricular hemorrhage. *J Neurol Surg A Cent Eur Neurosurg*. 2015;76(2):99–111. doi:10.1055/s-0034-1382778
64. Kumar G, Shahripour RB, Harrigan MR. Vasospasm on transcranial Doppler is predictive of delayed cerebral ischemia in aneurysmal subarachnoid hemorrhage: a systematic review and meta-analysis. *J Neurosurg*. 2016;124(5):1257–1264. doi:10.3171/2015.4.jns15428
65. Lysakowski C, Walder B, Costanza MC, et al. Transcranial doppler versus angiography in patients with vasospasm due to a ruptured cerebral aneurysm. *Stroke*. 2001;32(10):2292–2298. doi:10.1161/hs1001.097108
66. Vora YY, Suarez-Almazor M, Steinke DE, et al. Role of transcranial Doppler monitoring in the diagnosis of cerebral vasospasm after subarachnoid hemorrhage. *Neurosurgery*. 1999;44(6):1237–1248. doi:10.1097/00006123-199906000-00039
67. Lindegaard K, Bakke SJ, Sorteberg W, et al. A non-invasive Doppler ultrasound method for the evaluation of patients with subarachnoid hemorrhage. *Acta Radiol Suppl*. 1986;369:96–98.
68. Kumar G, Alexandrov AV. Vasospasm surveillance with transcranial doppler sonography in subarachnoid hemorrhage. *J Ultrasound Med*. 2015;34(8):1345–1350. doi:10.7863/ultra.34.8.1345
69. Lindegaard K-F, Nornes H, Bakke SJ, et al. Cerebral vasospasm diagnosis by means of angiography and blood velocity measurements. *Acta Neurochir (Wien)*. 1989;100(1):12–24. doi:10.1007/bf01405268
70. Sviri GE, Ghodke B, Britz GW, et al. Transcranial doppler grading criteria for basilar artery vasospasm. *Neurosurgery*. 2006;59(2):360–366. doi:10.1227/01.neu.0000223502.93013.6e
71. Washington CW, Zipfel GJ. Detection and monitoring of vasospasm and delayed cerebral ischemia: a review and assessment of the literature. *Neurocrit Care*. 2011;15(2):312. doi:10.1007/s12028-011-9594-8
72. Hoh BL, Carter BS, Ogilvy CS. Risk of hemorrhage from unsecured, unruptured aneurysms during and after hypertensive hypervolemic therapy. *Neurosurgery*. 2002;50(6):1207–1212. doi:10.1227/00006123-200206000-00006
73. Lannes M, Teitelbaum J, del Pilar Cortés M, et al. Milrinone and homeostasis to treat cerebral vasospasm associated with subarachnoid hemorrhage: the Montreal Neurological Hospital protocol. *Neurocrit Care*. 2012;16(3):354–362. doi:10.1007/s12028-012-9701-5
74. Patel AS, Griessenauer CJ, Gupta R, et al. Safety and efficacy of noncompliant balloon angioplasty for the treatment of subarachnoid hemorrhage–induced vasospasm: a multicenter study. *World Neurosurg*. 2017;98:189–197. doi:10.1016/j.wneu.2016.10.064
75. Rosenwasser RH, Armonda RA, Thomas JE, et al. Therapeutic modalities for the management of cerebral vasospasm: timing of endovascular options. *Neurosurgery*. 1999;44(5):975–979. doi:10.1097/00006123-199905000-00022

76. Gigante P, Hwang BY, Appelboom G, et al. External ventricular drainage following aneurysmal subarachnoid haemorrhage. *Br J Neurosurg.* 2010;24(6):625–632. doi:10.3109/02688697.2010.505989
77. Fountas K, Kapsalaki EZ, Machinis T, et al. Review of the literature regarding the relationship of rebleeding and external ventricular drainage in patients with subarachnoid hemorrhage of aneurysmal origin. *Neurosurg Rev.* 2006;29(1):14–18. doi:10.1007/s10143-005-0423-4

10 Complications of Cerebral Venous Thrombosis

Jessica D. Lee

KEY POINTS

- Cerebral venous thrombosis (CVT) is uncommon, responsible for approximately 0.5% to 1% of all strokes.
- The time from symptom onset to diagnosis ranges from 2 to 30 days in 56% of patients.
- Mortality in the acute phase of CVT occurs in about 4% of patients, usually due to associated mass effect from an intraparenchymal lesion and associated transtentorial herniation.
- Surgical interventions are occasionally needed in the management of CVT.

INTRODUCTION

Cerebral venous and dural sinus thrombosis (CVT) is a complex, and often unrecognized or underrecognized, cause of stroke. The disease may present with a wide range of clinical symptoms, ranging from headache to coma, and in a wide range of clinical settings, from the clinic to the emergency room, making the disease a diagnostic challenge.

Unlike venous thromboembolism and arterial ischemic stroke, CVT more commonly affects young people. CVT is caused by thrombosis of the dural sinuses or the cortical draining veins and may be acute, subacute, or chronic in nature. CVT is a serious, sometimes life-threatening, but potentially treatable disease that generally has a favorable outcome. There are numerous conditions that may predispose to or cause CVT (Box 10.1).

EPIDEMIOLOGY, MORBIDITY, AND MORTALITY

CVT is uncommon, responsible for approximately 0.5% to 1% of all strokes (1). Data from recent population-based studies indicate the actual estimated incidence of CVT ranges from 1.3 to 1.6 cases per 100,000 with a mortality of approximately 4% in the acute

 DOI: 10.1891/9780826124791.0010

Box 10.1 Associated Risk Factors

Prothrombotic Conditions

Acquired prothrombotic states

- Pregnancy and puerperium
- Nephrotic syndrome
- Malignancy

Genetic prothrombotic states

- Factor V Leiden gene mutation
- Prothrombin (factor II) gene mutation
- Elevated factor VIII activity
- Antithrombin III deficiency
- Protein C deficiency
- Protein S deficiency
- Hyperhomocysteinemia

Drugs

- Oral contraceptives
- Hormone replacement therapy
- Vitamin A
- IVIG

Autoimmune Disorders

- Antiphospholipid antibody syndrome
- Systemic lupus erythematosus
- Behçet disease
- Sjogren's syndrome
- Inflammatory bowel disease

Infection

- Meningitis
- Sinusitis
- Mastoiditis
- Other parameningeal infections

Hematological disorders

- Paroxysmal nocturnal hemoglobinuria
- Polycythemia vera
- Essential thrombocythemia

Mechanical Causes

- Trauma
- Lumbar puncture
- Invasive intracranial pressure monitoring

IVIG, intravenous immunoglobulin.

phase and up to 10% at long-term follow-up (2–4). The disease affects three times as many women as men (5). The reason for this is largely related to hormonal-related factors, including the use of oral contraceptives, pregnancy, and puerperium (6,7). The rate of CVT in pregnancy is an estimated 9 per 100,000 (8).

The prevalence of associated risk factors varies between different regions of the world, particularly in developed compared to underdeveloped countries. There is also likely some ethnic variability related to associated conditions, such as Behçet disease in Mediterranean and Middle Eastern countries (9).

A substantial decrease in the mortality of patients with CVT has been observed over the past 30 years, owing largely to a shift in risk factors and improvements in care (10). Mortality in the acute phase of CVT occurs in about 4% of patients, usually due to associated mass effect from an intraparenchymal lesion and associated transtentorial herniation (11,12). Status epilepticus and medical complications are other possible causes of early death. Between 5% and 10% of survivors of CVT have severe and permanent disability. Approximately 80% of patients recover without substantial functional disability, though many experience chronic symptoms such as headache or cognitive dysfunction (11,13).

ANATOMY

The cerebral veins function as the final collecting pathway for cerebral blood to exit the cranial vault and can be divided into three groups, the superficial cortical veins located in the pia mater, the deep venous system draining the internal structures, and the venous sinuses located within the dura. The cerebral veins also function to reabsorb cerebrospinal fluid via the arachnoid granulations within the superior sagittal sinus (SSS) and transverse sinuses.

The superficial cerebral veins have significant anatomic variability. These include the frontal, parietal, and occipital cerebral veins, which drain into the SSS, and the middle cerebral veins, which drain into the cavernous sinus. The anastomotic vein of Trolard connects the SSS to the middle cerebral veins, while the vein of Labbé connects the middle cerebral veins to the lateral (transverse + sigmoid) sinus.

The deep cerebral veins are anatomically more constant. These drain blood from the deep white matter of the cerebral hemispheres and from the basal ganglia. The internal cerebral veins receive blood from the choroidal, septal, and thalamostriate veins. The basal veins of Rosenthal, or central veins, join to form the great vein of Galen, which then drains into the straight sinus. The brainstem is drained by veins terminating in the inferior and transverse petrosal sinuses.

The occipital sinus, straight sinus, and SSS join below the occipital protuberance to form the confluence of sinuses, or torcular herophili. Often the brain may lack a complete confluence. The SSS continues as the right transverse sinus. The left transverse sinus is a continuation of the straight sinus (14).

The cortical draining veins are unique, in that they are thin-walled, and have no valves and no muscular layer. The venous sinuses (superior sagittal, inferior sagittal, transverse, and sigmoid) are located between two rigid layers of dura mater. This encasement prevents the sinuses' compression when intracranial pressure (ICP) increases in the absence of CVT.

PATHOPHYSIOLOGY

There are two possible pathophysiologic mechanisms of CVT: thrombosis within the cerebral veins producing local effects such as infarction and hemorrhage, and thrombosis within the venous sinuses resulting in increased ICP. As venous blood is forced back into small vessels and capillaries, an increase in venous and capillary pressure occurs (15,16). When recruitment of collateral venous drainage becomes insufficient, a disruption in the blood–brain barrier and decrease in cerebral perfusion pressure develops, leading to either or both cytotoxic edema or vasogenic edema, and often, intracerebral hemorrhage (ICH) (15,17,18). Venous infarction is characterized pathologically by dilation of the associated veins, vasogenic edema, and ischemic neuronal damage. Petechial or frank hemorrhage within the area of venous infarction may occur and is present in approximately 60% of patients with CVT (11,19,20).

Regardless of the predisposing factor, the disorders associated with the development of cerebral venous sinus thrombosis (CVST) act through the usual mechanisms of hypercoagulability, hemoconcentration, stasis, or inflammation of the vessel wall. In the past, CVT was more commonly associated with concomitant infection, particularly sinusitis, otitis, and mastoiditis. The frequency of septic CVST has declined significantly with the widespread use of antibiotics, though it remains higher in developing countries where access to healthcare and medications is limited (11).

The SSS, lateral sinus (transverse + sigmoid), and transverse sinus are the most common locations of CVST in decreasing order (Figures 10.1 and 10.2). In approximately two-thirds of CVST, more than one cerebral vein is involved (18).

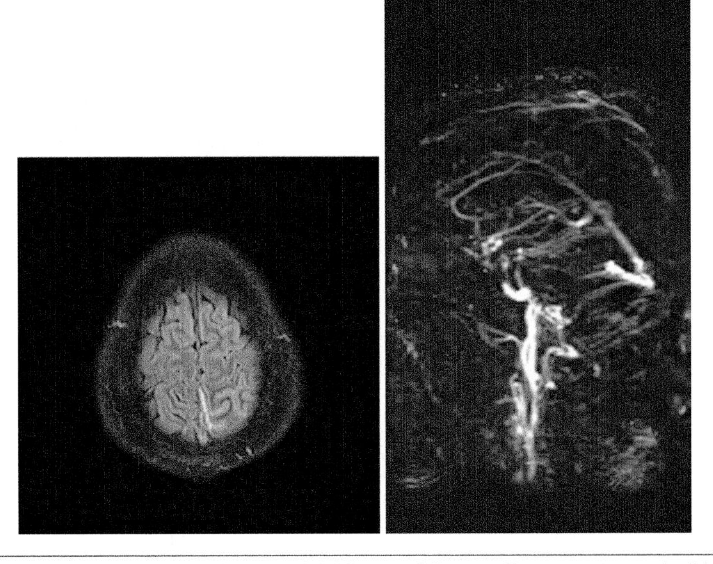

Figure 10.1 A 22-year-old man with history of Graves' disease, presented with three seizures in the setting of thyroid storm. Also complained of headache and blurred vision. MRI hyperintensity within the SSS on FLAIR (A) and mild vasogenic edema. MRV revealed thrombosis (B) of the SSS.

FLAIR, fluid-attenuated inversion recovery; MRV, magnetic resonance venogram; SSS, superior sagittal sinus.

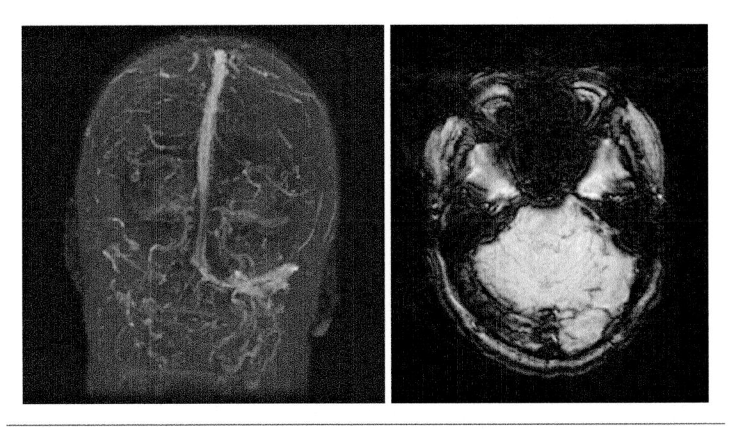

Figure 10.2 A 56-year-old woman with history of lupus, presented with a 5-day history of throbbing headache associated with nausea and vomiting. MRV (left) revealed right transverse and sigmoid sinus thrombosis. Susceptibility-weighted MRI also shows evidence of right transverse sinus thrombosis (right).

MRV, magnetic resonance venogram.

PREVENTION

The mainstay of prevention of neurological deterioration and long-term complications of CVT is early recognition and prompt initiation of anticoagulation. Antiepileptic drugs should be initiated as indicated in patients with seizures; however, their early use does not prevent the development of long-term seizures. Endovascular treatment, as described earlier, should be considered in select patients.

There is little evidence to support the widespread use of hyperosmotic agents to control cerebral edema. However, in patients with significant cerebral edema, their use may be appropriate.

In general, long-term anticoagulation is not needed for most patients with CVT as recurrence rates are low. However, in select patients with defined procoagulopathy, anticoagulation may be warranted.

IDENTIFICATION

Clinical Presentation

Clinical presentation of CVT may be quite varied and ranges from isolated headache to coma. The manifestation of clinical symptoms largely depends upon the anatomical location of the venous drainage that is affected, development of increased ICP, and the secondary injury of brain tissue related to venous infarction or hemorrhage. The time from symptom onset to diagnosis ranged from 2 to 30 days in 56% of patients, with a mean time of 18 days, according to the International Study on Cerebral Vein and Dural Sinus Thrombosis (ISCVT) (11).

Headache is the most common presenting symptom, present in nearly 90% of patients with CVT (4,11,18,21,22). The headache is generally diffuse and may be progressive over a period of days to weeks, often unrelenting. Isolated headache without focal symptoms or papilledema occurs in 25% of patients. The pattern of headaches may be lateralized or bilateral and no characteristic pattern distinguishes the headache associated with CVT from other primary or secondary headaches. Most commonly, the headaches are described as throbbing or aching (23). However, a change in headache pattern or severity should alert clinicians to the possibility of a secondary etiology (22). The mechanism of headache in CVT remains unclear. It has been postulated to be related to elevations in ICP, stretching of the sinus wall, presence of intraparenchymal or subarachnoid blood, or associated meningitis (24). Headache may be acute in onset, subacute and progressive in nature, or chronic.

Following headache, papilledema and diplopia are the main clinical signs and symptoms with CVT (24,25). Papilledema may be bilateral or unilateral. Sixth nerve palsies can result from elevated ICP and is often unilateral. The presence of associated papilledema or oculomotor palsy should prompt an ophthalmological consult.

Focal neurological deficits, occurring in up to 50% of patients, are dependent on the location of CVT and the presence of venous infarction or associated hemorrhage. Motor deficits and aphasia are common with superior and lateral sinus thrombosis (26,27). Rapid neurological deterioration may occur in patients with thrombosis of the deep cerebral venous system, in some cases progressing to coma or death.

Seizures are a common presenting symptom, as well as potential long-term complication, of CVT. Seizure is the initial clinical manifestation of CVST in 35% to 40% of patients. Seizures occurring within 2 weeks of diagnosis are present in 30% to 40% of patients, which is considerably higher than that seen with acute arterial stroke or spontaneous ICH. Focal seizures are not uncommon, again related to locality of the thrombosis (1,11,26,28).

Diagnostic Evaluation

Diagnostic evaluation should include a thorough neurological examination, including fundoscopy. Initial laboratory evaluation should include complete blood count, basic metabolic panel, urinalysis, prothrombin time, and activated partial thromboplastin time (1). While these tests are not specific to establish the diagnosis of CVT itself, they may contribute to the identification of underlying or associated conditions. Further laboratory investigation should be guided by the age of the patient and clinical history. This may include hypercoagulable and genetic laboratory tests (Box 10.2), particularly in young patients with no clear inciting event. Lumbar puncture should be reserved for those instances where an underlying central nervous system (CNS) infection is suspected (29).

Initial imaging should consist of noncontrast head CT as for any patient presenting with acute or progressive neurological symptoms; however, even experienced clinicians and radiologists may miss isolated CVT without infarct or hemorrhage on CT. Findings on noncontrast head CT may include hyperdensity of the dural or cortical veins (Figure 10.3) or the so-called "delta sign," which is hyperdensity within the torcular herophili (30,31).

The sensitivity of noncontrast head CT is approximately 30%, and the classic signs described earlier are not sufficiently specific for diagnosis of CVT (30,32). Thus, it is important to obtain more

Box 10.2 Additional Laboratory Studies to be Considered in the Diagnosis of CVT

Antiphospholipid antibodies
ESR
Homocysteine
Protein C activity
Protein S activity
Antithrombin III activity
Factor VIII activity
Prothrombin (factor II) gene mutation
Factor V Leiden gene mutation
Antinuclear antibody
Anti-SSA and anti-SSB
JAK-2 mutation

CVT, cerebral venous thrombosis; ESR, erythrocyte sedimentation rate.

detailed imaging with MRI. The presence of hemorrhage or ischemic lesions that do not respect typical arterial territories should raise suspicion of venous thrombosis. Early signs of CVT on basic MRI sequences include absence of the normal vascular flow void

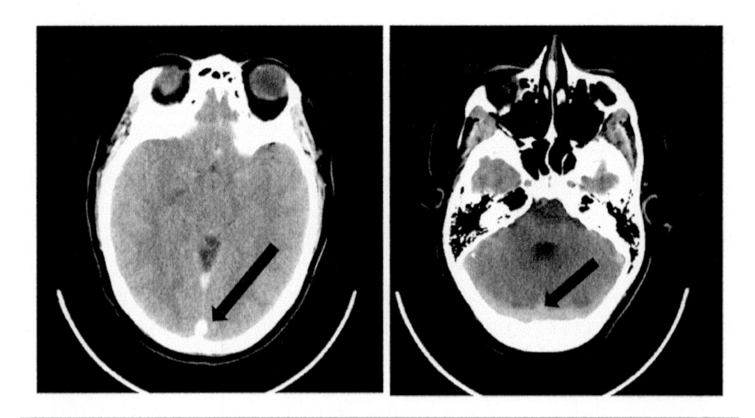

Figure 10.3 A 29-year-old woman, on oral contraceptives and estradiol due to menorrhagia, presented with 1-month history of headaches and 1-day history of altered mental status. Noncontrast CT of the head showed hyperdensity of the straight sinus (left), torcular herophili, and bilateral transverse sinuses (right).

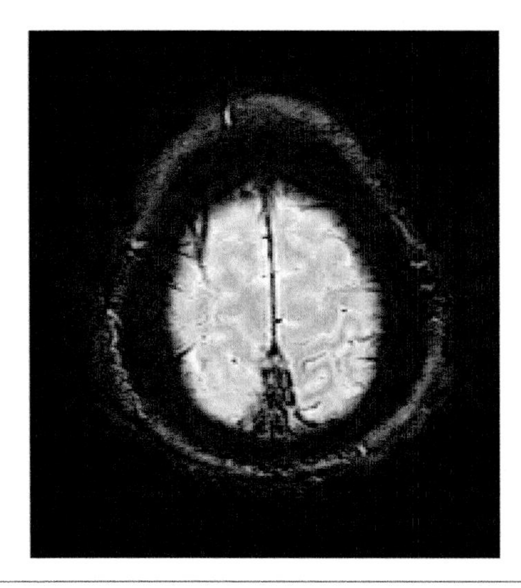

Figure 10.4 A 22-year-old man with superior sagittal sinus thrombosis, SWI.

SWI, susceptibility-weighted imaging.

seen on T2-weighted imagines, usually with corresponding hyperintensity. Correspondingly, there may be hypointensity seen in gradient echo and susceptibility-weighted images (Figure 10.4) (33–36).

Specific imaging of the venous drainage system can be obtained with magnetic resonance venogram (MRV) or CT venogram (CTV), bearing in mind that the bony anatomy may make interpretation of CTV somewhat challenging (Figure 10.5).

In studies comparing CTV and MRV, CTV is as accurate in diagnosing CVT as MRV. However, MRI has the advantage of showing the thrombus itself and being more sensitive in detecting parenchymal lesions (36–38). Contrast enhanced MRV is more sensitive than time of flight (TOF) MRV, particularly for sinuses with small diameter and/or slow blood flow (30). In selected cases, catheter-based venography may be useful.

COMPLICATIONS

As noted in the previous section on clinical manifestations, headache, seizures, altered mental status, and focal neurologic deficits may all be complications of acute or subacute CVT. Some degree of hydrocephalus occurs in approximately 15% of patients with CVT (22,39). Most of these cases are related to obstructive

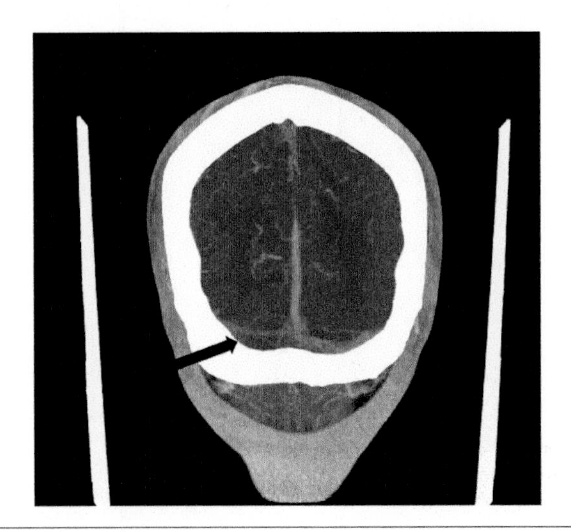

Figure 10.5 CT venogram demonstrating filling defect within the right transverse sinus.

hydrocephalus owing to edema of the basal ganglia and thalami, resulting from thrombosis of the deep venous system. The presence of hydrocephalus increases the risk of poor clinical outcome.

Transtentorial herniation is a severe complication that is the main cause of early death in patients with CVT. Transtentorial herniation most often occurs due to mass effect from a parenchymal lesion. In patients with clinical and radiological signs of impending herniation, decompressive surgery should be considered (1,37).

Other long-term complications include chronic headache, development of epilepsy, fatigue, and cognitive impairment. Long-term seizures occur in about 10% of all stroke patients (40), and in about 2% to 4% of ischemic stroke patients (41). In a study of the development of poststroke epilepsy with late presentation of seizures, approximately 26% of patients had history of venous infarction and CVT (40). Chronic headache, defined as headache more than once per week, occurs in about 20% of patients with CVT (42).

Recurrence of CVT and other thromboembolic events may also be a complication of CVT. Population-based studies have indicated an incidence of 1–5/200 patient-years for venous thromboembolism, including deep venous thrombosis and pulmonary embolism (42–44). The recurrence of CVT has been reported with an incidence of 1.5–2.2/100 patient-years (43,44).

MANAGEMENT

The mainstay of treatment of CVT remains anticoagulant therapy with either low molecular weight heparin or unfractionated heparin alone, or the former followed by vitamin K antagonists. Unfractionated heparin was first introduced as a treatment for venous thrombosis in the late 1930s. A meta-analysis of two small, randomized trials conducted in the 1990s showed a nonsignificant difference in clinical outcomes in favor of heparin, and more importantly, no occurrence of new ICHs in patients treated with heparin (45–47). Guidelines from both the European Federation of Neurological Societies and the American Heart Association recommend therapeutic anticoagulation with heparin as the primary treatment for CVT, regardless of the presence of ICH on baseline imaging (1,37). The duration of recommended anticoagulation is variable, ranging from 3 to 12 months (37). At present, there is very limited evidence to support the use of direct oral anticoagulants in the acute treatment of CVT.

In select patients, endovascular treatment may be indicated. Many case reports and case series have been published in recent years, but no randomized trials have been completed to date. Current endovascular techniques for the treatment of CVT include direct thrombolysis, in which a microcatheter is advanced into or through the thrombus, and a thrombolytic drug infused locally (48–51). Other techniques include balloon-assisted thrombectomy, aspiration thrombectomy, and the use of stent retrievers (52). Recanalization, either partial or complete, is reported in 70% to 90% of patients treated endovascularly; however, there is no uniform scoring system for the degree of recanalization (Figure 10.6).

Potential procedural complications include catheter-related complications, retroperitoneal hematoma, worsening ICH, or new ICH. In general, endovascular therapy is reserved for patients who do not respond to, or have a contraindication to, systemic anticoagulation or those with severe and progressive neurological deficits.

Surgical interventions are occasionally needed in the management of CVT. Although no randomized controlled trials have been performed evaluating the usefulness of decompressive surgery, that is, hemicraniectomy, it may be useful in select patients (1,37). In several case series and nonrandomized controlled studies, about 30% of patients undergoing decompressive surgery had a favorable recovery (modified Rankin Scale [mRS] <2) and about 5% had a severe dependency rate (mRS 4–5) (53,54). The average death or disability rate in these studies was 32.2% (37). Shunt procedures should only be considered in critical patients with obstructive

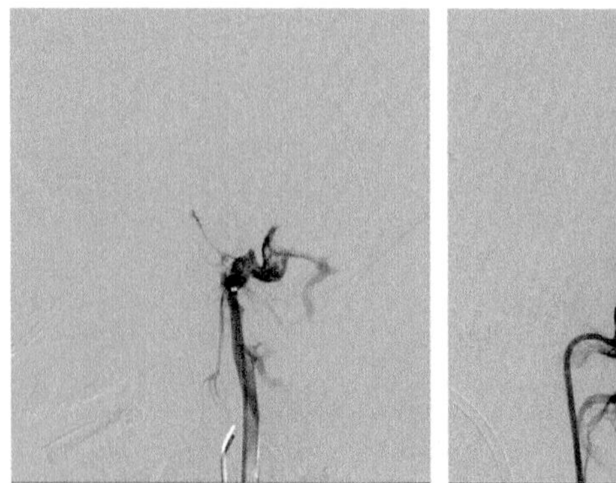
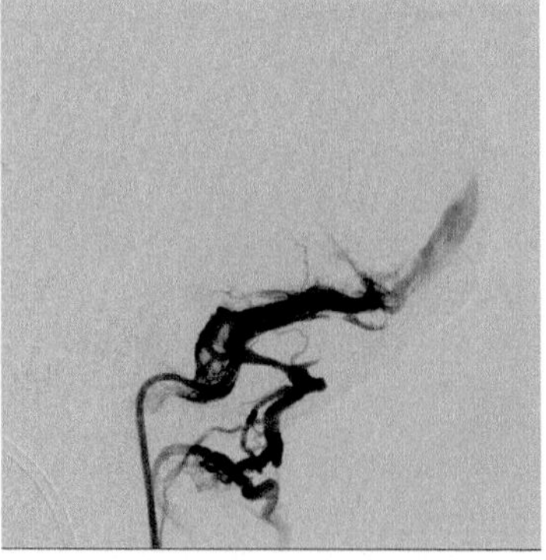

Figure 10.6 Right jugular venous injection on digital subtraction angiography, pre- (left) and post- (right) mechanical thrombectomy of transverse sinus thrombosis.

hydrocephalus, in whom no other condition aside from the hydrocephalus can explain the clinical state (39).

PROGNOSIS

Long-term outcomes are generally favorable. Good functional recovery (mRS <2) is achieved in 80% of patients (5,11,55). In prospective follow-up studies, outcomes did not significantly vary between early and late recanalization (good outcome in 88.3% early, 94.8% intermediate, 94.5% late, and 92.7% chronic, respectively) (5). Although the prevalence and associated risk factors may differ among developed or underdeveloped countries, there is no significant difference in outcomes among these patients (11).

Coma, presence of ICH, and malignancy are predictors of death or dependence (55–57). In addition, ISCVT identified male sex, age greater than37, involvement of the deep cerebral veins, and associated CNS infections as variables increasing the risk of death or dependence (11).

CONCLUSION

CVT is more common than previously thought, and may go unrecognized. The clinical presentation is quite varied, with headache being the most common presenting symptom. Prompt recognition and early initiation of anticoagulation is paramount. In some patients, advanced therapies such as direct thrombolysis and mechanical thrombectomy may be useful.

REFERENCES

1. Saposnik G, Barinagarrementeria F, Brown RD Jr, et al. American Heart Association Stroke Council and the Council on Epidemiology and Prevention. Diagnosis and management of cerebral venous thrombosis: a statement for healthcare professionals from the American Heart Association/American Stroke Association. *Stroke*. 2011;42(4):1158–1192. doi:10.1161/str.0b013e31820a8364
2. Coutinho JM, Zuurbier SM, Aramideh M, st al. The incidence of cerebral venous thrombosis: a cross-sectional study. *Stroke*. 2012;43(12):3375–3377. doi:10.1161/strokeaha.112.671453
3. Devasagayam S, Wyatt B, Leyden J, et al. Cerebral venous sinus thrombosis incidence is higher than previously thought: a retrospective population-based study. *Stroke*. 2016;47(9):2180–2182. doi:10.1161/strokeaha.116.013617
4. Silvis SM, de Sousa DA, Ferro JM, et al. Cerebral venous thrombosis. *Nat Rev Neurol*. 2017;13:555–565. doi:10.1038/nrneurol.2017.104
5. Rezoagli E, Martinelli I, Poli D, et al. The effect of recanalization on long-term neurological outcome after cerebral venous thrombosis. *J Thromb Haemost*. 2018;16(4):718–724. doi:10.1111/jth.13954
6. deBrujin SF, Stam J, Koopman MM, et al. Case-control study of risk of cerebral sinus thrombosis in oral contraceptive users and of who are carriers of hereditary prothrombotic conditions. The Cerebral Venous Sinus Thrombosis Study Group. *BMJ*. 1998;316(7131):589–592. doi:10.1136/bmj.316.7131.589
7. Cantu C, Barinagarrementeria F. Cerebral venous thrombosis associated with pregnancy and puerperium. Review of 67 cases. *Stroke*. 1993;24(12)1880–1884. doi:10.1161/01.str.24.12.1880
8. Swartz RH, Cayley ML, Foley N, et al. The incidence of pregnancy related stroke: a systematic review and meta-analysis. *Int J Stroke*. 2017;12(7):687–697. doi:10.1177/1747493017723271
9. Yesilot N, Bahar S, Yilmazer S, et al. Cerebral venous thrombosis in Behcet's disease compared to those associated with other etiologies. *J Neurol*. 2009;256(7):1134–1142. doi:10.1007/s00415-009-5088-4
10. Coutinho JM, Zuurbeir SM, Stam J. Declining mortality in cerebral venous thrombosis: a systematic review. *Stroke*. 2014;45(5):1338–1341. doi:10.1161/strokeaha.113.004666
11. Ferro JM, Canhao MD, Stam J, et al. ISCVT Investigators. Prognosis of cerebral vein and dural sinus thrombosis: results of the International Study on Cerebral Vein and Dural Sinus Thrombosis (ISCVT). *Stroke*. 2004;35(3):664–670. doi:10.1161/01.str.0000117571.76197.26
12. Canhao P, Ferro JM, lIndgren A, et al. ISCVT Investigators. Causes and predictors of death in cerebral venous thrombosis. *Stroke*. 2005;36(8):1720–1725. doi:10.1161/01.str.0000173152.84438.1c

13. Dentali F, Poli D, Scoditti U, et al. CErebral VEin Thrombosis International Study Investigators. Long-term outcomes of patients with cerebral vein thrombosis: a multicenter study. *J Thromb Haemost.* 2012;10(7):1297–302. doi:10.1111/j.1538-7836.2012.04774.x
14. Sokolof L. Anatomy of cerebral circulation. In: Welch KMA, Caplan LR, Reis DJ, et al., eds. *Primer on cerebrovascular diseases.* San Diego, US: Academic Press. Chapter 1; 1997:3–5.
15. Ueda K, Nakase H, Miyamoto K, et al. Impact of anatomical difference of the cerebral venous system on microcirculation in a gerbil superior sagittal sinus occlusion model. *Acta Neurochir (Wien).* 2000;142:75–82. doi:10.1007/s007010050010
16. Gotoh M, Ohmoto T, Kuyama H. Experimental study of venous circulatory disturbance by dural sinus occlusion. *Acta Neurochir (Wien).* 1993:124(2–4):120–126. doi:10.1007/bf01401133
17. Rottger C, Bachmann G, Gerriets T, et al. A new model of reversible sinus sagittalis superior thrombosis in the rat: magnetic resonance imaging changes. *Neurosurgery.* 2005;57(3):573–580. doi:10.1227/01.neu.0000170438.13677.22
18. Stam J. Thrombosis of the cerebral veins and sinuses. *N Engl J Med.* 2005;352(17):1791–1798. doi:10.1056/nejmra042354
19. Mullins ME, Grant PE, Wang B, et al. Parenchymal abnormalities associated with cerebral venous sinus thrombosis: assessment with diffusion-weighted MR imaging. *AJNR Am J Neuroradiol.* 2004;25(10):1666–1675.
20. Coutinho JM, van den Berg R, Zuurbier SM, et al. Small juxtacortical hemorrhages in cerebral venous thrombosis. *Ann Neurol.* 2014;75(6):908–916. doi:10.1002/ana.24180
21. Coutinho JM, Stam J, Canhao P, et al. ISCVT Investigators. Cerebral venous thrombosis in the absence of headache. *Stroke.* 2015;46(1):245–247. doi:10.1161/strokeaha.114.007584
22. Wasay M, Kojan S, Dai AI, et al. Headache in cerebral venous thrombosis: incidence, pattern and location in 200 consecutive patients. *J Headache Pain.* 2010;11:137–139. doi:10.1007/s10194-010-0186-3
23. Botta R, Donirpathi S, Yadav R, et al. Headache patterns in cerebral venous sinus thrombosis. *J Neurosci Rural Pract.* 2017;8(Suppl 1):S72–S77. doi:10.4103/jnrp.jnrp_339_16
24. Singh RJ, Saini J, Varadharajan S, et al. Headache in cerebral venous sinus thrombosis revisited: exploring the role of vascular congestion and cortical vein thrombosis. *Cephalalgia.* 2017;38(3):503–510. doi:10.1177/0333102417698707
25. Yagedari S, Jafari AK, Ashrafi E. Association of Ocular findings and outcome in cerebral venous thrombosis. *Oman J Ophthalmol.* 2017;20(3):173–176. doi:10.4103/ojo.ojo_39_2016
26. Bousser MG, Ferro JM. Cerebral venous thrombosis: an update. *Lancet Neurol.* 2007;6(2):162–170. doi:10.1016/s1474-4422(07)70029-7

27. Guenther G, Arauz A. Cerebal venous thrombosis: a diagnostic and treatment update. *Neurologia*. 2011;26:488–489. doi:10.1016/j.nrleng.2010.09.002
28. Ferro JM, Canhao P, Bousser MG, et al. ISCVT Investigators. Early seizures in cerebral vein and dural sinus thrombosis: risk factors and role of antiepileptics. *Stroke*. 2008;39(4):1152–1158. doi:10.1161/strokeaha.107.487363
29. Canhao P, Abreu LF, Ferro JM, et al. ISCVT Investigators. Safety of lumbar puncture in patients with cerebral venous thrombosis. *Eur J Neurol*. 2013;20(7):1075–1080. doi:10.1111/ene.12136
30. Leach JL, Fortuna RB, Jones BV, et al. Imaging of cerebral venous thrombosis: current techniques, spectrum of findings, and diagnostic pitfalls. *Radiographics*. 2006;26(Suppl 1):S19–S41; discussion S42–S43. doi:10.1148/rg.26si055174
31. Linn J, Ertl-Wagner B, Seelos KC, et al. Diagnostic value of multidetector-row CT angiography in the evaluation of thrombosis of the cerebral venous sinuses. *AJNR Am J Neuroradiol*. 2007;28(5):946–952.
32. Ford K, Sarwar M. Computed tomography of dural sinus thrombosis. *AJNR Am J Neuroradiol*. 1981;2(6):539–543.
33. Qu J, Yang M. Early imaging characteristics of 62 cases of cerebral venous sinus thrombosis. *Exp Ther Med*. 2013;5(1):233–236. doi:10.3892/etm.2012.796
34. Sagduyu A, Sirin H, Mulayim S, et al. Cerebral cortical and deep venous thrombosis without sinus thrombosis: clinical MRI correlates. *Acta Neurol Scand*. 2006;114:254–260. doi:10.1111/j.1600-0404.2006.00595.x
35. Favrole P, Guichard JP, Crassard I, et al. Diffusion-wedighted imaging of intravascular clots in cerebral venous thrombosis. *Stroke*. 2004;35(1):99–103. doi:10.1161/01.str.0000106483.41458.af
36. Ozsvath RR, Casey SO, Lustrin ES, et al. Cerebral venography: comparison of CT and MR projection venography. *AJR Am J Roentgenol*. 1997;169(6):1699–1707. doi:10.2214/ajr.169.6.9393193.
37. Ferro JM, Bousser MG, Canhao P, et al. European Stroke Organization. *Eur J Neurol*. 2017;24(10):1203–1213. doi:10.2214/ajr.169.6.9393193
38. Khandelwal N, Agarwal A, Kochhar R, et al. Comparison of CT venography with MR venography in cerebral sinovenous thrombosis. *AJR Am J Roentgenol*. 2006;187(6):1637–1643. doi:10.2214/ajr.05.1249
39. Zuurbier SM, van den Berg R, Troost D, et al. Hydrocephalus in cerebral venous thrombosis. *J Neurol*. 2015;262(4):931–937. doi:10.1007/s00415-015-7652-4
40. Benbir G, Ince B, Bozluolcay M. The epidemiology of post-stroke epilepsy according to stroke subtypes. *Acta Neurol Scand*. 2006;114:8–12. doi:10.1111/j.1600-0404.2006.00642.x
41. Camilo O, Goldstein LB. Seizures and epilepsy after ischemic stroke. *Stroke*. 2004;35(7):1769–1775. doi:10.1161/01.str.0000130989.17100.96

42. Hiltunen S, Putaala J, Haapaniemi E, Tatlisumak T. Long-term outcome after cerebral venous thrombosis of functional and vocational outcome, residual symptoms and adverse events in 161 patients. *J Neurol.* 2016;263:477–484. doi:10.1007/s00415-015-7996-9
43. Miranda B, Ferro JM, Canhao P, et al. ISCVT Investigators. Venous thromboembolic events after cerebral vein thrombosis. *Stroke.* 2010; 41(9):1901–1906. doi:10.1161/strokeaha.110.581223
44. Gosk-Bierska I, Wyoskinski W, Brown RD Jr, et al. Cerebral venous sinus thrombosis: incidence of venous thrombosis recurrence and survival. *Neruology.* 2006;67(5):814–819. doi:10.1212/01.wnl.0000233887.17638.d0
45. Coutinho J, de Brujin SF, Deveber G, et al. Anticoagulation for cerebral venous sinus thrombosis. *Cochrane Database Syst Rev.* 2011;(8):CD002005. doi:10.1002/14651858
46. de Brujin SF, Stam J, for the Cerebral Venous Sinus Thrombosis Study Group. Randomised, placebo-controlled trial of anticoagulant treatment with low-molecular weight heparin for cerebral sinus thrombosis. *Stroke.* 1999;30:484–488. doi:10.1161/01.str.30.3.484
47. Einhaupl KM, Villringer A, Meister W, et al. Heparin treatment in sinus venous thrombosis. *Lancet.* 1991;338:597–600. doi:10.1016/0140-6736(91)90607-q
48. Stam J, Majoie CV, van Deleden OM, et al. Endovascular thrombectomy and thrombolysis for severe cerebral sinus thrombosis: a prospective study. *Stroke.* 2008;39(5):1487–1490. doi:10.1161/strokeaha.107.502658
49. Frey JL, Muro GJ, McDougall CG, et al. Cerebral venous thrombosis: combined intrathrombus rtPA and intravenous heparin. *Stroke.* 1999;30(3):489–494. doi:10.1161/01.str.30.3.489
50. Li G, Zeng X, Hussain M, et al. Safety and validity of mechanical thrombectomy and thrombolysis on severe cerebral venous sinus thrombosis. *Neurosurgery.* 2013;72(5):730–738. doi:10.1227/neu.0b013e318285c1d3
51. Borhani Haghighi A, Mahmoodi M, Edgell RC, et al. Mechanical thrombectomy for cerebral venous sinus thrombosis: a comprehensive literature review. *Clin Appl Thromb Hemost.* 2014;20(5):507–515. doi:10.1177/1076029612470968
52. Ilyas A, Chen CJ, Raper DM, et al. Endovascular mechanical thrombectomy for cerebral venous sinus thrombosis: a systematic review. *J Neurointerv Surg.* 2017;9(11):1086–1092. doi:10.1136/neurintsurg-2016-012938
53. Ferro JM, Crassard I, Coutinho JM, et al. ISCVT 2 Investigators. Decompressive surgery in cerebrovenous thrombosis: a multicenter registry and a systematic review of individual patient data. *Stroke.* 2011;42(10):2825–2831. doi:10.1161/strokeaha.111.615393
54. Theaudin M, Crassard I, Bresson D, et al. Should decompressive surgery be performed in malignant cerebral venous thrombosis?: a series of 12 patients. *Stroke.* 2010;41(4):727–731. doi:10.1161/strokeaha.109.572909

55. Borhani Haghighi A, Edgell RC, Cruz-Flores S, et al. Mortality of cerebral venous-sinus thrombosis in a large national sample. *Stroke*. 2012;43(1):262–264. doi:10.1161/strokeaha.111.635664
56. De Brujin SF, de Haan RJ, Stam J. Clinical features and prognostic factors of cerebral venous sinus thrombosis in a prospective series of 59 patients. For The Cerebral Venous Sinus Thrombosis Study Group. *J Neurol Neurosurg Psychiatry*. 2001;70(1):105–108. doi:10.1136/jnnp.70.1.105
57. Beteau G, Mounier-vehier F, Godefroy O, et al. Cerebral venous thrombosis 3-year clinical outcome in 55 consecutive patients. *J Neurol*. 2003;250(1):29–35. doi:10.1007/s00415-003-0932-4

11 Delirium After Acute Stroke

Eugene L. Scharf and Alejandro A. Rabinstein

KEY POINTS

- Delirium is an acute neurocognitive disorder characterized by a fluctuating capacity to maintain attention and can be associated with psychomotor agitation, retardation, or both.
- Poststroke delirium is seen in approximately 25% of hospitalized stroke patients, particularly elderly, infected, and medically complex patients. Clinicians should be keenly sensitive to the development of this complication because it is associated with increased length of stay, higher rates of institutionalization, and greater mortality.
- Delirium is a preventable complication. Multimodal intervention with frequent reorientation, medication review, sensory stimulation, mobilization, and sleep hygiene have been shown in high-quality clinical trials to reduce incident delirium. Currently there is no high-level evidence for pharmacologic delirium prophylaxis in acute stroke patients.
- The Confusion Assessment Method (CAM) is a bedside clinical algorithm that can detect the presence of delirium with acceptable sensitivity and specificity. The Delirium Rating Scale (DRS) is validated to assess the severity of delirium.
- When delirium is detected, a broad investigation for common precipitants can often identify a cause; a thorough review of the medication administration record is particularly important.
- Current standards for the treatment of delirium apply universally across clinical contexts, and should consist of nonpharmacologic multimodal intervention, removal of offending medications, and improved sleep hygiene. Use of physical restraints and neuroleptic medication should be avoided unless there is agitation or violence. To date, there are no stroke-specific guidelines for the management of delirium and further research is necessary.

 DOI: 10.1891/9780826124791.0011

INTRODUCTION

Recognized since antiquity (1), delirium is an acute confusional state characterized by disorientation, inattention, and a fluctuating capacity to maintain a coherent thought process. This clinical syndrome is most commonly a complication of inpatient medicine and ICUs where it exerts a disproportionate effect on hospitalized elderly patients. A robust literature describes delirium in common clinical scenarios such as medical wards, postsurgical population, and medical and surgical ICUs (2). With the advent of dedicated stroke wards, delirium is now recognized as a complication of acute ischemic and hemorrhagic stroke. Delirium after an acute stroke can herald complications and portends worse functional outcome and increased short- and long-term mortality. Therefore, it is important for the practicing neurologist to understand this clinical syndrome so that it can be prevented, or quickly recognized and treated. This chapter provides an overview of the epidemiology, pathophysiology, prevention, diagnosis, and management of delirium when it is encountered in acute stroke.

EPIDEMIOLOGY, MORBIDITY, AND MORTALITY

Incidence

Delirium is common after an acute stroke but the exact incidence is unknown. The current understanding of delirium in acute stroke originates from inpatient observational cohorts. The reader is referred to recent reviews for concise summaries of existing observational data (3–5). The reported incidence of delirium in acute stroke varies widely depending on the patient sample and ranges from 2.3% to 61%. The largest retrospective cohort of delirium in acute ischemic stroke with over 640 patients estimated the incidence of delirium to be 19%; however, the assessment was completed by review of medical records (6). One prospective cohort of 113 ischemic stroke patients reported acute confusion on presentation or within 7 days of admission in 50% of acute stroke patients (7). The highest reported incidence of delirium after acute ischemic stroke (61%) was found in a cohort of patients with right middle cerebral artery infarction (8); yet another cohort of right hemispheric infarction had a reported incidence of delirium of only 4% (9). Generally, these studies are heterogeneous with respect to data collection methods, underlying stroke severity and localization, comorbidities, screening and assessment, and outcome criteria.

The reported incidence of delirium for patients with intracerebral hemorrhage is also wide-ranging, varying from 11% to 88%.

The largest prospective cohort of 114 patients with intracerebral hemorrhage reported a 27% incidence of delirium. Interestingly, 29 of the 31 patients diagnosed with delirium in this series were classified as hypoactive (10). A recent single-center prospective cohort of 90 patients with intracerebral hemorrhage reported a delirium incidence of 28% (11). Delirium is also observed in subarachnoid hemorrhage. A retrospective analysis of 646 patients with aneurysmal subarachnoid hemorrhage described delirium as a presenting clinical feature in 1.4% (12). In one prospective cohort of 68 patients hospitalized for subarachnoid hemorrhage, 11 patients (16%) were diagnosed with delirium; its occurrence was associated with Hunt–Hess scores ≥2, decreased alertness, and aphasia. Approximately half of this cohort had aneurysmal subarachnoid hemorrhage (13). It is currently unknown whether the etiology of subarachnoid hemorrhage influences the incidence of delirium and further research is necessary to explore this area.

Predictors of Delirium

Several risk factors have been identified as independent predictors for the development of delirium in acute ischemic stroke. Older age, infection, and medical complexity are almost universally reported as independent risk factors. Other risk factors that have been identified are poor vision and spatial neglect (14,15), preexisting cognitive impairment (16), aphasia (17), anticholinergic medication (17), urinary retention (18), chest infection (18), posterior circulation strokes (18), unsafe swallow (19), elevated C-reactive protein (19), apnea-related hypoxemia (20), low body mass index (BMI <27 kg/m^2) (20), stroke severity (21), and hearing impairment (21). Additionally, anterior circulation infarcts were found to be more associated with the development of delirium (18,22,23). One important methodological limitation that should be noted is that these series did not stratify the risk of delirium based on the severity of specific neurologic deficits (e.g., aphasia, hearing loss, visual loss).

A predictive model for delirium stratifies the risk of delirium to less than 5%, 5% to 20%, and greater than 20% based on the patient's age, presence of infection, severity of National Institutes of Health Stroke Scale (NIHSS), and location and severity of infarction (total anterior circulation, partial anterior circulation, posterior circulation, and lacunar infarction) with a reported sensitivity of 79% and specificity of 81% (21). Clinicians should however be aware that delirium can occur even in the absence of these common predisposing clinical and demographic factors.

Risk factors for the development of delirium in intracerebral hemorrhage were explored in a recent single-center cohort, and found that hematoma localized to the right hemisphere, and/or parahippocampal gyri was an independent risk factor; this series excluded patients whose underlying etiology was traumatic, secondary to a vascular malformation, or structural mass lesion (11).

Morbidity and Mortality

Delirium in acute stroke is associated with increased morbidity and mortality. Observational data consistently show that delirium in acute stroke is associated with medical complications (24), increased hospital length of stay, higher inpatient mortality, post-hospital institutionalization, worse functional outcomes (15,18,25), higher mortality at both 6 and 12 months (23), and worse long-term survival (6). One large prospective cohort of 314 stroke patients found delirium was associated with increased length of stay (mean 45 vs. 22 days), greater proportion discharged to a nursing home (62% vs. 11.2%), greater proportion institutionalized at 6 months (60% vs. 12.5%) and at 12 months (65% vs. 13%), and higher inpatient mortality (18% vs. 2.2%) and 1-year mortality (30% vs. 7.4%). However, it must be noted that delirious patients were older, had more medical complexity and more severe strokes (NIHSS 16.8 vs. 6.5) than patients who did not develop delirium (18). A large systematic review of over 2,000 patients with acute stroke supports the conclusion that delirium is associated with increased length of stay, increased likelihood of discharge to an institution, and higher mortality both as in-hospital and at 1 year, although these data were not risk adjusted for underlying confounders such as stroke severity or comorbidities (5). Also, delirium can assume a chronic and fluctuating course over several weeks. These patients with prolonged delirium often develop variable degrees of persistent cognitive impairment.

PATHOPHYSIOLOGY

The pathophysiology of delirium is multifactorial and results from the interaction of concurrent biological processes (26–28). In acute stroke, the processes that precipitate a delirium are likely pathophysiological responses to cerebral ischemia that overwhelm a weakened cognitive substrate. There are three domains of inquiry that have attempted to describe the complex pathophysiology of delirium: dysfunction of the hypothalamic–pituitary–adrenal axis leading to states of excessive cortisol secretion, deleterious effects of inflammation and immune cell infiltration of the injured brain, and alteration in neurotransmission.

Hypothalamic–Pituitary–Adrenal Axis Dysfunction

Abnormal elevations in plasma cortisol were first observed in delirious postsurgical patients (29). In the setting of ischemic stroke, it has been shown that delirium is associated with increased sensitivity to adrenocorticotropin, loss of normal glucocorticoid diurnal rhythm, and loss of sensitivity to glucocorticoid mediated feedback inhibition (30). In a cohort of 83 patients admitted for ischemic stroke, inappropriately elevated cortisol levels after dexamethasone were independently associated with delirium (31). The adverse effects of chronic elevated glucocorticoid exposure to the central nervous system (CNS) have been explored in the setting of depression, but the effects of short-term acute elevations, particularly in the setting of cerebral insults, are still undefined. However, these data suggest that excessive adrenal stress response to an acute stroke may contribute to the pathogenesis of delirium.

Neuroinflammation

Cerebral ischemia results in a complex cascade of immune cell responses (32). The systemic inflammatory response may have direct adverse effects on higher order cognitive functioning (33). In cerebral ischemia, the blood–brain barrier is breached both by degradation of cellular structure secondary to hypoxic/ischemic insult and proinflammatory signaling that upregulates cellular adhesion molecule expression on vascular endothelial cells permitting passage of immune cells into the brain parenchyma. Immune cell infiltration, cytokine and chemokine upregulation, proinflammatory arachidonic acid lipid signaling, native CNS microglial activation, and widespread reactive oxygen species are thought to create a susceptible environment to the development of delirium. Proinflammatory cytokines interleukin 1 and prostaglandin E(2) have been described to stimulate adrenocorticotropic hormone (ACTH) secretion through effects on hypothalamic neurons secreting corticotropin releasing hormone in rodent models, although this mechanism has not been confirmed in clinical settings (34). Immunosuppressive agents to reduce CNS immune cell trafficking have been tested as neuroprotective strategies for acute ischemic stroke in clinical trials but have not resulted in improved functional outcomes; although measures of global cognitive functioning were exploratory end points, incident delirium was not assessed in these trials (35–37).

Abnormal Neurotransmission: Cholinergic Deficit and Dopamine Excess

Acetylcholine drives critical brain networks that sustain arousal, attention, memory, and rapid eye movement (REM) sleep. Cholinergic neurons originating from the nucleus basalis project to the reticular formation, thalamus, striatum, and forebrain. Deficiencies in acetylcholine neurotransmission have been suggested as a cause of delirium after acute stroke (38). In an animal model of cerebral ischemia, a transient increase followed by decreased acetylcholine has been demonstrated in the striatum (39). Autoradiography studies of rodent brains have shown postischemic alterations in acetylcholine receptor density following cerebral ischemia in multiple striatal structures, even outside the vascular distribution of the ischemic insult (40). It is hypothesized that a primary substrate for neuronal acetylcholine synthesis, acetyl coenzyme A, is reduced in the setting of ischemia and hypoxia, and results in shunting of this neurotransmitter precursor to serve the demands of oxidative metabolism in the citric acid cycle (41). The role of acetylcholine deficiency in the development of delirium is also supported by the well-known delirium precipitating effects of anticholinergic medications (42).

Dopaminergic and cholinergic pathways overlap in the striatum and have opposing functions. Surges of dopamine inhibit acetylcholine signaling exacerbating the cholinergic deficits. Serotonin and melatonin have been implicated in the genesis of delirium, but there is no generally accepted mechanism to date.

There are no biomarkers or neuroimaging indicators of delirium. The scientific community is only beginning to understand the multifactorial pathophysiology of delirium. It is unknown whether the pathophysiology of delirium is similar in the myriad clinical contexts in which it is encountered, and whether independent, overlapping, or still undefined mechanisms contribute to delirium in acute stroke. Further investigation is needed.

PREVENTION

Recently published systematic reviews by the Cochrane Library guide our understanding in preventing delirium for long-term care facility and non-ICU hospitalized patients (43,44). Strategies for the prevention of delirium include nonpharmacological multimodal interventions, pharmacologic therapy directed at correcting the suspected neurotransmitter dysfunction, melatonin for promotion of sleep hygiene, alternative anesthetics in surgical patients, and anesthetic monitoring with bispectral index. There is strong evidence to support the use of multimodal intervention for the prevention of delirium. The Hospital Elder Life Program (HELP) reduced incident delirium from 15% to 10% in a nonrandomized controlled clinical trial of non-ICU general medical elderly patients who received multimodal interventions including reorientation, reduction of psychoactive medication use, early mobilization, proper sleep hygiene, and assessment and treatment of vision and hearing deficits (45). Several more interventional trials employing variations of this program have confirmed the efficacy of the multimodal approach for the primary prevention of delirium. This intervention has been shown to be cost-saving when implemented in a community hospital setting (46).

Several trials have evaluated pharmacological options for the prevention of delirium. Prophylactic administration of cholinesterase inhibitors, antipsychotic medications, or melatonin and melatonin agonists was not found to reduce the incidence, duration, or severity of delirium, or decrease length of stay in clinical studies completed to date. However, methodological limitations, lack of complete outcomes, and bias may have impacted the results of these trials. On the basis of the current evidence, routine pharmacological prophylaxis for delirium is not recommended; yet each treatment decision should be individualized to the clinical context.

IDENTIFICATION

Clinical Presentation

Delirium is a clinical diagnosis. As a general rule, a clinician should routinely assess for delirium in any older age hospitalized patient. It is a neurocognitive disorder defined in the fifth edition of the American Psychiatric Association's *Diagnostic and Statistical Manual of Mental Disorders* (5th ed.; *DSM-5*; American Psychiatric Association, 2013) by the following key features: a deterioration in attention and awareness developing acutely over hours to days and usually precipitated by a medical condition, infection, medication, or metabolic disturbance (Table 11.1) (47).

Additional clinical features may include emotional disturbances and sleep–wake reversal. Delirium with concomitant psychomotor agitation or retardation is termed hyperactive (or agitated) and hypoactive delirium respectively. When patients present with both hyperactive and hypoactive components, it is termed mixed delirium. Subsyndromal delirium is a novel concept that describes incomplete or partial criteria for delirium; however, this concept has no accepted definition and requires a more in-depth exploration in the stroke population (48).

Once delirium is suspected, a brief screening tool can assist in diagnosis. Numerous bedside screening methods have been developed to assist in determining diagnosis and severity (49). The most common diagnostic algorithm for delirium is the CAM, which had a reported sensitivity of 94% to 100% and a specificity of 90%

Table 11.1 Diagnostic Criteria for Delirium

A. A disturbance in attention (i.e., reduced ability to direct focus sustain and shift attention) and awareness (reduced orientation to the environment).
B. The disturbance develops over a short period of time usually hours to a few days), represents a change from baseline attention and awareness, and tends to fluctuate in severity during the course of a day.
C. An additional disturbance in cognition (e.g., memory deficit, disorientation, language, visual spatial ability, or perception).
D. The disturbance in criteria A and C are not better explained by another pre-existing, established, or evolving neuro cognitive disorder and do not occur in the context of a severely reduced level of arousal, such as coma.
E. There is evidence from history, physical examination, or laboratory findings that the disturbances a direct physiological consequence of another medical condition, substance intoxication or withdrawal (i.e., due to the drug of abuse or to medication), or exposure to a toxin, or is due to multiple etiologies.

Specify if:

A. Hyperactive: The individual demonstrates increased psychomotor activity including agitation, distress, anger, and/or uncooperativeness.
B. Hypoactive: The individual demonstrates reduced psychomotor activity appearing lethargic, apathetic, and/or sluggish.
C. Mixed level of activity: The individual demonstrates either normal or fluctuating psychomotor function accompanied by disturbances in attention and awareness.

Source: Adapted from American Psychiatric Association. (2013). *Diagnostic and Statistical Manual of Mental Disorders* (5th ed.). Arlington, VA: American Psychiatric Association Publishing.

to 95% in its initial description (50). This instrument consists of a four-part assessment of the key criteria of delirium: (a) acute onset with fluctuating course, (b) inattention, (c) disorganized thinking, and (d) altered level of consciousness. A diagnosis of delirium can be inferred if parts 1 and 2 are present in addition to either part 3 or 4. This screening method has been expanded to include the patients in the ICU (51). The severity of delirium is typically measured using the DRS (52).

Assessment

Any acute neurological deterioration or mental status change observed in an acute stroke patient should prompt an immediate evaluation consisting of an abbreviated history, measurement of vital signs, and focused neurological exam. The next decision is whether immediate intracranial imaging and/or advanced diagnostic neuroimaging is indicated to assess for new or progressive ischemia, hemorrhage, or symptomatic cerebral edema. Medical systemic complications should be considered (e.g., sepsis, deep venous thrombosis, pulmonary embolism, gastrointestinal hemorrhage, acute coronary syndrome) (Figure 11.1).

In the absence of an emergency, the clinician should obtain a detailed history establishing the baseline level of cognitive function because delirium is much more common among patients with preexistent cognitive impairment. Information on recent illnesses, fevers, behavioral changes, medication adjustments, illicit substance use, and recent hospitalizations can also be very valuable. A full review of systems will often elicit relevant historical details not otherwise volunteered with open-ended questioning. Often, an informed history can only be taken from family, friends, caregivers,

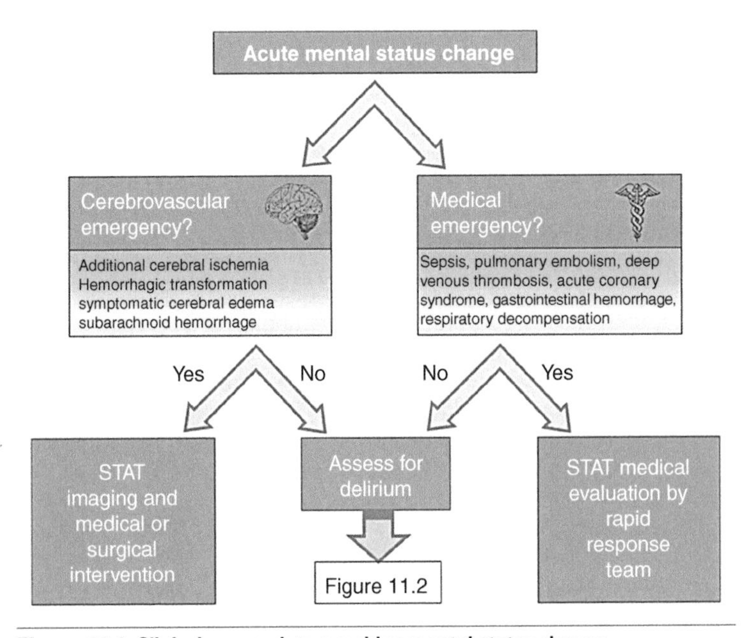

Figure 11.1 Clinical approach to a sudden mental status change.

Cerebrovascular patients who develop sudden changes in mental status must be assessed immediately at the bedside for cerebrovascular and medical complications with an abbreviated history and physical. If no immediate complication is present, a formal assessment for delirium can proceed (described in Figure 11.2)

and bedside medical personnel. It is necessary to directly inquire about alcohol use and, if present, when was the last drink or whether there is a history of withdrawal. A comprehensive review of the medication administration record should be performed with attention to frequency and dosing of narcotic, sedative, anesthetic, neuroleptic, anticholinergic, benzodiazepine, antihistaminergic, and context dependent neurotoxic medications (e.g., neurotoxic antimicrobials). A review of existing laboratory evaluations should assess for potential etiological clues or direct precipitants of delirium such as renal failure with uremia, liver failure, electrolyte imbalances, and altered gas exchange. A review of the fluid balance should be completed as dehydration, urinary retention, or constipation can cause delirium.

Next, a physical exam should be performed to look for signs of dehydration, skin breakdown, urine retention, constipation, abdominal pain, joint pathology, or other abnormal findings. During the physical examination note whether there are signs of pain (e.g., hip or shoulder pathology) that may be contributing to the presentation. A neurological exam should be performed with attention to the patient's mental status. Take note of the patient's level of alertness, content of consciousness, muscle tone, and presence of adventitious movements such as myoclonus, akathisia, dystonia, dyskinesia, tremor, asterixis, or clonus. Useful bedside maneuvers for assessing attentional deficits involve reverse order sequencing (i.e., stating the days of the week or months of the year in reverse; or counting backward by 7 from 100).

Additional laboratory and radiological investigations are crucial for a complete evaluation. Recommended investigations for delirious patients include comprehensive metabolic panel, serum lactate, complete blood cell count with differential, and assays of liver and renal function (including blood urea nitrogen [BUN] and ammonia). Arterial blood gases should be obtained if hypercapnia is suspected or oxygen saturation is low. Creatine kinase, urinalysis, urine toxicology, bladder scanning, chest radiography, and ECG may be pertinent in many instances. Tests should be repeated where clinically indicated. Additional infectious evaluations such as blood cultures or sputum cultures should be guided by the results of the initial survey.

A critical component of the evaluation is excluding the several neurologic conditions that present as delirium. Unexplained fevers, leukocytosis, meningismus, new obtundation, bizarre behavior, or headache should prompt consideration for cerebrospinal fluid analysis to assess for encephalitis, meningitis, or subarachnoid hemorrhage. Delirium accompanied by fever and autonomic instability in the setting of neuroleptic use should prompt concern for neuroleptic malignant syndrome. Agitated delirium with fever, autonomic instability, tremor, clonus, hyperreflexia, and/or diarrhea should prompt concern for serotonin syndrome. A fluctuating mental status or a subtle clonus should prompt concern for nonconvulsive status epilepticus, and EEG is a highly effective diagnostic tool that can differentiate this delirium mimic (53,54). Sundowning is an acute behavioral disorder characterized by confusion late in the day and is a poorly understood phenomenon of neurodegenerative diseases. Lewy body dementia, a neurodegenerative alpha-synucleinopathy characterized by fluctuations in mental status and hallucinations, should be considered in the differential diagnosis of delirium in the appropriate context.

MANAGEMENT

The clinical management of delirium has considerable overlap with its prevention and consists of two primary aims: treating any precipitant of delirium (e.g., infection, organ failure, metabolic abnormality) and treating delirium itself. Delirium-specific treatments are nonpharmacological multimodal interventions and pharmacological therapy. As discussed earlier, multimodal interventions have been shown to be efficacious for preventing delirium, but may also reduce its duration and severity once it occurs. There are no stroke-specific guidelines for the management of delirium to date.

Multimodal Intervention

The following components of multimodal intervention should be instituted by an interdisciplinary team guided by a hospital protocol. Frequent reorientation, social interaction, and the presence of familiar persons and objects (e.g., pictures of loved ones) exert a stabilizing effect on attention and awareness and reduce anxiety. Improvements to sleep hygiene can be achieved by minimizing nonessential nursing checks, blood draws, and other interruptions during the conventional sleep period. Use of nonbenzodiazepine sleep aids such as melatonin or melatonin receptor agonists should be considered to maintain normal diurnal rhythm. When safe, immobility should be avoided by minimizing bed rest orders, gradual mobilization, physical and occupational therapy, and off-floor visits to public areas within the institution. Physical restraints should also be avoided because their use can prolong delirium (55). Sensory deprivation can be addressed by using adjuncts such as eyeglasses, hearing aids, music (if preferred), massage, or other complementary modalities. Delirium education of family and caregivers is beneficial (56). Finally, pain severity and hydration status should be routinely assessed.

Pharmacologic Therapy

There are no cerebrovascular-specific guidelines for the pharmacological management of delirium. Generally, pharmacologic therapy for treatment of delirium should be reserved for specific contexts such as agitation, alcohol withdrawal or severe and prolonged psychomotor retardation, or the ICU. A possible benefit from cholinesterase inhibitors for acute stroke patients with delirium was suggested by a case report (57) and a pilot study (58). However, cholinesterase inhibitors were not found helpful for the treatment of delirium in clinical trials involving critically ill patients (59). In a systematic review of 17 randomized controlled trials including over 2,800 intensive care patients treated for delirium, pharmacologic drug therapy was shown to shorten duration of delirium, although there was no short-term mortality benefit in the treatment arms (60). Gabapentin, methylprednisolone, non-steroidal anti-inflammatory drugs (NSAIDS), and ketamine have been investigated in clinical trials and their use was not associated with improved outcomes in patients with non-ICU delirium (44). Judicious use of neuroleptic medication for the treatment of delirium is reasonable to control violent or harmful agitation. Atypical neuroleptic medications such as olanzapine or quetiapine have been shown to reduce length of delirium, and lessen violent or uncontrollable delirium in intensive care settings (61,62). Stimulant therapy for hypoactive delirium can be considered in select circumstances such as multiorgan failure (63) or advanced cancer (64), but has not been evaluated for delirium related to acute stroke. A general approach to the assessment and management of delirium is shown in Figure 11.2.

CONCLUSION

Delirium in hospitalized patients is associated with increased hospital length of stay, higher rate of institutionalization, worse patient functional outcomes, and ultimately, greater mortality. Although frequent after cerebrovascular events, delirium is understudied in this patient population. Generally accepted predictors of delirium can guide selection of candidates for more intensive screening and implementation of a primary prevention program consisting of multimodal, nonpharmacologic strategies. Delirium management should be based on these multimodal interventions with drug therapy use restricted to select cases.

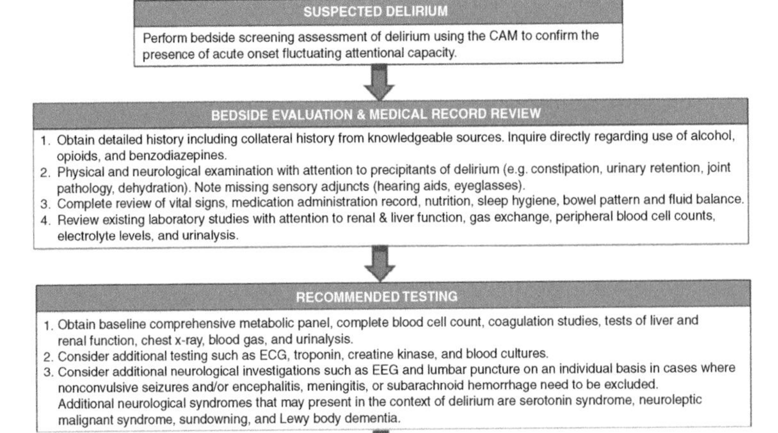

Figure 11.2 Clinical assessment and management of delirium.

CAM, confusion assessment method.

Our understanding of delirium in stroke patients is only just beginning to grow, and much remains to be discovered. One key epidemiological question is whether delirium itself is detrimental or whether it is a marker of greater stroke severity, worse brain reserve, and more comorbidities that are truly responsible for the worse outcome in delirious patients. Methodologically rigorous controlled prospective studies are needed to address this fundamental question. Identification of delirium biomarkers has not been successful because our understanding of the pathophysiology of delirium is incomplete. Key research priorities for delirium treatment in acute stroke should include clinical trials of drug therapy for poststroke delirium and expanding nonpharmacological interventions including physical and occupational therapy and optimizing the restorative aspects of sleep. Despite the unknown, one fact is clear: early recognition and management of delirium is critical to provide optimal care to patients with cerebrovascular disease.

REFERENCES

1. Adams F. *The genuine works of hippocrates.* New York, NY; William Wood and Company; 1886.
2. Inouye SK. The dilemma of delirium: clinical and research controversies regarding diagnosis and evaluation of delirium in hospitalized elderly medical patients. *Am J Med.* 1994;97(3):278–288. doi:10.1016/0002-9343(94)90011-6
3. Klimiec E, Dziedzic T, Kowalska K, et al. Knowns and unknowns about delirium in stroke: a review. *Cogn Behav Neurol.* 2016;29(4):174–189. doi:10.1097/wnn.0000000000000110
4. Oldenbeuving AW, de Kort PL, Jansen BP, et al. Delirium in acute stroke: a review. *Int J Stroke.* 2007;2(4):270–275. doi:10.1111/j.1747-4949.2007.00163.x
5. Shi Q, Presutti R, Selchen D, et al. Delirium in acute stroke: a systematic review and meta-analysis. *Stroke.* 2012;43(3):645–649. doi:10.1161/strokeaha.111.643726
6. Melkas S, Laurila JV, Vataja R, et al. Post-stroke delirium in relation to dementia and long-term mortality. *Int J Geriatr Psychiatry.* 2012;27(4):401–408. doi:10.1002/gps.2733
7. Gustafson Y, Olsson T, Eriksson S, et al. Acute confusional states (delirium) in stroke patients. *Cerebrovasc Dis.* 1991;1(5):257–264. doi:10.1159/000108852
8. Mori E, Yamadori A. Acute confusional state and acute agitated delirium. Occurrence after infarction in the right middle cerebral artery territory. *Arch Neurol.* 1987;44(11):1139–1143. doi:10.1001/archneur.1987.00520230029009
9. Schmidley JW, Messing RO. Agitated confusional states in patients with right-hemisphere infarctions. *Stroke.* 1984;15(5):883–885. doi:10.1161/01.str.15.5.883
10. Naidech AM, Beaumont JL, Rosenberg NF, et al. Intracerebral hemorrhage and delirium symptoms. Length of stay, function, and quality of life in a 114-patient cohort. *Am J Respir Crit Care Med.* 2013;188(11):1331–1337. doi:10.1164/rccm.201307-1256oc
11. Naidech AM, Polnaszek KL, Berman MD, et al. Hematoma locations predicting delirium symptoms after intracerebral hemorrhage. *Neurocrit Care* . 2016;24(3):397–403. doi:10.1007/s12028-015-0210-1
12. Reijneveld JC, Wermer M, Boonman Z, et al. Acute confusional state as presenting feature in aneurysmal subarachnoid hemorrhage: frequency and characteristics. *J Neurol.* 2000;247(2):112–116. doi:10.1007/pl00007791
13. Caeiro L, Menger C, Ferro JM, et al. Delirium in acute subarachnoid haemorrhage. *Cerebrovasc Dis.* 2005;19(1):31–38. doi:10.1159/000081909

14. Caeiro L, Ferro JM, Albuquerque R, et al. Delirium in the first days of acute stroke. *J Neurol.* 2004;251(2):171–178. doi:10.1007/s00415-004-0294-6
15. McManus J, Pathansali R, Stewart R, et al. Delirium post-stroke. *Age Ageing.* 2007;36(6):613–618. doi:10.1093/ageing/afm140
16. Henon H, Lebert F, Durieu I, et al. Confusional state in stroke: relation to preexisting dementia, patient characteristics, and outcome. *Stroke.* 1999;30(4):773–779. doi:10.1161/01.str.30.4.773
17. Carin-Levy G, Mead GE, Nicol K, et al. Delirium in acute stroke: screening tools, incidence rates and predictors: a systematic review. *J Neurol.* 2012;259(8):1590–1599. doi:10.1007/s00415-011-6383-4
18. Miu DK, Yeung JC. Incidence of post-stroke delirium and 1-year outcome. *Geriatr Gerontol Int.* 2013;13(1):123–129. doi:10.1111/j.1447-0594.2012.00871.x
19. McManus J, Pathansali R, Hassan H, et al. The course of delirium in acute stroke. *Age Ageing.* 2009;38(4):385–389. doi:10.1093/ageing/afp038
20. Sandberg O, Franklin KA, Bucht G, et al. Sleep apnea, delirium, depressed mood, cognition, and ADL ability after stroke. *J Am Geriatr Soc.* 2001;49(4):391–397. doi:10.1046/j.1532-5415.2001.49081.x
21. Oldenbeuving AW, de Kort PLM, van Eck van der Sluijs JF, et al. An early prediction of delirium in the acute phase after stroke. *J Neurol Neurosurg Psychiatry.* 2014;85(4):431–434. doi:10.1136/jnnp-2013-304920
22. Kostalova M, Bednarik J, Mitasova A, et al. Towards a predictive model for post-stroke delirium. *Brain Inj.* 2012;26(7–8):962–971. doi:10.3109/02699052.2012.660510
23. Sheng AZ, Shen Q, Cordato D, et al. Delirium within three days of stroke in a cohort of elderly patients. *J Am Geriatr Soc.* 2006;54(8):1192–1198. doi:10.1111/j.1532-5415.2006.00806.x
24. Dostovic Z, Dostovic E, Smajlovic D, et al. Predictors for post-stroke delirium outcome. *Mater Sociomed.* 2016;28(5):382–386. doi:10.5455/msm.2016.28.382-386
25. Oldenbeuving AW, de Kort PL, Jansen BP, et al. Delirium in the acute phase after stroke: incidence, risk factors, and outcome. *Neurology.* 2011;76(11):993–999. doi:10.1212/wnl.0b013e318210411f
26. Bogovic TZ, Tonkovic D, Sekulic A, et al. Pathophysiology of delirium. *Acta Med Croatica.* 2012;66(1):61–66.
27. van der Mast RC. Pathophysiology of delirium. *J Geriatr Psychiatry Neurol.* 1998;11(3):138–145; discussion 157–138. doi:10.1177/089198879801100304
28. Hshieh TT, Fong TG, Marcantonio ER, et al. Cholinergic deficiency hypothesis in delirium: a synthesis of current evidence. *J Gerontol A Biol Sci Med Sci.* 2008;63(7):764–772. doi:10.1093/gerona/63.7.764

29. McIntoshTK, Bush HL, Yeston NS, et al. Beta-endorphin, cortisol and post-operative delirium: a preliminary report. *Psychoneuroendocrinology.* 1985;10(3):303–313.
30. Olsson T. Activity in the hypothalamic-pituitary-adrenal axis and delirium. *Dement Geriatr Cogn Disord.* 1999;10(5):345–349. doi:10.1159/000017168
31. Olsson T, Marklund N, Gustafson Y, et al. Abnormalities at different levels of the hypothalamic-pituitary-adrenocortical axis early after stroke. *Stroke.* 1992;23(11):1573–1576. doi:10.1161/01.str.23.11.1573
32. Wang Q, Tang XN, Yenari MA. The inflammatory response in stroke. *J Neuroimmunol.* 2007;184(1–2):53–68. doi:10.1016/j.jneuroim.2006.11.014
33. Cunningham C, MacLullich AMJ. At the extreme end of the psychoneuroimmunological spectrum: delirium as a maladaptive sickness behaviour response. *Brain Behav Immun.* 2013;28:1–13. doi:10.1016/j.bbi.2012.07.012
34. Furuyashiki T, Narumiya S. Roles of prostaglandin E receptors in stress responses. *Curr Opin Pharmacol.* 2009;9(1):31–38. doi:10.1016/j.coph.2008.12.010
35. Elkins J, Veltkamp R, Montaner J, et al. Safety and efficacy of natalizumab in patients with acute ischaemic stroke (ACTION): a randomised, placebo-controlled, double-blind phase 2 trial. *Lancet Neurol.* 2017;16(3):217–226. doi:10.1016/s1474-4422(16)30357-x
36. Enlimomab Acute Stroke Trial I. Use of anti-ICAM-1 therapy in ischemic stroke: results of the Enlimomab Acute Stroke Trial. *Neurology.* 2001;57(8):1428–1434. doi:10.1212/wnl.57.8.1428
37. Krams M, Lees KR, Hacke W, et al. Acute Stroke Therapy by Inhibition of Neutrophils (ASTIN): an adaptive dose-response study of UK-279,276 in acute ischemic stroke. *Stroke.* 2003;34(11):2543–2548. doi:10.1161/01.str.0000092527.33910.89
38. Trzepacz PT. Anticholinergic model for delirium. *Semin Clin Neuropsychiatry.* 1996;1(4):294–303. doi:10.1053/SCNP00100294
39. Bertrand N, Ishii H, Beley A, et al. Biphasic striatal acetylcholine release during and after transient cerebral ischemia in gerbils. *J Cereb Blood Flow Metab.* 1993;13(5):789–795. doi:10.1038/jcbfm.1993.100
40. Nagasawa H, Araki T, Kogure K. Alteration of muscarinic acetylcholine binding sites in the postischemic brain areas of the rat using in vitro autoradiography. *J Neurol Sci.* 1994;121(1):27–31. doi:10.1016/0022-510x(94)90152-x
41. Gibson GE, Blass JP, Huang HM, et al. The cellular basis of delirium and its relevance to age-related disorders including Alzheimer's disease. *Int Psychogeriatr.* 1991;3(2):373–395. doi:10.1017/s1041610291000820
42. Campbell N, Boustani M, Limbil T, et al. The cognitive impact of anticholinergics: a clinical review. *Clin Interv Aging.* 2009;4:225–233. doi:10.2147/cia.s5358

43. Clegg A, Siddiqi N, Heaven A, et al. Interventions for preventing delirium in older people in institutional long-term care. *Cochrane Database Syst Rev.* 2014;(1):CD009537. doi:10.1002/14651858.cd009537.pub2

44. Siddiqi N, Harrison JK, Clegg A, et al. Interventions for preventing delirium in hospitalised non-ICU patients. *Cochrane Database Syst Rev.* 2016;3:CD005563. doi:10.1002/14651858.cd005563.pub3

45. Inouye SK, Bogardus ST Jr, Charpentier PA, et al. A multicomponent intervention to prevent delirium in hospitalized older patients. *N Engl J Med.* 1999;340(9):669–676. doi:10.1056/nejm199903043400901

46. Rubin FH, Neal K, Fenlon K, et al. Sustainability and scalability of the hospital elder life program at a community hospital. *J Am Geriatr Soc.* 2011;59(2):359–365. doi:10.1111/j.1532-5415.2010.03243.x

47. Association AP. *Diagnostic and statistical manual of mental disorders.* 5th ed. Arlington, VA: American Psychiatric Publishing; 2013.

48. Klimiec E, Dziedzic T, Kowalska K, et al. PRospective Observational POLIsh Study on post-stroke delirium (PROPOLIS): methodology of hospital-based cohort study on delirium prevalence, predictors and diagnostic tools. *BMC Neurol.* 2015;15:94. doi:10.1186/s12883-015-0351-z

49. Adamis D, Sharma N, Whelan PJ, et al. Delirium scales: a review of current evidence. *Aging Ment Health.* 2010;14(5):543–555. doi:10.1080/13607860903421011

50. Inouye SK, van Dyck CH, Alessi CA, et al. Clarifying confusion: the confusion assessment method. A new method for detection of delirium. *Ann Intern Med.* 1990;113(12):941–948. doi:10.7326/0003-4819-113-12-941

51. Ely EW, Margolin R, Francis J, et al. Evaluation of delirium in critically ill patients: validation of the Confusion Assessment Method for the Intensive Care Unit (CAM-ICU). *Crit Care Med.* 2001;29(7):1370–1379. doi:10.1097/00003246-200107000-00012

52. Trzepacz PT, Mittal D, Torres R, et al. Validation of the Delirium Rating Scale-revised-98: comparison with the delirium rating scale and the cognitive test for delirium. *J Neuropsychiatry Clin Neurosci.* 2001;13(2):229–242. doi:10.1176/jnp.13.2.229

53. Brenner RP. Utility of EEG in delirium: past views and current practice. *Int Psychogeriatr.* 1991;3(2):211–229. doi:10.1017/s1041610291000686

54. Naeije G, Depondt C, Meeus C, et al. EEG patterns compatible with nonconvulsive status epilepticus are common in elderly patients with delirium: a prospective study with continuous EEG monitoring. *Epilepsy Behav.* 2014;36:18–21. doi:10.1016/j.yebeh.2014.04.012

55. Inouye SK, Zhang Y, Jones RN, et al. Risk factors for delirium at discharge: development and validation of a predictive model. *Arch Intern Med.* 2007;167(13):1406–1413. doi:10.1001/archinte.167.13.1406

56. Bull MJ, Boaz L, Jerme M. Educating family caregivers for older adults about delirium: a systematic review. *Worldviews Evid-Based Nurs.* 2016;13(3):232–240. doi:10.1111/wvn.12154
57. Kobayashi K, Higashima M, Mutou K, et al. Severe delirium due to basal forebrain vascular lesion and efficacy of donepezil. *Prog Neuro-Psychoph.* 2004;28(7):1189–1194. doi:10.1016/j.pnpbp.2004.06.021
58. Oldenbeuving AW, de Kort PL, Jansen BP, et al. A pilot study of rivastigmine in the treatment of delirium after stroke: a safe alternative. *BMC Neurol.* 2008;8:34. doi:10.1186/1471-2377-8-34
59. van Eijk MMJ, Roes KCB, Honing MLH, et al. Effect of rivastigmine as an adjunct to usual care with haloperidol on duration of delirium and mortality in critically ill patients: a multicentre, double-blind, placebo-controlled randomised trial. *Lancet.* 2010;376(9755):1829–1837. doi:10.1016/s0140-6736(10)61855-7
60. Al-Qadheeb NS, Balk EM, Fraser GL, et al. Randomized ICU trials do not demonstrate an association between interventions that reduce delirium duration and short-term mortality: a systematic review and meta-analysis. *Crit Care Med.* 2014;42(6):1442–1454. doi:10.1097/ccm.0000000000000224
61. Gilchrist NA, Asoh I, Greenberg B. Atypical antipsychotics for the treatment of ICU delirium. *J Intensive Care Med.* 2012;27(6):354–361. doi:10.1177/0885066611403110
62. Wang HR, Woo YS, Bahk WM. Atypical antipsychotics in the treatment of delirium. *Psychiatry Clin Neurosci.* 2013;67(5):323–331. doi:10.1111/pcn.12066
63. Morita T, Otani H, Tsunoda J, et al. Successful palliation of hypoactive delirium due to multi-organ failure by oral methylphenidate. *Support Care Cancer.* 2000;8(2):134–137. doi:10.1007/s005200050028
64. Gagnon B, Low G, Schreier G. Methylphenidate hydrochloride improves cognitive function in patients with advanced cancer and hypoactive delirium: a prospective clinical study. *J Psychiatr Neurosci.* 2005;30(2):100–107.

12 Cardiac Complications After Acute Stroke

Brian Silver

KEY POINTS

- Cardiac complications after stroke include direct myocardial injury and arrhythmias, and occur in approximately 20% of patients.
- Cardiac complications after stroke can be immediate or may occur years after stroke.
- Cardiac complications after stroke are believed to be due to catecholamine surges and systemic inflammatory response.
- Detection of cardiac complications after acute stroke includes measurement of troponin levels, obtaining an ECG, and performing telemetry.
- Management of complications is frequently done in collaboration with cardiology.

INTRODUCTION

Cardiac complications following ischemic and hemorrhagic stroke occur frequently. The time frame for these complications includes the days following the event. In addition, patients who suffer from stroke also have an increased risk of cardiovascular morbidity and mortality in the months and years following stroke. Complications include myocardial infarction and cardiac arrhythmias. In this chapter, the frequency of these events, their diagnosis, and potential prevention are discussed.

EPIDEMIOLOGY, MORBIDITY, AND MORTALITY

Myocardial Injury

In a study conducted in the 1970s and prior to the routine use of CT scans, myocardial injury occurred in 12.7% of stroke patients within 72 hours after stroke (1). In 71% of these patients, no clinical symptoms occurred and the diagnosis was made based on ECG and/or

 DOI: 10.1891/9780826124791.0012

enzyme studies. Mortality was substantial in this study, speaking to the gains made in reducing mortality after stroke. Nevertheless, 1-year mortality was significantly greater in those with combined stroke and myocardial infarction compared with those with stroke alone (64% vs. 42%).

A study of 200 patients, published over 30 years later, found ECG changes consisting of T-wave inversions and ST-segment depressions in 20.4% of patients tested and elevation of troponin I in 13% of patients tested (2). No patients had ST-segment elevation on ECG. In-hospital mortality was 8% in the entire group; however, troponin elevation and ischemic ECG changes were associated with 38% and 17% in-hospital mortality, respectively. Troponin elevation was more common in those with National Institutes of Health Stroke Scale (NIHSS) greater than 10 compared to those with NIHSS ≤10 (21.4% vs. 6.8%, respectively), and ischemic changes on ECG were also more common in those with NIHSS greater than 10 (26.8% vs. 12.1%). In-hospital mortality was 17.9% versus 4.5% in these respective groups. Whether mortality was entirely due to a more severe stroke or partially augmented by myocardial injury was not explored in this study. Nonetheless, abnormal findings on ECG or troponin I suggest an increased risk for death during hospitalization.

A separate study of troponin T of 181 patients with acute ischemic stroke found abnormal elevations in 17% of patients (3). Troponin T elevation was associated with a 40% in-hospital mortality compared with 13% in those who did not have troponin elevation. At 60 days, mortality differences persisted. A multivariate analysis, which included age, altered level of consciousness, and raised troponin T concentrations, found all three variables to be independent predictors of mortality. Other measures of stroke severity, included in the multivariable analysis, were not predictors in this study. Similar to the aforementioned studies, most patients were not symptomatic.

The risk of myocardial injury persists for years after ischemic stroke and transient ischemic attack. A meta-analysis of 39 studies, which included 65,996 patients, followed for a mean of 3.5 years found that annual rates of non-fatal and fatal myocardial infarction were 0.9% and 1.1%, respectively (4). The annual risk of myocardial infarction at approximately 2% per year remained linear over time. In patients with intracerebral hemorrhage, similar risks of myocardial injury as seen in ischemic stroke are also found. A study of 235 patients found that approximately 16% had elevation of troponin I within 24 hours of onset (5). Among patients with troponin I elevations, mortality was 58% compared with 34% who did not have troponin elevations. In this study, troponin I greater than 0.4 was an independent predictor of death. Among patients with subarachnoid hemorrhage, a meta-analysis of 12 studies involving 2,214 patients found a rate of 30% with elevated troponin levels at admission (6). Troponin elevation was associated with delayed cerebral ischemia, poor outcome, and death.

Cardiac Arrhythmias

Abnormalities on ECG following stroke have been known since the 1940s (7). Changes, including T-wave abnormalities and QT prolongation, occur in up to 70% of stroke patients (8). Most of these changes are not associated with immediate life-threatening events; however, ventricular arrhythmias can result in sudden death (9). Cardiac arrhythmias are seen in approximately 25% of acute stroke patients within 72 hours of admission (10). Atrial fibrillation is the most common arrhythmia occurring in approximately 60% of all patients identified as having any arrhythmia. The next most common arrhythmias are focal atrial tachycardia, Mobitz type II atrioventricular block, and asystole/sinoatrial block. Insular infarction, in particular, appears to confer an increased risk of these arrhythmias in prospective studies (11,12). However, data from randomized controlled trials of prolonged cardiac monitoring failed to show an increased risk of atrial fibrillation based on infarction in different brain regions (13). Long-term cardiac monitoring of patients with ischemic stroke by means of an implanted cardiac monitor suggests that nearly a third of patients with cryptogenic stroke will ultimately be found to have atrial fibrillation by 3 years (14).

A retrospective cross-sectional study of 200 acute ischemic stroke patients identified an in-hospital mortality rate of 8%. Of the 200 patients 28.5% had an ejection fraction less than 50%, 20.4% had ischemic changes on ECG with T-wave inversions or ST-segment depressions, 10.5% presented with atrial fibrillation, 13% had serum troponin I elevation, and 1.1% had potentially lethal arrhythmias on telemetry. In-hospital mortality was more prevalent among those with systolic dysfunction, troponin elevation, atrial fibrillation, and ischemic changes on ECG. Following subarachnoid hemorrhage, any ECG change can occur in 50% or more of patients; however, clinically significant arrhythmias occur in 4% of these patients (15). Approximately 75% of these arrhythmias are atrial fibrillation and atrial flutter. Predictors of a significant arrhythmia include older age, abnormal ECG at admission, and a history of arrhythmia. In this population, significant arrhythmias predict myocardial ischemia, hyperglycemia, herniation, death, and severe disability.

PATHOPHYSIOLOGY

Potential mechanisms underlying myocardial injury and electrical abnormalities detected on ECG include hypothalamic–pituitary–adrenal axis alteration, alterations in immune system function, and gut microbiome dysbiosis (16). The catecholamine surge theory postulates that release of catecholamines from the adrenal glands during stress such as acute stroke can lead to myocardial injury. During brain death, and possibly stroke, an increase in circulating catecholamines occurs as well as a significant increase in the amount of catecholamines released from myocardial nerve endings (17). In turn, this leads to damage to the adjacent myocardium (18). Experimental animal studies corroborate this relationship in stroke (19). In subarachnoid hemorrhage, the surge in catecholamines can lead to prolongation of the QT interval and myocardial injury (20).

The location of injury may also play a role in cardiac involvement after stroke. Ischemia involving the insula increases the risk of cardiac complications including arrhythmias and myocardial injury (21). Some studies suggest that laterality is also important. Because of differential control of the autonomic nervous system, with the right hemisphere controlling sympathetic function and the left hemisphere controlling parasympathetic function, different complications are seen (19). Autonomic derangement has been observed after right insular infarction and is associated with arrhythmias and increased mortality (12), while left hemisphere infarctions are associated with an increased risk of myocardial events and wall motion abnormalities (22). Increased sympathetic activity during subarachnoid hemorrhage is also associated with myocardial injury (23).

Blood–brain barrier disruption leads to entry of inflammatory cytokines, macrophages, and neutrophils into the brain (24). Further disruption of the blood–brain barrier as a result of the increased inflammatory activity leads to augmentation of the peripheral immune response. Release of tumor necrosis factor-alpha leads to the breakdown of troponin I and results in impaired cardiac contractility (25). A systemic inflammatory response syndrome is found in approximately 50% of patients with subarachnoid hemorrhage at admission and the vast majority of patients within a week of onset (26). An increase in the number of circulating monocytes occurs after myocardial infarction and is associated with poor cardiac function and reduced left ventricular function (27).

A new concept regarding the relationship between brain and cardiac function includes an intermediary organ, the gastrointestinal tract. The brain–gut axis, which includes signaling neuropeptides, can affect the immune response and worsen outcome after stroke when microflora are altered (28). Ischemic stroke patients with increased bacterial counts of *Lactobacillus ruminis* have elevated systemic inflammatory markers and altered metabolism (29). In turn, these changes can lead to or worsen cardiac function (30). Choline, trimethylamine N-oxide, and betaine are gut microflora-dependent metabolites and are associated with cardiovascular disease (31). The interactions between brain, heart, and the gastrointestinal tract and their simultaneous effects on brain and cardiac function after stroke require further investigation.

PREVENTION

Prevention of arrhythmias after stroke has not been studied to the same extent as arrhythmias after myocardial infarction. In the 1980s and 1990s, lidocaine drips were frequently used to treat premature ventricular contractions but were ultimately found not to be beneficial for the reduction of fatal arrhythmic events. Some studies suggested that patients taking beta-blockers and angiotensin-converting enzyme (ACE) inhibitors had reduced occurrences of sudden death, but these studies have not been confirmed further. In patients with subarachnoid hemorrhage, one study found that preadmission use of beta-blockers was associated with a reduced risk of left ventricular dysfunction and cerebral vasospasm (32). At this time, the use of antiarrhythmic agents for the prevention of arrhythmias following stroke is not supported by existing literature and guidelines. Further study is needed to better elucidate the potential role of antiarrhythmics in patients perceived to be at higher risk, such as strokes affecting the insular cortex.

Prevention of myocardial infarction after stroke, which occurs in at least 10% of patients by 5 years, has not been studied in a randomized trial. And in some cases, exercise-induced ischemia led to the identification of those with significant coronary artery disease and eventual stenting. If these findings are confirmed in larger cohorts, cardiac stress test for stroke patients may prove essential to identify those with increased future risk for myocardial injury and death. Depending on its effect size, the reduction in mortality could exceed that of some acute interventions. However, other routine evaluations, such as cardiologist workup for patients with asymptomatic carotid artery disease, do not appear to reduce the risk of myocardial infarction in that patient population. Prior studies of cardiac rehabilitation in stroke patients found improvement in lipid profile, aerobic capacity, and body mass index, as well as reductions in smoking rates (33), providing additional potential mechanisms for a mortality benefit.

IDENTIFICATION

Identification of arrhythmias immediately following stroke is accomplished by monitoring patients on telemetry. Current guidelines support routine monitoring of stroke patients within the first 24 hours after stroke (34), though the effect on mortality remains unknown. Additionally, the duration of monitoring in hospital is also uncertain without data to support specific durations. The main advantage of continuous monitoring is the identification of atrial arrhythmias among those either not initially known to have atrial fibrillation or detected on ECG tracing at admission, which is at least 4 seconds duration. Posthospitalization, monitoring for arrhythmias can be performed with various Holter devices for 24 hours to 30 days (35), and implantable loop recorders for as long as 2 to 3 years (14). In general, the longer the duration of monitoring, the greater the likelihood of atrial arrhythmia detection. Use of these devices has not been shown to reduce mortality at this time, though cardiac outcomes were not a specific focus of original studies.

Evidence of myocardial injury is accomplished through serologic and electrophysiological testing. Serologic studies typically include a serum troponin at admission and are recommended in acute stroke guidelines (34). If there is evidence of elevated troponin at admission, troponin levels are trended over 24 hours, similar to what is done in patients who are admitted with chest pain. ECG is also routinely done at admission to evaluate for concomitant myocardial injury or ischemia.

MANAGEMENT

When an elevated troponin is identified in the setting of acute stroke, correlation with ECG is performed to determine whether it represents an ST-segment myocardial infarction versus a non–ST-segment myocardial infarction. A cardiology consultation should be obtained in these circumstances to determine further cardiac care. Occasionally, the goals of cardiac care may be in conflict with those of stroke care. For example, the recommendations may be to maintain both a systolic blood pressure below 140 mmHg to reduce cardiac afterload and a higher pressure to adequately perfuse the brain. In these situations, a compromise is often made to target a systolic blood pressure that represents a compromise between these two competing goals. Another situation that arises is the request to use heparin in patients with ST-segment myocardial infarction. When there is a large ischemic stroke, it may be considered a higher risk to introduce an anticoagulant. Risks versus benefits of initiating an anticoagulant in the face of two opposing needs should be considered. In addition to ST-segment and non–ST-segment myocardial infarction, a third situation may occur in which a mild elevation of troponin is not sufficient to be deemed infarction and is termed "demand ischemia" (36). In these cases, no specific intervention is typically required and cardiac consultation usually suggests monitoring of troponin levels.

For patients who are identified as having atrial fibrillation, appropriate anticoagulation in suitable patients is recommended (34). For those with atrial fibrillation who are not candidates for anticoagulation, use of antiplatelet therapy is recommended. Concomitant use of anticoagulants and antiplatelet agents is frequently done in patients with comorbid atrial fibrillation and coronary artery disease, but the evidence supporting this practice is uncertain (34). Other therapeutic considerations include clinical trials of left atrial appendage closure or ligation.

Patients who are identified as having potentially lethal arrhythmias are very uncommon. However, when these events do occur, consultation with cardiology is recommended to determine appropriate antiarrhythmic treatment. For patients with rapid ventricular response atrial fibrillation, diltiazem is often used in the acute setting to lower heart rate. A low dose ($\leq$0.2 mg/kg) might be as effective as a standard (0.2–0.3 mg/kg) and high dose ($\geq$0.3 mg/kg) with less risk of hypotension (37).

CONCLUSION

Cardiac complications after acute ischemic stroke, intracerebral hemorrhage, and subarachnoid hemorrhage are common and include arrhythmias as well as myocardial injury. The timing of these events may be immediately after cerebral injury or delayed with events happening months later. The effects of these complications can range from minor with no residual lingering effect to fatal. Though the mechanism of these events is not entirely understood, surges in catecholamine and differential modulation of the sympathetic and parasympathetic nervous systems likely play a role. Furthermore, a systemic inflammatory response may also contribute. Detection of complications can be accomplished through serologic testing for myocardial biomarkers and rhythm monitoring. Identification of these events can lead to alteration in management, particularly in the identification of atrial fibrillation, and a change in antithrombotic treatment. Myocardial infarction is typically managed in collaboration with cardiology. Treatments include beta-blockade, antiplatelet treatment, and statin use, most of which overlap with acute ischemic stroke treatment. Future studies are needed to identify early interventions that may reduce the likelihood of these events.

REFERENCES

1. Chin PL, Kaminski J, Rout M. Myocardial infarction coincident with cerebrovascular accidents in the elderly. *Age Ageing.* 1977;6:29–37. doi:10.1093/ageing/6.1.29
2. Wira CR 3rd, Rivers E, Martinez-Capolino C, et al. Cardiac complications in acute ischemic stroke. *West J Emerg Med.* 2011;12:414–420. doi:10.5811/westjem.2011.2.1785
3. James P, Ellis CJ, Whitlock RM, et al. Relation between troponin T concentration and mortality in patients presenting with an acute stroke: observational study. *BMJ.* 2000;320:1502–1504. doi:10.1136/bmj.320.7248.1502
4. Touze E, Varenne O, Chatellier G, et al. Risk of myocardial infarction and vascular death after transient ischemic attack and ischemic stroke: a systematic review and meta-analysis. *Stroke.* 2005;36:2748–2755. doi:10.1161/01.STR.0000190118.02275.33
5. Hays A, Diringer MN. Elevated troponin levels are associated with higher mortality following intracerebral hemorrhage. *Neurology.* 2006;66:1330–1334. doi:10.1212/01.wnl.0000210523.22944.9b
6. Zhang L, Wang Z, Qi S. Cardiac troponin elevation and outcome after subarachnoid hemorrhage: a systematic review and meta-analysis. *J Stroke Cerebrovasc Dis.* 2015;24:2375–2384. doi:10.1016/j.jstrokecerebrovasdis.2015.06.030
7. Byer E, Ashman R, Toth LA. Electrocardiograms with large, upright T waves and long Q-T intervals. *Am Heart J.* 1947;33:796–806. doi:10.1016/0002-8703(47)90025-2
8. Korpelainen JT, Sotaniemi KA, Huikuri HV, et al. Circadian rhythm of heart rate variability is reversibly abolished in ischemic stroke. *Stroke.* 1997;28:2150–2154. doi:10.1161/01.STR.28.11.2150
9. Oppenheimer SM, Cechetto DF, Hachinski VC. Cerebrogenic cardiac arrhythmias. Cerebral electrocardiographic influences and their role in sudden death. *Arch Neurol.* 1990;47:513–519. doi:10.1001/archneur.1990.00530050029008

10. Kallmunzer B, Breuer L, Kahl N, et al. Serious cardiac arrhythmias after stroke: incidence, time course, and predictors—a systematic, prospective analysis. *Stroke*. 2012;43:2892–2897. doi:10.1161/STROKEAHA.112.664318
11. Abboud H, Berroir S, Labreuche J, et al. Insular involvement in brain infarction increases risk for cardiac arrhythmia and death. *Ann Neurol*. 2006;59:691–699. doi:10.1002/ana.20806
12. Colivicchi F, Bassi A, Santini M, et al. Prognostic implications of right-sided insular damage, cardiac autonomic derangement, and arrhythmias after acute ischemic stroke. *Stroke*. 2005;36:1710–1715. doi:10.1161/01.STR.0000173400.19346.bd
13. Bernstein RA, Di Lazzaro V, Rymer MM, et al. Infarct topography and detection of atrial fibrillation in cryptogenic stroke: results from CRYSTAL AF. *Cerebrovasc Dis*. 2015;40:91–96. doi:10.1159/000437018
14. Sanna T, Diener HC, Passman RS, et al. Cryptogenic stroke and underlying atrial fibrillation. *N Engl J Med*. 2014;370:2478–2486. doi:10.1056/NEJMoa1313600
15. Frontera JA, Parra A, Shimbo D, et al. Cardiac arrhythmias after subarachnoid hemorrhage: risk factors and impact on outcome. *Cerebrovasc Dis*. 2008;26:71–78. doi:10.1159/000135711
16. Chen Z, Venkat P, Seyfried D, et al. Brain-heart interaction: cardiac complications after stroke. *Circ Res*. 2017;121:451–468. doi:10.1161/CIRCRESAHA.117.311170
17. Mertes PM, Carteaux JP, Jaboin Y, et al. Estimation of myocardial interstitial norepinephrine release after brain death using cardiac microdialysis. *Transplantation*. 1994;57:371–377. doi:10.1097/00007890-199402150-00010
18. Jacob WA, Van Bogaert A, De Groodt-Lasseel MH. Myocardial ultrastructure and haemodynamic reactions during experimental subarachnoid haemorrhage. *J Mol Cell Cardiol*. 1972;4:287–298. doi:10.1016/0022-2828(72)90076-4
19. Hachinski VC, Smith KE, Silver MD, et al. Acute myocardial and plasma catecholamine changes in experimental stroke. *Stroke*. 1986;17:387–390. doi:10.1161/01.STR.17.3.387
20. Cruickshank JM, Neil-Dwyer G, Stott AW. Possible role of catecholamines, corticosteroids, and potassium in production of electrocardiographic abnormalities associated with subarachnoid haemorrhage. *Br Heart J*. 1974;36:697–706. doi:10.1136/hrt.36.7.697
21. Sander D, Winbeck K, Klingelhofer J, et al. Prognostic relevance of pathological sympathetic activation after acute thromboembolic stroke. *Neurology*. 2001;57:833–838. doi:10.1212/WNL.57.5.833
22. Laowattana S, Zeger SL, Lima JAC, et al. Left insular stroke is associated with adverse cardiac outcome. *Neurology*. 2006;66:477–483. doi:10.1212/01.wnl.0000202684.29640.60

23. Masuda T, Sato K, Yamamoto S-I, et al. Sympathetic nervous activity and myocardial damage immediately after subarachnoid hemorrhage in a unique animal model. *Stroke*. 2002;33:1671–1676. doi:10.1161/01.STR.0000016327.74392.02
24. Gelderblom M, Leypoldt F, Steinbach K, et al. Temporal and spatial dynamics of cerebral immune cell accumulation in stroke. *Stroke*. 2009;40:1849–1857. doi:10.1161/STROKEAHA.108.534503
25. Adams V, Linke A, Wisloff U, et al. Myocardial expression of Murf-1 and MAFbx after induction of chronic heart failure: effect on myocardial contractility. *Cardiovasc Res*. 2007;73:120–129. doi:10.1016/j.cardiores.2006.10.026
26. Dhar R, Diringer MN. The burden of the systemic inflammatory response predicts vasospasm and outcome after subarachnoid hemorrhage. *Neurocrit Care*. 2008;8:404–412. doi:10.1007/s12028-008-9054-2
27. Tsujioka H, Imanishi T, Ikejima H, et al. Impact of heterogeneity of human peripheral blood monocyte subsets on myocardial salvage in patients with primary acute myocardial infarction. *J Am Coll Cardiol*. 2009;54:130–138. doi:10.1016/j.jacc.2009.04.021
28. Benakis C, Brea D, Caballero S, et al. Commensal microbiota affects ischemic stroke outcome by regulating intestinal gammadelta T cells. *Nat Med*. 2016;22:516–523. doi:10.1038/nm.4068
29. Yamashiro K, Tanaka R, Urabe T, et al. Gut dysbiosis is associated with metabolism and systemic inflammation in patients with ischemic stroke. *PLoS One*. 2017;12:e0171521. doi:10.1371/journal.pone.0171521
30. Nagatomo Y, Tang WH. Intersections between microbiome and heart failure: revisiting the gut hypothesis. *J Card Fail*. 2015;21:973–980. doi:10.1016/j.cardfail.2015.09.017
31. Wang Z, Klipfell E, Bennett BJ, et al. Gut flora metabolism of phosphatidylcholine promotes cardiovascular disease. *Nature*. 2011;472:57–63. doi:10.1038/nature09922
32. Chalouhi N, Daou B, Okabe T, et al. Beta-blocker therapy and impact on outcome after aneurysmal subarachnoid hemorrhage: a cohort study. *J Neurosurg*. 2016;125:730–736. doi:10.3171/2015.7.JNS15956
33. Prior PL, Hachinski V, Unsworth K, et al. Comprehensive cardiac rehabilitation for secondary prevention after transient ischemic attack or mild stroke: I: feasibility and risk factors. *Stroke*. 2011;42:3207–3213. doi:10.1161/STROKEAHA.111.620187
34. Powers WJ, Rabinstein AA, Ackerson T, et al. 2018 Guidelines for the early management of patients with acute ischemic stroke: a guideline for healthcare professionals from the American Heart Association/American Stroke Association. *Stroke*. 2018;49(3):e46–e110. doi:10.1161/STR.0000000000000158

35. Gladstone DJ, Spring M, Dorian P, et al. Atrial fibrillation in patients with cryptogenic stroke. *N Engl J Med.* 2014;370:2467–2477. doi:10.1056/NEJMoa1311376
36. Tanindi A, Cemri M. Troponin elevation in conditions other than acute coronary syndromes. *Vasc Health Risk Manag.* 2011;7:597–603. doi:10.2147/VHRM.S24509
37. Lee J, Kim K, Lee CC, et al. Low-dose diltiazem in atrial fibrillation with rapid ventricular response. *Am J Emerg Med.* 2011;29:849–854. doi:10.1016/j.ajem.2010.03.021

13 Pulmonary Complications After Acute Ischemic and Hemorrhagic Stroke

Daniel Agustín Godoy and Ali Seifi

KEY POINTS

- Respiratory compromise is highly prevalent in the acute phase of stroke.
- Potential pulmonary complications are dynamic, varied, and evolving.
- Stroke physiopathology is complex, but there is clearly an interaction between the lungs and the brain.
- The most consistent predisposing factors for pulmonary complications are consciousness level, stroke severity, stroke location, dysphagia, and mechanical ventilation (MV).
- The predominant respiratory complications associated with stroke are pneumonia, dysphagia, gastric content aspiration, and abnormal ventilatory patterns during sleep.
- For diagnosing different respiratory complications, clinical examination, chest radiography, and assessing gas exchange are essential.
- Respiratory complications increase the possibility of poor results.
- Preventive measures play a critical role in the management of respiratory complications.

INTRODUCTION

Individuals suffering from acute stroke, whether ischemic or hemorrhagic, are at risk for developing a broad spectrum of respiratory complications (1–6). The impact of these complications depends on a number of factors, including the severity, location, and extent of stroke (1,4–6). Respiratory complications increase a patient's risk for compromised lung function via ventilatory pattern alteration and upper airway obstruction; this can eventually lead to infection, atelectasis, pulmonary embolism (PE), or acute respiratory distress

 DOI: 10.1891/9780826124791.0013

syndrome (ARDS) (1,4–6). Patients with compromised consciousness often require artificial airways and mechanical ventilatory support to maintain a stable condition, which elevates their risk for damage induced by therapeutic modalities (1,6). Respiratory compromise of any origin causes the appearance of secondary insults, such as hypoxemia, hypercapnia, and/or hypocapnia; that must be managed in order to prevent the aggravation of primary injury (1–6).

EPIDEMIOLOGY, MORBIDITY, AND MORTALITY

Nearly two-thirds of stroke patients have an episode of hypoxemia lasting more than 5 minutes (2,3). The prevalence of respiratory complications in this population is generally high, but the precise numbers vary according to stroke etiology (1,4,7). Among patients with spontaneous intracerebral hemorrhage (ICH), 30% develop pulmonary complications, especially during the early phase of evolution (5). The incidence is lower among patients with subarachnoid hemorrhage (SAH), averaging 15% to 20%; under these conditions, complications emerge more frequently after the patient's second week (6). Among individuals with ischemic stroke, the prevalence of respiratory complications is lowest: 5% to 10% (7). Respiratory compromise brought about by any type of complication prolongs hospital stay and contributes to a patient's final result (7). One study reported that the mere presence of respiratory compromise increases a patient's risk of death by three times (7).

The following conditions are considered risk factors for the development of respiratory complications (5–11):

- Low levels of consciousness
- National Institutes of Health (NIH) scale score greater than 15 points
- Stroke of the posterior circulation
- Dysphagia
- Mechanical ventilation
- Nasogastric tube

Less consistently reported risk factors include age, dysarthria, hyperglycemia, basal ganglia involvement, hemorrhagic transformation of infarct, and the use of proton pump inhibitors or H_2 receptor blockers (5–11).

PATHOPHYSIOLOGY

Abnormal ventilatory patterns cause pharyngeal and laryngeal musculature dysfunction. Because the contraction of these muscle groups keeps the upper airways open by increasing anteroposterior and transverse diameters, this dysfunction ultimately results in airflow obstruction. When swallowing, gag, or cough reflexes are compromised along with the sighing mechanism, pharyngeal secretions can accumulate and provoke atelectasis, which subsequently triggers hypoxemia by altering the ventilation–perfusion ratio (V/Q) and increasing the shunt fraction (1–11). These mechanisms decrease vital capacity, promote air trapping, and can cause the lungs to become overdistended. These phenomena cause mechanical alterations in total lung compliance and airway resistance, which increases the work of breathing and predisposes the patient to respiratory muscle fatigue (1–11).

Simultaneously, the compromise of the aforementioned defensive reflexes creates the necessary conditions for gastric content aspiration; this increases the prevalence of infectious complications, primarily pneumonia (1–12). Certain severe subtypes of stroke cause the sympathetic nervous system (SNS) to become overactive and flood the bloodstream with catecholamines. The surge of catecholamines elicits pulmonary hypertension and the extravasation of fluids into the pulmonary interstitial tissue, which triggers neurogenic pulmonary edema (NPE) because of the increased permeability of the alveolar–capillary barrier (1,4–6). Prolonged immobilization, another relevant sequela of stroke, increases the incidence of deep vein thrombosis (DVT) and PE (1,4–6). Therapeutic modalities can also play a role in disease progression: MV, when used inappropriately, causes the release of inflammation mediators that are capable of perpetuating neurological damage and causing/aggravating lung involvement (13–17) (Figures 13.1 and 13.2).

IDENTIFICATION

Although many physicians employ the use of a high respiratory rate alarm to detect potential respiratory issues, in most situations gas exchange assessment, chest radiography, and the patient's overall clinical picture will provide sufficient evidence of any respiratory complications (1–11). Signs of lung function deterioration include state of consciousness alterations, disorientation, agitation, restlessness, or progressive somnolence, which can lead to coma in severe cases (1–11). Signs that require close monitoring include accumulation of secretions in the pharynx cavity (pharyngeal lake), weak or ineffective cough, and dysphagia. Knowledge of respiratory semiology is especially helpful when assessing a patient's condition. Tachypnea, tachycardia, changes in sputum characteristics (greater quantity, purulence), or fever combined with alterations in

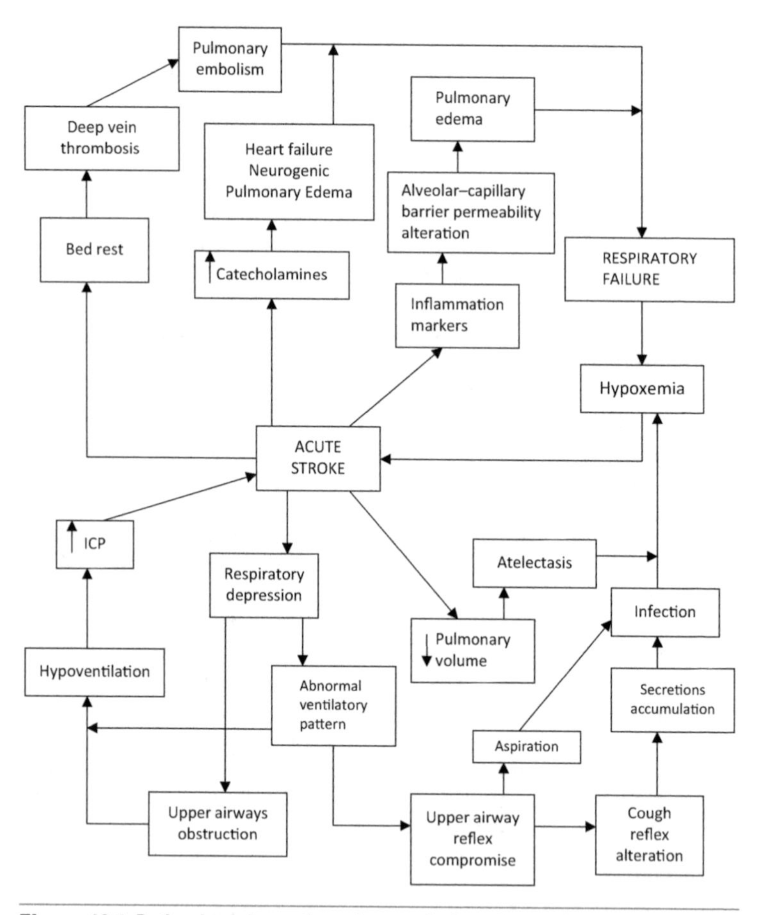

Figure 13.1 Pathophysiology of respiratory dysfunction during stroke.

arterial gases or arterial saturation (pulse oximetry) indicate a need to establish a quick diagnosis (11). The presence of nasal flaring, the use of accessory muscles of ventilation (sternocleidomastoid, trapezius), diaphragmatic paradox, and cyanosis all indicate muscular fatigue and imminent respiratory arrest (1–11).

Gas exchange can sufficiently be determined using noninvasive continuous pulse oximetry and the pressures of arterial blood gasses. These include PaO_2, $PaCO_2$, and derived indices, the most widely used being the PaO_2/FiO_2 ratio (1–11). Simple chest radiography can be used to detect most reported complications when the results are analyzed within the general clinical context.

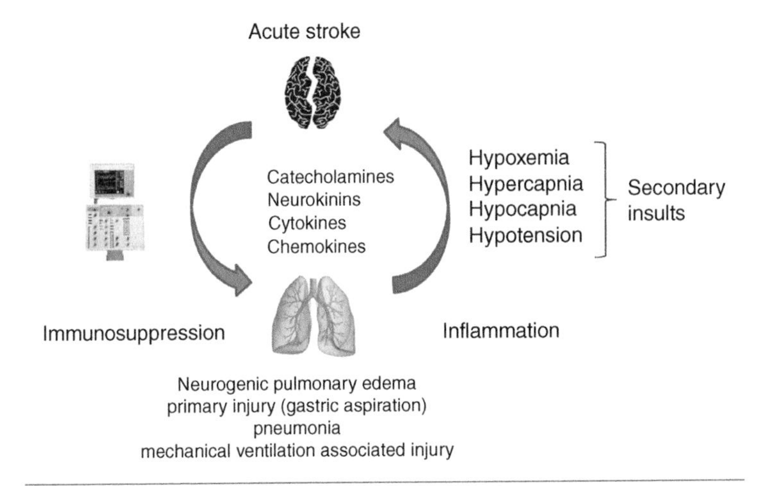

Figure 13.2 Brain–lung interaction.

Occasionally, it is recommended that physicians perform CT or CT angiography (CTA) of the thorax (1–11). Complementary studies that cover the diagnostic spectrum include cultures of respiratory secretions or pleural effusions, airway endoscopy, Doppler of the lower limbs, radioscopy (for dysphagia or diaphragmatic evaluation), electromyography, and polysomnography (1–11).

EVOLUTIONARY CLASSIFICATION OF RESPIRATORY COMPLICATIONS OF STROKE

Respiratory complications that can occur after stroke (according to chronology of appearance):

a) **Immediate** (first 48 hours)

   Abnormal ventilatory patterns

   Dysphagia/Aspiration of gastric content/Chemical pneumonitis

   atelectasis

   Neurogenic pulmonary edema

b) Mediate (>72 hours <14 days)

   Pneumonia

   ARDS

   Neurogenic/Cardiogenic pulmonary edema

   Pulmonary injury induced by MV

c) **Delayed** (>14 days)
   Upper airway lesions (orotracheal tube, tracheostomy)
   Polyneuromyopathy
   DVT/PE
   Sleep disordered breathing

ABNORMAL VENTILATORY PATTERNS

Stroke alters ventilatory pattern in 18% to 88% of cases (1,4). These alterations are usually seen in individuals with severe stroke who have a compromised state of consciousness or spinal cord infarction (1,4). Examples of abnormal ventilatory patterns that have been described in the literature include apneusis, ataxia, Cheyne–Stokes breathing, periodic breathing, and agonal breathing (gasping) (1,4). These patterns are more likely to be discovered when the patients are asleep because voluntary control tends to compensate for the alterations during the waking state. Patients will frequently demonstrate a mix of abnormal patterns rather than a single type.

Cardiac instability is associated with all types of abnormal ventilatory patterns. Generally speaking, abnormal ventilatory patterns lack predictive significance and do not necessarily indicate the compromise of any specific anatomical site (1,4). Sustained central neurogenic hyperventilation is the only abnormal ventilatory pattern with a clearly established prognostic value (1,4).

The diagnosis of abnormal ventilatory pattern is clinical (1,4). Complementary studies are not necessary!

DYSPHAGIA–ASPIRATION OF GASTRIC CONTENTS

Swallowing disorders are prevalent in stroke patients, but they are especially common in patients who have suffered brainstem or hemispheric infarction (1,4,8,12,18–22). The numbers vary according to the method of detection, but the reported incidence ranges from 22% to 65% (1,4,8,12,18–22). Swallowing disorders increase a patient's risk for infection, malnutrition, and mortality; they also prolong a patient's length of stay in critical care units and their overall hospital stay (1,4,8,12,18–22). In more than 80% of cases, swallowing disorders are functional and transient; patients usually recover after 2 to 4 weeks.

To determine if a patient might have a swallowing disorder, evaluate their ability to ingest 5 mL of water at the bedside (12,18–22). Possible signs and symptoms include weak cough, cough when swallowing, nasal voice or nasal regurgitation, hoarse voice, absence of nausea reflexes, prolonged swallowing, and accumulation of secretions or food in pharynx (1,4,8,12,18–22). Video fluoroscopy or endoscopy can also be used to evaluate complex cases (8,18–22). We have included an algorithm (Figure 13.3) to assist in the assessment of these disorders.

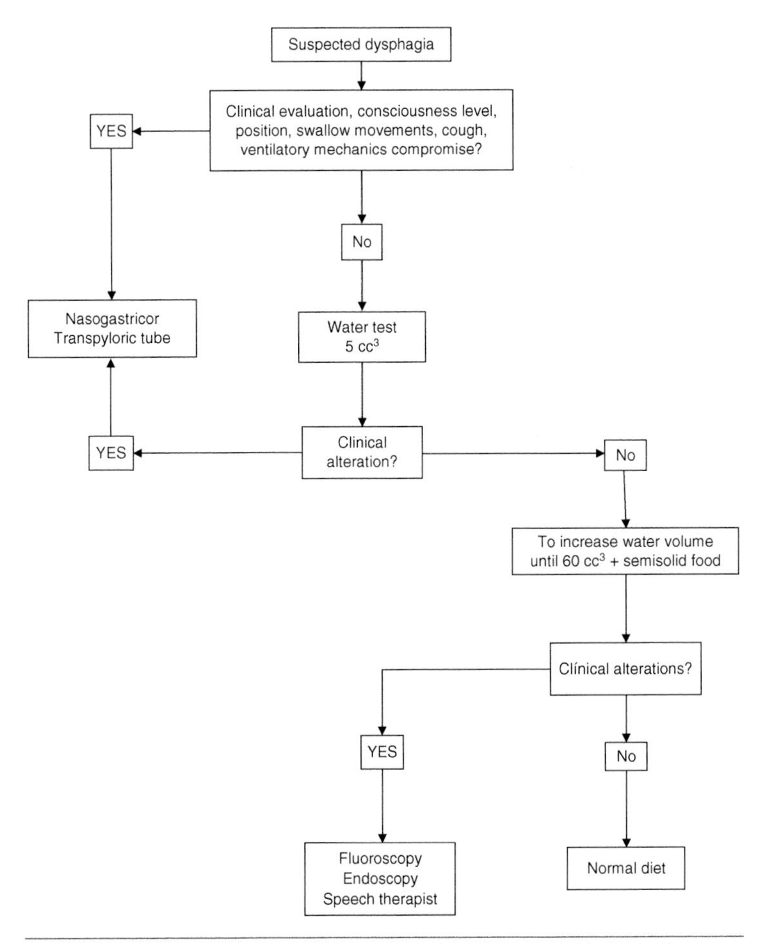

Figure 13.3 Algorithm for dysphagia evaluation at the bedside in stroke patients.

PNEUMONIA

Pneumonia is one of the most severe and prevalent complications seen in stroke patients (1,4,12,23–35) (Figure 13.4). Its incidence ranges from 5% to 9% (1,4,12,23–35). In the first 48 hours of stroke, pneumonia is the most frequent cause of fever (1,4,12,23–35). Among stroke-related deaths, 34% are due to pneumonia.

Population-based cohort studies have established several modifiable, predisposing factors for pneumonia, including alcoholism, the aspiration of gastric content (present in 21%–42% of cases), the use of a nasogastric or bladder catheter, the use of antihistamine antacids (ranitidine), the use of proton pump blockers, and the presence of atrial fibrillation (1,4,12,23–35). Some examples of predisposing factors for pneumonia that cannot be managed or modified are age, stroke severity, dysphagia, and dysarthria (1,4,12,23–35). Therapies and care associated with the management of pneumonia (such as MV) increase the possibility of poor outcomes. Those factors also make it more difficult to establish a differential or definitive diagnosis (1,4,12,23–35). Under those circumstances, it will often be necessary to use more sophisticated, invasive techniques, such as alveolar bronchial lavage by fibrobronchoscopy, in order to better assess the patient's case.

Pneumonias primarily affect the dependent lung; the germs responsible for infection usually originate from the oral cavity or the pharyngeal cavity. Haemophilus influenzae, streptococcus pneumoniae, and staphylococcus aureus are all examples of

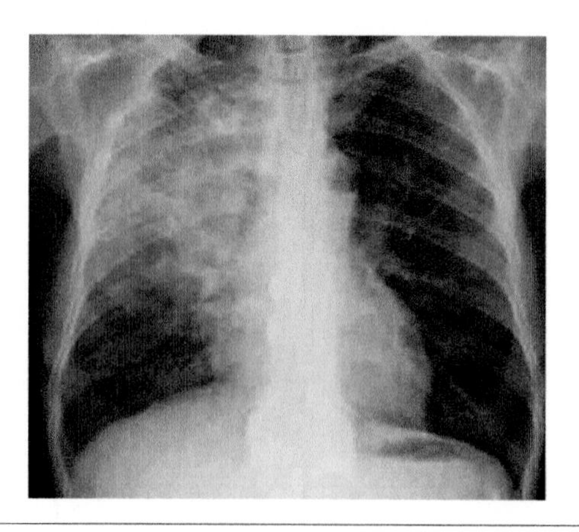

Figure 13.4 Pneumonia.

potentially responsible culprits. If a patient stays in the ICU for longer than 48 hours, there is greater chance that gram-negative bacilli will enter the lungs through their respiratory tract and dominate their pharyngeal flora (1,4,12,23–35).

NEUROGENIC PULMONARY EDEMA

NPE is a rare clinical syndrome linked to severe injury occurring at a nonspecific location. It most often associated with poor grade SAH or severe forms of spontaneous ICH (36–38). NPE usually appears at the beginning of the injury; it can resolve or be fatal, depending on the evolution of neurological damage (36–38). The pathophysiology of the syndrome is not completely understood. A concomitant increase in intravascular/interstitial pressure and capillary permeability appears to be the driving mechanism at work. It is hypothesized that SNS hyperactivity occurs due to hypothalamic stress; this causes a massive increase in catecholamine production that subsequently injures the pulmonary capillaries by increasing hydrostatic pressure and the permeability of the alveolar–capillary barrier (36–38). Diagnosing NPE requires one to rule out any cardiogenic causes of pulmonary edema (36–38).

PULMONARY INJURY INDUCED BY MV

MV is a crucial component of acute brain injury management; however, it is not free of complications (13–15,36–43). In a large-scale, epidemiological study conducted in America, the authors reported that MV was used in 12.5% of individuals who suffered stroke; within that population, according to stroke type, 8% were ischemic, 30% were ICH, and 38.5% were SAH (43). The mortality of stroke patients requiring MV was 52% (43).

The inappropriate use of MV causes the release of mediators that initiate a systemic inflammatory state; this inflammation can induce or perpetuate damage to the lungs and other organs (13–17,35). The excessive tension and repeated lung deformation caused by MV affect the fibroskeleton, microvasculature, small airways, and interstitial tissue via different mechanisms of damage (13–17):

- Volutrauma: excessive stretching and rupture of the alveolar wall
- Barotrauma: excessive airway pressures
- Atelectrauma: constant opening and closing of the alveolar space
- Biotrauma: release of inflammatory mediators

Protective ventilation combined with low tidal volumes and adequate positive end-expiratory pressure (PEEP) levels diminishes the patient's likelihood of developing complications and reduces the relative risk of death by 22% (13–17).

ACUTE RESPIRATORY DISTRESS SYNDROME

ARDS is one of the most severe forms of acute respiratory failure presentation. It generally develops 2 or 3 days after a precipitating event (44–48). Although stroke is an infrequent cause, incidences of 4% secondary to ischemic stroke and 20% to 30% after SAH have been reported (4,44–48). The most relevant predisposing factors for ARDS are the aspiration of gastric contents, pneumonia, and sepsis (4,44–48). The pathophysiological progression of ARDS begins with lung inflammation, the loss of alveolar–capillary membrane permeability, and pulmonary surfactant reduction followed by the appearance of hemorrhagic lesions, hyaline membrane formation, and fibrosis in the late stage (44–48). The predominant mechanism at work is refractory hypoxemia secondary to increased shunt fraction (48). The diagnosis is clinical–radiological (47,48).

According to the Berlin definition, a description of ARDS proposed in 2011 by a panel of international experts convened by the European Society of Intensive Care Medicine, ARDS can be recognized as an acute, diffuse inflammatory lung injury that develops within the first 7 days of a known clinical insult or new or worsening respiratory symptoms; it leads to increased pulmonary vascular permeability, increased lung weight, and aerated lung tissue loss (45). Clinical hallmarks of ARDS include hypoxemia and bilateral radiographic opacities, increased venous admixture, increased physiological dead space, decreased lung compliance, and, most notably in acute cases, diffuse alveolar damage (45). The severity of gas exchange compromise can be determined by using the PaO_2/FiO_2 ratio; severe forms of ARDS have a PaO_2/FiO_2 less than 100 mmHg (47,48) (Figure 13.5).

THROMBOEMBOLIC DISEASE (TD)

TD, including DVT and PE, has within the context of stroke, a 40% incidence without prophylaxis (4). The highest prevalence of TD is observed secondary to ischemic stroke (4) (Table 13.1).

The mortality rate associated with PE ranges from 9% to 50% (49–58). The presence of profound hemiplegia, brainstem injuries, and the craniectomy recovery period all predispose patients to PE (4,49–58). Although it may seem unintuitive, there is no evidence to suggest that immobility, by itself, is a risk factor (4–7). It has been

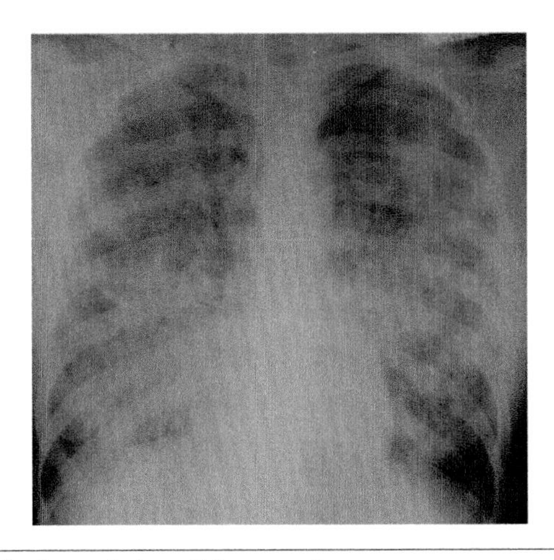

Figure 13.5 Acute respiratory distress syndrome.

postulated that stroke predisposes patients to TD by creating a prothrombotic state via fibrinolytic mechanism compromise (4,49–54). Some therapies that have been developed with this interaction in mind include the use of recombinant human factor VII, the use of tranexamic acid in ICH, and the use of antifibrinolytics during prolonged acute phases of SAH (4,58).

TD is generally a late-onset entity that should be suspected with the sudden onset of restlessness, tachypnea, tachycardia, and hypoxemia (4,49–58). Diagnostic certainty is difficult. The D-dimer test is limited in that it only has a reliable negative predictive value and the results of a ventilation–perfusion scan can be difficult to interpret (4,49–58). Doppler ultrasound scans of the lower limbs

Table 13.1 Prevalence of Venous Thromboembolic Disease Among Stroke Subtypes

Stroke Subtype	DVT	PE
Ischemic	2%–20%	10%–20%
ICH	2%	1%
SAH	5%–7%	1%

DVT, deep vein thrombosis; ICH, intracerebral hemorrhage; PE, pulmonary embolism; SAH, subarachnoid hemorrhage.

can be used to investigate DVT and helicoidal angiotomography can also provide physicians with valuable information (4,49–58) (Figure 13.6).

PREVENTION AND MANAGEMENT OF RESPIRATORY COMPLICATIONS

Most therapies for respiratory complications can be avoided with a rigorous prevention plan. It is of prime importance to begin by evaluating the patient's cough and swallow reflexes (1,4,8,9,12). If they are altered, it is advisable to stop oral feeding and insert a nasogastric or nasojejunal catheter (1,4,8,9,12). Afterward, promptly initiate swallowing rehabilitation (1,4,8,9,12). Glycemic control should also be established to ensure that either hypo- or hyperglycemia does not worsen the patient's condition (59).

Early enteral feeding maintains trophism of the intestinal villi and prevents bacterial translocation while enhancing defensive mechanisms or natural defense barriers. There is no better gastric protector than enteral nutrition, given that both proton pump inhibitors and H_2 receptor blockers have been associated with the development of pneumonia (1,4,7–9,23,24). Contact antacids, such as sucralfate, can be employed to provide gastric protection. However, there exists only low-level evidence of their efficacy.

The patient's head should be positioned at 30 degrees from the horizontal, especially during feeding periods, to reduce the

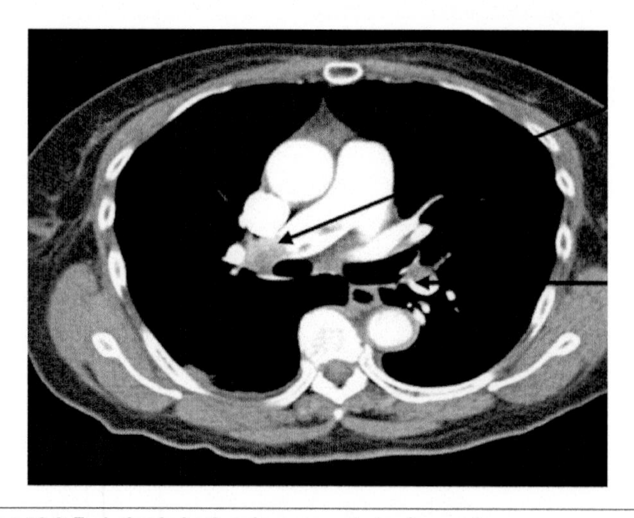

Figure 13.6 Embolus in both pulmonary arteries (arrows).

possibility of gastric content aspiration (1,4,7–9,23,24). Oral hygiene with chlorhexidine and handwashing must be performed at regular intervals and with strict adherence (1,4,7–9,23,24). If pneumonia ensues, secretion cultures and pleural effusions should be used to determine the cause so that the predominant flora can be targeted with antibiotics (1,4,7–9,23,24).

Physiotherapy, bronchodilators, and early mobilization prevent the development of atelectasis, favor the drainage of secretions, and improve gas exchange. When the latter is compromised, the use of supplementary oxygen with high-flow cannulas, continuous positive airway pressure (CPAP), or noninvasive ventilation is necessary (1,4,7–9,23,24). Hyperoxia should be avoided; it increases oxidative stress, causes lung damage via airway inflammation, and promotes atelectasis by resorption (1,4). If the state of consciousness is altered or the ability to protect airway permeability is lost, it is necessary to create an artificial airway (40–42). For coma patients with Glasgow scale scores less than or equal to 8 points, orotracheal intubation is mandatory (40–42). MV is required when the respiratory system is unable to maintain adequate oxygenation to meet tissue demands; among neurocritical patients, normalizing carbon dioxide levels is also relevant because hypercapnia triggers cerebral vasodilation and increases intracranial pressure (1,4,13–17,40–42,45).

MV is indicated in the following situations:

- Severe impairment of neurological status
- Intracranial hypertension
- Respiratory insufficiency that does not respond to conventional oxygen therapy
- Abnormal ventilatory patterns
- Weakness of respiratory muscles
- Apnea

To minimize MV and artificial airway time, use protective ventilation (low tidal volumes with adequate levels of PEEP) and implement a program of sedoanalgesia holidays once the clinical-neurological situation has stabilized (1,4,13–17,40–42,45). Monitor cuff inflation pressure closely and maintain it within an optimal range; if indicated, an early tracheostomy should be performed. Check fluids levels regularly to ensure that negative balances are achieved; if that goal is not met, consider using diuretics (1,4). Secretions should be aspirated only when necessary and only via sterile techniques. Suction probes and ventilator units should both be closed systems.

To minimize the risk of acquiring muscle weakness in the ICU, establish strict glycemic control by avoiding sepsis, steroids, amino glycosides, and muscle relaxants (60). Prophylaxis ofTD should be achieved by mechanical means (elastic stockings, pneumatic intermittent inflation systems) or pharmacological intervention (low molecular weight heparins) depending on the individual circumstances of the case (58). Drafting and executing an infection control plan will help by reducing the risk of exposure to pathogens and providing a clear hierarchy of clinical responsibilities to supervisors and team members (1,4,13–17,40–42,45).

CONCLUSION

Stroke is one of the leading causes of death in developing countries. Stroke survivors often experience some medical complications and long-term disability. Disturbances in respiratory system function are common after stroke. The nature of these disorders depends on the severity and localization of injury. Alterations in breathing control, respiratory mechanics, and breathing pattern are common and may lead to gas exchange abnormalities, hypoxemia, hypercapnia, or hypocapnia, all secondary insults with strong negative impact in outcome. MV is sometimes necessary. Stroke can lead to sleep disordered breathing such as central or obstructive sleep apnea. Both disorders may also play a role in the pathogenesis of cerebral infarction. Venous thromboembolism, swallowing abnormalities, aspiration, and pneumonia are among the most common respiratory complications of stroke. NPE occurs less often. Close clinical observation and monitoring of the stroke patient for these potential disturbances and quick implementation of prophylactic measures can prevent significant morbidity and mortality.

REFERENCES

1. Rochester CL, Mohsenin V. Respiratory complication of Stroke. *Sem Resp Crit Care Med.* 2002;23:248–260. doi:10.1055/s-2002-33033
2. Roffe C: Hypoxia and Stroke. *Age Ageing.* 2002;31(S2):10–12. doi:10.1093/ageing/31.suppl_2.10
3. Ferdinand P, Roffe C. Hypoxia after stroke: a review of experimental and clinical evidence. *Exp Transl Stroke Med.* 2016;8:9. doi:10.1186/s13231-016-0023-0
4. Lee K, Rincon F. Pulmonary complications in patients with severe brain injury. *Crit Care Res Pract.* 2012;2012:1–8. doi:10.1155/2012/207247
5. Maramattom BV, Weigand S, Reinalda M, et al. Pulmonary complications after intracerebral hemorrhage. *Neurocrit Care.* 2006;5:115–119. doi:10.1385/NCC:5:2:115

6. Bruder N, Rabinstein A. Participants in the International Multi-Disciplinary Consensus Conference on the Critical Care Management of Subarachnoid Hemorrhage. Cardiovascular and pulmonary complications of aneurysmal subarachnoid hemorrhage. *Neurocrit Care.* 2011;15:257–269. doi:10.1007/s12028-011-9598-4
7. Matz K, Seyfang L, Dachenhausen A, et al. Post-stroke pneumonia at the stroke unit - a registry based analysis of contributing and protective factors. *BMC Neurol.* 2016;16:107. doi:10.1186/s12883-016-0627-y
8. Kumar S, Selim MH, Caplan LR. Medical complications after stroke. *Lancet Neurol.* 2010;9:105–118. doi:10.1016/S1474-4422(09)70266-2
9. Alberti A, Agnelli G, Caso V, et al. Non-neurological complications of acute stroke: frequency and influence on clinical outcome. *Intern Emerg Med.* 2011;Suppl 1:119–123. doi:10.1007/s11739-011-0675-7
10. Koivunen RJ, Haapaniemi E, Satopää J, et al. Medical acute complications of intracerebral hemorrhage in young adults. *Stroke Res Treat.* 2015;2015:1–7. doi:10.1155/2015/357696
11. Johnston KC, Li JY, Lyden PD, et al. Medical and neurological complications of ischemic stroke: experience from the RANTTAS trial. RANTTAS Investigators. *Stroke.* 1998;29:447. doi:10.1161/01.STR.29.2.447
12. Cohen DL, Roffe C, Beavan J, et al. Post-stroke dysphagia: a review and design considerations for future trials. *Int J Stroke.* 2016;11:399–411. doi:10.1177/1747493016639057
13. Gattinoni L, Protti A, Caironi P, et al. Ventilator-induced lung injury: the anatomical and physiological framework. *Crit Care Med.* 2010;38(10 Suppl):S539–S548. doi:10.1097/CCM.0b013e3181f1fcf7
14. Biehl M, Kashiouris MG, Gajic O. Ventilator-induced lung injury: minimizing its impact in patients with or at risk for ARDS. *Respir Care.* 2013;58:927–937. doi:10.4187/respcare.02347
15. Beitler JR, Malhotra A, Thompson BT. Ventilator-induced lung injury. *Clin Chest Med.* 2016;37:633–646. doi:10.1016/j.ccm.2016.07.004
16. Quílez ME, López-Aguilar J, Blanch L. Organ crosstalk during acute lung injury, acute respiratory distress syndrome, and mechanical ventilation. *Curr Opin Crit Care.* 2012;18:23–28. doi:10.1097/MCC.0b013e32834ef3ea
17. Mazzeo AT, Fanelli V, Mascia L. Brain-lung crosstalk in critical care: how protective mechanical ventilation can affect the brain homeostasis. *Minerva Anestesiol.* 2013;79:299–309.
18. Smithard DG. Swallowing and stroke: neurological effects and recovery. *Cerebrovasc Dis.* 2002;14:1–8. doi:10.1159/000063716
19. Ramsey DJC, Smithard DG, Kalra L. Early assessments of dysphagia and aaspiration risk in acute stroke patients. *Stroke.* 2003;34:1252–1257. doi:10.1161/01.STR.0000066309.06490.B8
20. Gordon C, Langton Hewer R, et al. Dysphagia in acute stroke. *BMJ.* 1987;295:411–414. doi:10.1136/bmj.295.6595.411

21. Smithard DG, O'Neill PA, Park C, et al. Complications and outcome after acute stroke: does dysphagia matter? *Stroke.* 1996;27:1200–1204. doi:10.1161/01.STR.27.7.1200
22. Smithard DG, O'Neill PA, England RE, et al. The natural history of dysphagia following stroke. *Dysphagia.* 1997;12:188–193. doi:10.1007/PL00009535
23. Finlayson O, Kapral M, Hall R, et al. Risk factors, inpatient care, and outcomes of pneumonia after ischemic stroke. *Neurology.* 2011;77:1338. doi:10.1212/WNL.0b013e31823152b1
24. Yuan MZ, Li F, Tian X, et al. Risk factors for lung infection in stroke patients: a meta-analysis of observational studies. *Expert Rev Anti Infect Ther.* 2015;13:1289–1298. doi:10.1586/14787210.2015.1085302
25. Ingeman A, Andersen G, Hundborg HH, et al. In-hospital medical complications, length of stay, and mortality among stroke unit patients. *Stroke.* 2011;42:3214. doi:10.1161/STROKEAHA.110.610881
26. Hilker R, Poetter C, Findeisen N, et al. Nosocomial pneumonia after acute stroke: implications for neurological intensive care medicine. *Stroke.* 2003;34:975. doi:10.1161/01.STR.0000063373.70993.CD
27. Miller CM, Behrouz R. Impact of infection on stroke morbidity and outcomes. *Curr Neurol Neurosci Rep.* 2016;16:83. doi:10.1007/s11910-016-0679-9
28. Smith CJ, Kishore AK, Vail A, et al. Diagnosis of stroke-associated pneumonia: recommendations from the pneumonia in stroke consensus group. *Stroke.* 2015;46:2335–2340. doi:10.1161/STROKEAHA.115.009617
29. Dziewas R, Ritter M, Schilling M, et al. Pneumonia in acute stroke patients fed by nasogastric tube. *J Neurol Neurosurg Psychiatry.* 2004;75:852. doi:10.1136/jnnp.2003.019075
30. Silver FL, Norris JW, Lewis AJ, et al. Early mortality following stroke: a prospective review. *Stroke.* 1984;15:492. doi:10.1161/01.STR.15.3.492
31. Grau AJ, Buggle F, Schnitzler P, et al. Fever and infection early after ischemic stroke. *J Neurol Sci.* 1999;171:115. doi:10.1016/S0022-510X(99)00261-0
32. Bravata DM, Ho SY, Meehan TP, et al. Readmission and death after hospitalization for acute ischemic stroke: 5-year follow-up in the Medicare population. *Stroke.* 2007;38:1899. doi:10.1161/STROKEAHA.106.481465
33. Sellars C, Bowie L, Bagg J, et al. Risk factors for chest infection in acute stroke: a prospective cohort study. *Stroke.* 2007;38:2284. doi:10.1161/STROKEAHA.106.478156
34. Busl KM. Nosocomial infections in the neurointensive care unit. *Neurol Clin.* 2017;35:785–807. doi:10.1016/j.ncl.2017.06.012
35. Herzig SJ, Doughty C, Lahoti S, et al. Acid-suppressive medication use in acute stroke and hospital-acquired pneumonia. *Ann Neurol.* 2014;76:712. doi:10.1002/ana.24262

36. Busl KM, Bleck TP. Neurogenic pulmonary edema. *Crit Care Med.* 2015;43:1710–1715. doi:10.1097/CCM.0000000000001101
37. Šedý J, Kuneš J, Zicha J. Pathogenetic mechanisms of neurogenic pulmonary edema. *J Neurotrauma.* 2015;32:1135–1145. doi:10.1089/neu.2014.3609
38. Balofsky A, George J, Papadakos P. Neuropulmonology. *Handb Clin Neurol.* 2017;140:33–48. doi:10.1016/B978-0-444-63600-3.00003-9
39. Wijdicks EF, Scott JP. Causes and outcome of mechanical ventilation in patients with hemispheric ischemic stroke. *Mayo Clin Proc.* 1997;72:210. doi:10.4065/72.3.210
40. Stevens RD, Lazaridis C, Chalela JA. The role of mechanical ventilation in acute brain injury. *Neurol Clin.* 2008;26:543–563. doi:10.1016/j.ncl.2008.03.014
41. Seder DB, Bösel J. Airway management and mechanical ventilation in acute brain injury. *Handb Clin Neurol.* 2017;140:15–32. doi:10.1016/B978-0-444-63600-3.00002-7
42. Gujjar AR, Deibert E, Manno EM, et al. Mechanical ventilation for ischemic stroke and intracerebral hemorrhage: indications, timing, and outcome. *Neurology.* 1998;51:447. doi:10.1212/WNL.51.2.447
43. Lahiri S, Mayer SA, Fink ME, et al. Mechanical ventilation for acute stroke: a multi-state population-based study. *Neurocrit Care.* 2015;23:28–32. doi:10.1007/s12028-014-0082-9
44. Zhao J, Liu Y, Li HC. Aspiration-related acute respiratory distress syndrome in acute stroke patient. *PLoS One.* 2015;10(3):e0118682. doi:10.1371/journal.pone.0118682
45. ARDS Definition Task Force, Ranieri VM, Rubenfeld GD, et al. Acute respiratory distress syndrome: the Berlin Definition. *JAMA.* 2012;307:2526–2533.
46. Veeravagu A, Chen YR, Ludwig C, et al. Acute lung injury in patients with subarachnoid hemorrhage: a nationwide inpatient sample study. *World Neurosurg.* 2014;82:e235–e241. doi:10.1016/j.wneu.2014.02.030
47. Rincon F, Maltenfort M, Dey S, et al. The prevalence and impact of mortality of the acute respiratory distress syndrome on admissions of patients with ischemic stroke in the United States. *J Intensive Care Med.* 2014;29:357–364. doi:10.1177/0885066613491919
48. Thompson BT, Chambers RC, Liu KD. Acute respiratory distress syndrome. *N Engl J Med.* 2017;377:562–572. doi:10.1056/NEJMra1608077
49. Kappelle LJ. Preventing deep vein thrombosis after stroke: strategies and recommendations. *Curr Treat Options Neurol.* 2011;13:629–635. doi:10.1007/s11940-011-0147-4
50. André C, de Freitas GR, Fukujima MM. Prevention of deep venous thrombosis and pulmonary embolism following stroke: a systematic review of published articles. *Eur J Neurol.* 2007;14:21–32. doi:10.1111/j.1468-1331.2006.01536.x

51. Masotti L, Di Napoli M, Godoy DA, et al. The practical management of intracerebral hemorrhage associated with oral anticoagulant therapy. *Int J Stroke*. 2011;6:228–240. doi:10.1111/j.1747-4949.2011.00595.x
52. Caprini JA. Mechanical methods for thrombosis prophylaxis. *Clin Appl Thromb Hemost*. 2010;16:668–673. doi:10.1177/1076029609348645
53. Lacut K, Bressollette L, Le Gal G, et al. Prevention of venous thrombosis in patients with acute intracerebral hemorrhage. *Neurology*. 2005;65:865–869. doi:10.1212/01.wnl.0000176073.80532.a2
54. Dennis M, Sandercock PA, Reid J, et al. Effectiveness of thigh-length graduated compression stockings to reduce the risk of deep vein thrombosis after stroke (CLOTS trial 1): a multicentre, randomised controlled trial. *Lancet*. 2009;373:1958–1965. doi:10.1016/S0140-6736(09)60941-7
55. CLOTS (Clots in Legs or Stockings after Stroke) Trial Collaboration. Thigh-length versus below-knee stockings for deep venous thrombosis prophylaxis after stroke: a randomized trial. *Ann Intern Med*. 2010;153:553–562. doi:10.7326/0003-4819-153-9-201011020-00280
56. Masotti L, Godoy DA, Napoli MD, et al. Pharmacological prophylaxis of venous thromboembolism during acute phase of spontaneous intracerebral hemorrhage: what do we know about risks and benefits? *Clin Appl Thromb Hemost*. 2012;18:393–402. doi:10.1177/1076029612441055
57. Ageno W, Gallus AS, Wittkowsky A, et al. Oral anticoagulant therapy: Antithrombotic Therapy and Prevention of Thrombosis, 9th ed: American College of Chest Physicians Evidence-Based Clinical Practice Guidelines. *Chest*. 2012;141:e44S–e88S. doi:10.1378/chest.11-2292
58. Nyquist P, Jichici D, Bautista C, et al. Prophylaxis of venous thrombosis in neurocritical care patients: an executive summary of evidence-based guidelines a statement for healthcare professionals from the neurocritical care society and society of critical care medicine. *Crit Care Med*. 2017;45:476–479. doi:10.1097/CCM.0000000000002247
59. Godoy DA, Behrouz R, Di Napoli M. Glucose control in acute brain injury: does it matter? *Curr Opin Crit Care*. 2016;22:120–127. doi:10.1097/MCC.0000000000000292
60. Kramer CL. Intensive care unit-acquired weakness. *Neurol Clin*. 2017;35:723–736. doi:10.1016/j.ncl.2017.06.008

14 Metabolic Complications After Acute Stroke

Kanita Beba Abadal and Katharina M. Busl

KEY POINTS

- After acute stroke, a wide array of metabolic changes can lead to secondary damage to ischemic areas and negatively impact clinical outcomes.
- Disorders of sodium homeostasis are the most frequent electrolyte abnormality in hospitalized patients and both hypo- and hypernatremia have been shown to increase inpatient mortality in ischemic stroke patients.
- Dehydration is remarkably common in stroke patients, and has been associated with a significant increase in poor outcomes.
- Acute kidney injury is associated with worse outcomes in both ischemic and hemorrhagic stroke patients, and may increase in-hospital death by more than threefold.
- New-onset hyperglycemia in the setting of acute stroke is thought to be reactive or stress hyperglycemia, and may lead to increased infarct size, exacerbate stroke severity in both ischemic and hemorrhagic strokes, and lead to more poststroke complications.
- The delivery of oxygen to the brain is dependent on cerebral blood flow and arterial oxygen content. A state of decreased blood hemoglobin levels may impair oxygen delivery to the brain during an acute stroke.
- There are multiple factors associated with the development of undernutrition in acute stroke patients, including the presence of dysphagia, cognitive and physical deficits that may impair the patient's ability to self-feed, increased metabolic demand due to elevation of stress hormones, infections, mechanical ventilation, and certain commonly used medications.

© Springer Publishing Company DOI: 10.1891/9780826124791.0014

- The excess of the neurotransmitter glutamate leads to a type of neurotoxicity referred to as excitotoxicity, and is implicated in neuronal degeneration following stroke.

INTRODUCTION

After acute stroke, a wide array of metabolic changes can occur. These metabolic complications may have implications on clinical and neurological course, and affect outcomes. In this chapter, we review the occurrence and impact of electrolyte disturbances, changes in fluid balance, acute kidney injury, disturbance in glucose homeostasis, anemia, and complications of nutritional deficits in acute stroke patients. Furthermore, we review the intrinsic and molecular metabolic complications of glutamate excitotoxicity as pertaining to acute forms of stroke.

ELECTROLYTE DISTURBANCES

Electrolyte disturbances are common in clinical practice and occur in the setting of a variety of frequently encountered diseases and stroke risk factors, including diabetes mellitus, hypertension, and heart failure. Disorders of sodium homeostasis are the most frequent electrolyte abnormality in hospitalized patients (1). Both hypo- and hypernatremia have been shown to increase inpatient mortality (1,2). In acute stroke patients, a disturbance of sodium homeostasis may occur due to the major role of the central nervous system (CNS) in water homeostasis (3).

Hyponatremia

Among patients with acute brain injury, hyponatremia is the most common electrolyte disturbance (4). It can lead to worsening of the existing neurological deficits, but can also mimic signs and symptoms of neurological disease. In stroke patients, vomiting, poor intake, adrenal insufficiency, hypothyroidism, use of osmotic agents, diuretics, and other drugs may all contribute to hyponatremia, but hyponatremia is often primarily related to the syndrome of inappropriate antidiuretic hormone secretion (SIADH) or cerebral salt-wasting (CSW) (5,6). Stroke and acute neurological injuries may result in a stress response that may result in the dysregulation of the hypothalamic–pituitary–adrenal (HPA) axis. SIADH occurs in CNS disorders, carcinomas, pulmonary disorders, and secondary to a variety of drugs including analgesics, antidepressants, barbiturates, carbamazepine, and oral hypoglycemic. SIADH is the result of a persistent production of antidiuretic hormone (ADH) despite body fluid hypotonicity and an expanded effective circulatory volume, with failure of the negative feedback mechanism that usually controls ADH secretion, and continued ADH release. CSW is defined as hyponatremia due to excessive natriuresis in the setting of cerebral disease, with extracellular volume depletion and dehydration with or without high urinary sodium concentration, and normal adrenal and thyroid functions (7). The exact pathophysiologic mechanism of CSW is not known. CSW and SIADH may share common features of hyponatremia, low serum osmolality, high urinary osmolality, and urinary sodium, and distinction is often difficult. Evidence of dehydration by clinical exam and laboratory tests (raised hematocrit and blood urea), and high urinary output (>3 L) may suggest CSW (8), but the clinical assessment of volume status in patients with hyponatremia has a limited sensitivity and specificity, with only about 50% correct identification (9). To this end, various studies have reported either CSW (10) or SIADH (11) as the more frequent etiology of hyponatremia.

Reported incidence and prevalence of poststroke hyponatremia varies, likely due to differences in inclusion criteria, ethnicity, and sample size in different studies, and ranges from 7% to 43% (10,12,13). In one of the larger series, hyponatremia was attributed to drugs or associated gastrointestinal symptoms in 33% of patients (10). Hyponatremia may be more common in cortical ischemic stroke compared with brainstem or infratentorial stroke (14), and less common in anterior circulation infarcts (10).

Hyponatremia in stroke patients correlates with markers of stroke severity including National Institutes of Health Stroke Scale (NIHSS) score and the Barthel index score (15), and systemic inflammatory response syndrome (SIRS), Glasgow Coma Scale (GCS) score, and duration of hospitalization (10). Interestingly, some studies reported a more significant link to poor outcome for the presence of CSW as opposed to alternative etiologies of hyponatremia (11).

Poststroke hyponatremia has been associated with poor outcomes (15). A relationship between hyponatremia and long-term mortality after ischemic stroke has been consistently found (13,15,16). However, evidence on the effect of hyponatremia on in-hospital mortality is conflicting (13,15), with some data indicating an association of hyponatremia with higher in-hospital mortality (15), and other data not finding increased short-term mortality after stroke (13).

Additionally, hyponatremia was found to be a significant predictor for overall higher medical costs in ischemic stroke patients (17).

Hypernatremia

Pathogenesis, occurrence, and outcomes associated with hypernatremia are less well studied in acute stroke patients. Poststroke hypernatremia may be the consequence of central diabetes insipidus, but rarely, it can also occur due to hypodipsia secondary to lesions of the hypothalamic thirst center (18). In one series of stroke patients, hypernatremia was found in 6%, and both hypernatremia and hyponatremia in 4% of patients (10). However, most commonly, hypernatremia is iatrogenic due to the use of hypertonic and osmolar agents to manage increased cerebral edema and decrease intracranial pressure (19). Hypertonic saline, in various concentrations, is one of the most commonly used agents. Sodium chloride is completely excluded from the intact blood–brain barrier and hence, theoretically, is a better osmotic agent than mannitol (20). Continuous infusion of hypertonic saline in neurocritically ill patients is generally perceived as safe, without increased risk of infection, deep venous thrombosis, or renal failure, as long as sodium levels are carefully monitored (21). While hypertonic saline can enhance cerebral blood flow and oxygen delivery (22), hypernatremia also has been associated with early neurological worsening (23). Higher concentrations of hypertonic saline have been found to increase infarct volumes in animal models, and hypertonic saline therapy leading to significant hypernatremia can increase tissue damage after vascular occlusion and focal cerebral ischemia (24). For patients with subarachnoid hemorrhage (SAH), hypernatremia has been found associated with higher mortality, poorer outcome, and adverse cardiac events (25). In one recent large series of stroke patients, there was a significant association of hypernatremia with mortality (10), but broad outcome data on acute ischemic stroke and hypernatremia are lacking.

Hypochloremia

Serum chloride is another important extracellular anion serving many functions, including the maintenance of osmotic pressure, acid–base balance, and the movement of water between fluid compartments (26). Hypochloremia is known to be associated with higher mortality in patients with heart failure, chronic kidney disease, hypertension, and in the postoperative setting (27–30). More recently, hypochloremia has been evaluated in a study of 3,314 stroke patients and was found to be associated with a 2.43-fold increase in risk of in-hospital mortality (31), with an indication that chloride levels may perhaps have a stronger prognostic role than sodium levels (31).

Other Electrolyte and Metabolic Disturbances

Metabolic changes pose an immediate stroke risk as evidenced by patients with end-stage renal disease (ESRD) on hemodialysis (HD), with a large proportion experiencing neurologic changes and acute ischemic strokes during HD (32), but data are scarce for the various other possible electrolyte disturbances in acute ischemic stroke.

Magnesium, a mineral implicated with neuroprotective properties, has been found to be associated with reduced risk of stroke in epidemiological studies (33). While previous data on hypomagnesemia in acute stroke patients and its association with outcome were conflicting (34–36), a recent larger study evaluating low magnesium admission levels for patients with acute ischemic stroke endorsed a significant association between lower magnesium levels and in-hospital mortality (37). A recent study evaluating magnesium levels in acute intracerebral hemorrhage (ICH) found that lower admission magnesium levels were associated with larger hematoma volumes and hematoma growth, as well as poor functional outcomes at 3 months (38), supporting the notion that magnesium may play an important role in hemostasis in ICH. Hypokalemia and hyponatremia have been found to be significant predictors for higher cost in ischemic stroke patients (17). Poststroke hypokalemia was also found to be associated with an increased risk of mortality (39).

FLUID BALANCE

Euvolemia is crucial in acutely ill patients. Fluids serve as the solvent for vitamins, minerals, glucose and other nutrients, are a medium for waste products through the body, and may be important in wound healing (40). Several markers of volume contraction are used in the literature, including blood urea nitrogen (BUN)/creatinine ratio, urine specific gravity, and plasma osmolality. BUN/creatinine ratio is commonly used clinically, especially in patients with normal renal function (41,42). Using serum osmolality as a marker of dehydration, a study suggests that it is present in over a third of older adults admitted to the hospital for medical emergencies, and that nearly two-thirds of these patients remain dehydrated on admission 48 hours later (43). Along with older age, the risk of dehydration on presentation increases with polypharmacy, mental and physical disability, and other medical comorbidities (43). Contributing factors to fluid loss during a hospitalization include elevated temperature, vomiting, profuse sweating, diarrhea, and heavily draining wounds (40).

For stroke patients, dehydration has been associated with a significant increase in poor outcomes. Dehydrated patients were found to have higher rates of death, placement in hospice, and placement in nursing homes within 30 days of admission (42). Risk of in-hospital mortality was six times greater as compared to patients who were euvolemic, independent of key confounders such as age, gender, comorbidities, or illness severity (43). Dehydration on admission has also been linked to higher scores on the NIHSS in patients presenting with an acute stroke (44). In addition to unfavorable association with outcomes, healthcare costs were higher in stroke patients with dehydration (41).

At the time of an acute stroke there is impairment of autoregulation of cerebral vasculature, leaving the brain vulnerable to fluctuations in blood pressure. Cerebral blood flow becomes less responsive to changes in arterial CO_2 and shifts to passively following changes in systemic blood pressure (45). Dehydration is known to cause decreased blood pressure, increased blood viscosity, reduced cardiac stroke volume, impaired collateral flow, and reduced cerebral perfusion (41). Hypovolemia may predispose to hypoperfusion and exacerbate the existing ischemic brain injury (46). At the time of an acute stroke, brain areas still at risk for ischemia become especially dependent on collateral blood flow, which can be adversely affected by hypotension (47,48). A low mean blood pressure may limit blood flow to the ischemic penumbra, and lead to greater infarct size (49). This impact of blood pressure on cerebral perfusion pressure was corroborated by a study of acute ischemic stroke patients that found the risk of all-cause mortality to be significantly increased in those with admission mean blood pressure below 100 mmHg, and discharge systolic blood pressure below 120 mmHg (50). Another study evaluated blood pressure trends in acute stroke and found that reductions in systolic and diastolic blood pressures of greater than 20 mmHg during the first 24 hours were associated with a higher frequency of early neurologic deterioration, increased infarct volume, and worse outcome at 3 months poststroke (48). Given that dehydration reduces cardiac output and increases systemic vascular resistance (51), adequate hydration and avoidance of wide fluctuations in blood pressure should be part of supportive care for acute stroke patients, as it can help to maintain collateral blood flow to ischemic areas of the brain. Recent findings on regional cerebral blood flow in patients with

SAH support the notion that both intravascular volume and rheological effects are of importance (52).

Studies have shown that dehydration also has a detrimental effect on cognition. Dehydration of as little as 2% of body weight led to an impairment in physical and cognitive performance in one study (53). Data from a study that investigated hemispatial neglect demonstrated that dehydration is associated with more severe hemispatial neglect. This is significant because patients with neglect tend to have a worse functional status, owing in part to more difficult time in participating in rehabilitation and longer stays in rehabilitation facilities (44).

Another concern of dehydration is the tendency to develop thromboembolic complications. Stroke patients who are in a volume contracted state tend to have more recurrent embolic strokes and thrombotic events including venous thromboembolism (42), with dehydration as an independent risk factor for deep venous thrombosis after stroke (54).

Infection is the most common medical complication after an acute stroke. Between 23% and 65% of patients acquire an infection during their admission, with urinary tract infection and pneumonia being the most common (55). There is an intentional suppression of systemic immunity by the nervous system during the acute stroke period to protect the brain from secondary injury resulting from inflammation. This, however, could increase the susceptibility to infections in acute stroke patients (55). Dehydration has also been found to worsen infections during acute illness, and the inflammatory response that results from infection could lead to further secondary damage to ischemic brain areas (56,57).

Hypervolemia is likewise undesirable during the acute stroke period. It may exacerbate brain edema caused by strokes and increase stress on the heart (46). In one study assessing fluid intake after acute stroke, intake of greater than 1,650 mL or 28 mL/kg/day was significantly and independently associated with the development of malignant brain edema (58). The cause and effect relationship between hydration and outcome in acute stroke is not clear. Current stroke guidelines recommend rapid repletion of intravascular volume for patients who are hypovolemic on admission, followed by maintenance intravenous fluids. Caution should be exercised with rapid repletion of patients who are prone to intravascular volume overload, such as those with poor cardiac ejection fraction or renal failure. In patients with SAH, cumulative evidence suggests that hypervolemia is associated with poor outcomes (59), and more restrictive fluid management is recommended.

The overall accepted goal of care should be to achieve and maintain euvolemia. Maintenance intravenous fluids should be initiated in patients who are euvolemic at presentation (46), with careful titration to maintain this status.

ACUTE KIDNEY INJURY

Acute kidney injury is defined as an abrupt deterioration in kidney function, evidenced by a decrease in urine output, increase in serum creatinine, or both. The increase in serum creatinine is often described as a percentage increase of at least 50% from baseline (138,139). Kidney injury is seen in about 14% of patients with ischemic stroke (138) and associated with worse outcomes in both ischemic and hemorrhagic infarcts. A study in ischemic and hemorrhagic stroke patients demonstrated in-hospital death to be more than threefold higher in patients who had acute kidney injury during their hospitalization compared to those who did not (138). Acute renal failure is also associated with higher likelihood of severe disability and mortality in patients with intracerebral hemorrhage (140, 141). There are various risk factors for developing kidney injury in the acute stroke period. Some of these are a result of interventions performed to minimize the risk of expansion or complications of ischemic strokes or hemorrhages, and include volume depletion, rapid blood pressure reduction to prevent hemorrhage expansion, contrast exposure for CT scans, and mannitol administration to decrease intracerebral edema and intracranial pressure (141). The underlying mechanism of neuronal injury following acute kidney injury is incompletely understood. Data from animal studies demonstrate that renal failure leads to an increase in cytokine levels, augmenting the inflammatory response that is already under way due to the stroke, and leading to subsequent functional changes in the brain (142,143). Patients experiencing acute kidney injury also tend to have higher rates of other comorbidities that may lead to higher risk of complications and morbidity—such as venous thromboembolism, urinary tract infections, sepsis, myocardial infarctions, and gastrointestinal hemorrhage (144).

CT contrast should be used with caution in patients with acute kidney injury. Magnetic resonance (MR) angiography is preferred for vessel imaging in these patients, especially since it can be performed without contrast. While very uncommon, MR gadolinium contrast reactions can be very dangerous. Nephrogenic systemic fibrosis, thought to be caused by gadolinium based contrast, is a serious syndrome resembling diffuse scleroderma and is the reason gadolinium-based MR contrast media should be avoided in patients with estimated glomerular filtration rate <30 mL/min/ 1.73 m^2 (46,145). Involving nephrologists early in the hospitalization in patients with acute kidney injury could alter the course of the disease by a number of mechanisms. Nephrologists can give a proper volume assessment, recognize other systemic disease affecting the kidneys, and adjust medications to prevent further hemodynamic or toxic injury to the kidney (146).

DISTURBANCE IN GLUCOSE HOMEOSTASIS

Blood glucose abnormalities are a common problem in stroke patients. Admission blood glucose levels were found to be elevated in up to 40% of patients presenting with an acute ischemic stroke (60). A significant portion of these patients, between 25% and 50%, have not been previously diagnosed with diabetes or demonstrated prior evidence of glucose intolerance. This new onset hyperglycemia in the setting of acute stroke is thought to be reactive, or stress, hyperglycemia (61). In SAH, hyperglycemia has long been postulated to be a result of elevated blood catecholamine levels secondary to HPA axis activation (62). The activation of the HPA axis and sympathetic autonomic nervous system in the acute stroke period leads to an increase in catecholamines and cortisol blood levels, hormones that enhance a variety of reactions (e.g., glycogenolysis, gluconeogenesis, proteolysis, and lipolysis), all leading to excess glucose in the blood (63).

Multiple studies have shown high admission blood glucose levels to be strongly and independently associated with poor functional outcome after an acute ischemic stroke (63,64). Interestingly, hyperglycemia was not required to be severe in order to lead to some of the disparities in outcome between euglycemic and hyperglycemic stroke patients. Even slightly elevated admission blood glucose levels, 125 to 130 mg/dL, were associated with increased infarct volume and worse functional outcome (65). Hypoglycemia, on the other hand, is usually iatrogenic in acute stroke patients, related to antidiabetic medications. If severe enough, however, it can cause neurological symptoms. Severe prolonged hypoglycemia can lead to permanent brain damage and low levels (<60 mg/ dL) should be treated emergently (46). For patients with SAH, one large cohort study demonstrated admission hyperglycemia to be associated with poor outcomes in the short term, with a particularly increased mortality in previously nondiabetic patients (66). A prospective study in nondiabetic patients with SAH demonstrated that hyperglycemia within the first 14 days of hemorrhage was not only associated with poor short-term outcomes, but also associated with increased 1-year mortality (67).

In addition to being associated with an overall worse functional outcome and increased mortality after acute stroke, hyperglycemia has also been shown to exacerbate stroke severity in both ischemic and hemorrhagic strokes, and to lead to more poststroke complications. A retrospective review of stroke patients showed that the patients who also presented with hyperglycemia developed more pronounced cerebral edema, midline shift, or ventricular compression (68). In a study wherein continuous glucose monitoring was performed throughout the duration of admission following acute stroke, persistent hyperglycemia was associated with a higher likelihood of expansion of infarct size (65). Not only has hyperglycemia on admission been associated with an increased risk of hemorrhagic transformation in patients who received intravenous thrombolysis, but also with a higher risk of symptomatic hemorrhagic conversion in patients not treated with thrombolytic therapy (69–72). In SAH, there is evidence that hyperglycemia on admission leads to an increased risk of vasospasm (73). In a recent rat model study, hyperglycemia exacerbated cerebral vasospasm after SAH, presumably through dysregulation of the nitric oxide pathway (74). Hyperglycemia may even have adverse effects on stroke by altering the coagulation pathway. In one small sample study in young, healthy, nondiabetic patients, induced prolonged hyperglycemia was thought to cause activation of the tissue factor pathway, reflected by increases in plasma coagulation factors (75). Admission hyperglycemia was also found to be independently associated with the occurrence of poststroke infections. One possible reasoning behind this is that hyperglycemia exacerbates the already immunocompromised state in the acute ischemic stroke period (76), but it is also possible that hyperglycemia and poststroke infections are both a result of sympathetic nervous system activation rather than being causally related (77).

The mechanism by which hyperglycemia contributes to neuronal injury during acute stroke is not clear, but animal models suggest that it might be through accentuated tissue acidosis and lactate generation (65). In the ischemic penumbra, or the at-risk area surrounding the evolving infarct, aerobic metabolism switches to anaerobic metabolism and leads to production of lactate and unbuffered protons. The persistent anaerobic metabolism leads to a heterogeneous distribution of intracellular acidosis and may result in irreversible neuronal injury through expansion of the infarct core into the penumbra. If the patient is also hyperglycemic at the time of this process, anaerobic glycolysis is stimulated, and results in further lactic acidosis and additional neuronal injury (61). A study in rats that were made hyperglycemic prior to a cerebral ischemia event showed them to develop elevated cerebral lactate levels compared to controls, and they had poorer recovery of cortical neuronal tissue (61). Another study, using a rabbit stroke model, confirmed the development of a pronounced intracellular acidosis and retardation of N-acetyl dehydrogenase regeneration in animals that were made hyperglycemic (78). In addition to intracellular acidosis, hyperglycemia in animal models has been shown to stimulate vascular inflammation and increase blood–brain barrier permeability (60). Hyperglycemia furthermore induces progressive cerebrovascular changes through arterial remodeling (79).

There are several retrospective studies that have demonstrated a decreased mortality rate after normalization of blood glucose levels following acute ischemic stroke. In one such study, normalization of blood glucose to less than 130 mg/dL during the first 48 hours of hospitalization led to a markedly decreased mortality, even after controlling for age, stroke severity, and other potentially confounding conditions (60). Lowering blood glucose levels may reduce the cerebral edema and oxidative injury initially caused by the hyperglycemia after stroke. There is currently no evidence that targeting blood glucose to particular levels will improve functional outcomes in acute stroke. Although multiple different insulin management protocols exist, these have not been compared to each other in acute stroke patients (46). There is only one randomized efficacy trial of hyperglycemia treatment in acute stroke (GIST-UK) to date (80). The trial compared intravenous insulin, vitamin K, and glucose with saline in patients not previously treated with insulin, within the first 24 hours of admission for acute stroke. While it showed no difference in clinical outcomes between the two groups, there were several shortcomings of the trial. It was stopped early, underpowered to detect possible treatment effect, had a relatively short duration of treatment (24 hours), and a small contrast in mean glucose levels between the intervention and control groups (0.57 mmol/L). There is a clear need for further research in this area. In the meantime, current guidelines of the American Heart Association suggest treating hyperglycemia to achieve blood glucose levels in a range of 140 to 180 mg/dL (46), considering that there is strong evidence indicating that persistent in-hospital hyperglycemia is associated with worse outcomes than normoglycemia. This should be exercised with caution, however, as intensive insulin therapy can be accompanied by an increase in hypoglycemic episodes, which can be detrimental as well (63).

ANEMIA

Anemia is an important but less commonly discussed complication after acute stroke. The prevalence of anemia is thought to be as high as 30% on admission in acute stroke patients (81). The delivery of oxygen to the brain is dependent on cerebral blood flow and arterial oxygen content, the latter being largely determined by blood hemoglobin concentrations. A state of decreased blood hemoglobin levels, therefore, may further impair oxygen delivery to the brain during an acute stroke (82). Anemia on admission was found to be associated with an increased mortality risk in both hemorrhagic and ischemic stroke in a cohort of greater than 8,000 acute stroke patients (83). Multiple other studies have corroborated this finding. A prospective study of 1,176 patients showed admission anemia to be an independent predictor of death both at discharge and at 13 months postdischarge. A subsequent meta-analysis of 3,810 patients concurred (81). Low hemoglobin levels are also associated with increased stroke severity, older age, higher prestroke disability, and increased risk of comorbidities (83). The relationship between admission hemoglobin and mortality in acute stroke was not found to be linear, however. Mortality was found to be increased at both extremes of hemoglobin in acute stroke (84). Higher than normal blood hemoglobin has also been found as an independent risk factor for reduced reperfusion and greater infarct size after an ischemic stroke, in a randomized control trial that showed a strong inverse relationship between hematocrit and reperfusion. This is thought to be secondary to the association between elevated hematocrit and blood viscosity with carotid artery stenosis and stroke (85). In acute ICH, the presence of anemia was found to be an independent predictor of larger volume of hemorrhage (86).

While there is abundant evidence in the literature in support of maintaining higher hemoglobin levels in acute stroke, there is still no current standard for threshold of blood transfusion. Current guidelines suggest that anemia should be avoided, but aggressive transfusions are not recommended (87). In current practice, there continues to be a fairly restrictive approach to blood transfusions, and data on detrimental effect of blood transfusions complicate this matter. There are, however, large multicenter trials under way to further investigate a more standardized approach (88). In hemorrhagic strokes, the benefit of transfusions has been elucidated more. A study of over 500 nontraumatic ICH patients demonstrated that anemia develops in the majority of patients with ICH and that packed red blood transfusions were associated with an improved outcome (89).

In aneurysmal SAH, anemia is also common—between 39% and 57% of patients will develop a hematocrit less than 30% during their hospitalization (90). A recent study found a hemoglobin concentration less than 11.1 g/dL to be associated with an unfavorable outcome after acute SAH (91). Based on data indicating a possible benefit in SAH patients to aim for a higher hemoglobin threshold than generally standard in critically ill patients, modification of anemia has been regarded as a potential factor to improve outcome. Patients experiencing vasospasm, lower mean hemoglobin values were an independent predictor of the need for intra-arterial vasospasm therapy (e.g., vasodilators, balloon angioplasty, and cerebral blood flow augmentation devices) and poor discharge modified Rankin Scale scores (92). In another study of patients with aneurysmal SAH who were surgically treated, outcomes suggested that maintaining the hemoglobin concentration at a particular level (11–12 g/dL) may reduce the incidence of symptomatic cerebral vasospasm (93). This is significant because approximately 50% of patients with cerebral vasospasm have delayed neurologic ischemic deficits, and 15% to 20% of those result in stroke or death (94). However, data are not unequivocal: while some studies have shown potential benefit in aiming for higher hemoglobin levels, others have shown detrimental effect of blood transfusions, and the benefit of transfusion is unproven, as transfused blood may not effectively increase oxygen delivery and can be associated with clinical complications (90). Red blood cell transfusions have been associated with unfavorable neurologic outcomes in patients with SAH (95). Interestingly, blood transfusions, in some studies, have also been associated with an increased risk of vasospasm and poor outcome (96), and also with an increased risk of thrombotic events in a dose-dependent manner (86). Overall, the acceptable degree of anemia as well as appropriate transfusion thresholds remain controversial and practice varies widely (90). Society guidelines include the option for transfusions without specifying exact transfusion goals and levels (97).

Although anemic hypoxia is not an independent factor leading to ischemic stroke, there are several case reports of severe anemia resulting in stroke or transient ischemic attack (TIA) in patients with underlying vascular stenosis. Hsiao presented a case of a patient with severe anemia and vertebral artery insufficiency who presented with symptoms of posterior circulation stroke, which worsened with declining hemoglobin levels and completely resolved with correction of anemia by blood transfusion (98). Another paper reported two patients with carotid artery stenosis and anemia, in whom neurological deficits appeared whenever the hemoglobin level fell below a particular threshold and resolved with the correction of the anemia (99). In all of these cases, the patients had high-grade vessel obstruction and severe anemia, where neither factor alone produced neurological impairment, but the combination of both led to brain tissue hypoxia. A separate study of clinical performance showed a relationship between low hemoglobin levels and worse scores on certain functional tasks, suggesting a relationship between anemia and worse unilateral spatial neglect (100).

Anemia alone is thought to be insufficient to lead to significant neurologic problems, because under normal conditions, cerebral homeostasis adjusts to meet the brain oxygen requirements even during situations of profound anemia. However, organs in an already compromised condition, such as the brain in an acute stroke, may be aggravated by anemic hypoxia (98). Anemia and hemodilution can adversely affect cerebrovascular autoregulation and lead to fluctuation and decrease in cerebral perfusion (101,102). The resultant hyperdynamic circulation has been shown to trigger an inflammatory response and expression of adhesion molecules on vascular endothelial cells, both of which may lead to thrombus formation in a process similar to atherosclerosis (103,104). Anemia has also been shown to be associated with an upregulation of production of inducible nitric oxide synthase and chemokine receptors (105), inflammatory mediators that may worsen outcomes in stroke and which have been associated with neuronal damage (106,107). Furthermore, there are studies demonstrating prolonged bleeding time in patients with anemia, suggesting altered mechanism of hemostasis with lowered red blood counts (108). This could be a potential explanation for why low hemoglobin correlates with increased ICH volumes. Current and future research is set out to clarify the role of anemia further, and shed light on optimal hemoglobin levels and transfusion strategies.

NUTRITION

Undernutrition is an important and often underrecognized complication of acute stroke. The true prevalence of undernutrition in patients hospitalized with acute stroke is uncertain, and the literature reports ranges varying from 8% to 49% in hospitalized stroke patients (109). This wide range is attributed to heterogeneity of patient populations, and, more notably, to a great variation in nutrition assessment methods (109).

There are multiple factors associated with the development of undernutrition in acute stroke patients. Some patient populations, especially older adults, those with impaired functional capacity, and those living in aged care facilities, are more susceptible to undernutrition even prior to being hospitalized with a stroke (110). Studies have shown that on admission, 16% to 49% of patients with acute stroke are already malnourished (110,111). Once the patient is admitted with a stroke, dysphagia is very common and may contribute to the development of undernutrition. According to one review of studies of malnutrition in stroke, the presence of dysphagia ranged from 24% to 53%, and the odds of being malnourished were increased with the presence of dysphagia following stroke (109). The particular area of the brain infarcted may also have an impact on nutritional status. Cognitive deficits such as visual neglect, upper extremity paresis, apraxia, and decreased food intake associated with depression may affect the patient's ability to self-feed (112–114). Patients who have elevated intracranial pressures can have delayed gastric emptying. They may encounter problems with nasogastric tube feeding initially and require postpyloric feeding instead (112). After any neurological insult, elevation of stress hormones such as catecholamines, cortisol, glucagon, and acute-phase proteins and certain interleukins leads to an alteration of metabolic demands and may further exacerbate malnutrition (115). Some amino acids such as arginine and glutamine become conditionally essential during periods of severe stress (40). Subsequently during the hospitalization, infections, severity of stroke, comorbidities, medications, and requirement of mechanical ventilation can all alter caloric requirements (112). It is also important to be cognizant of the commonly used medications that may affect nutritional demands. Phenytoin, a commonly used anticonvulsant in patients who experience seizures after strokes, may decrease medication absorption when given in patients who are on enteral tube feeds. Narcotic pain medications can cause constipation and ileus, and concomitant use of prophylactic stool softeners is advisable. Barbiturates decrease caloric requirement, and the fat content of propofol may necessitate a diet with adjusted fat content to prevent overfeeding (112). For these reasons, nutrition interventions should be implemented early to prevent or correct nutritional deficits. If possible, clinical nutrition specialists should be consulted to frequently reassess nutritional requirements.

Enteral nutrition should be initiated as soon as possible. In a study of the impact of early enteral nutrition on the short-term prognosis of stroke, early nasogastric nutrition improved nutritional status and reduced complications in patients with acute stroke and dysphagia (116).

Recognizing and correcting undernutrition is integral to the comprehensive care of stroke patients. Studies have shown a highly significant increase in mortality with increasing risk of malnutrition (117). Prehospital undernutrition was found to be an independent risk factor for poor stroke outcomes (110). This is significant because it implies that patients who are predisposed to having strokes may be able to influence their survival or level of independence after a stroke by maintaining good baseline nutrition. Studies have shown undernutrition after stroke to be associated with increased mortality and dependence both at 1 month (118,119) and 6 months after a stroke (117,120). Malnutrition in stroke patients is also related to increased length of stay and decreased progress during rehabilitation. Early treatment of undernutrition could significantly affect a patient's ability to effectively participate in rehabilitation, functional activities, and to be able to complete activities of daily living (113). Adequate nutrition is also important in maintaining tissue integrity and preventing tissue breakdown. Consuming sufficient calories, proteins, fluids, minerals, and vitamins is necessary for the prevention and treatment of pressure ulcers in hospitalized patients (40). Study findings have also suggested that malnutrition increases the risk of infections, gastrointestinal bleeding, cardiac insufficiency, and acquired immune dysfunction (113,120). In a study where 760 patients with both adequate nutritional status and undernutrition on admission were followed for a 10-month period, the patients who became malnourished during the hospitalization were found to have even worse functional outcomes than those who were malnourished at baseline on admission. This study suggests that it is equally important, if not more, to monitor for deteriorating nutritional status during hospitalization (121).

Even though the literature and current guidelines support screening of all stroke patients for malnutrition at the time of admission and during hospitalization, there are currently no standardized screening tools for stroke patients (117). Nutritional parameters and definitions of undernutrition differ among studies, and the time points of assessment are often variable as well (122). Nutritional assessment methods include the monitoring of serum laboratory values such as albumin, prealbumin, and transferrin;

anthropometric measurements such as triceps skin fold thickness and arm muscle circumference, or both (112). Serum albumin can be a useful marker in the absence of infection and other causes of inflammation (112). Hypoalbuminemia has been shown to be an independent predictor of mortality (123), poststroke complications, and poor clinical outcome in stroke patients (122). There are limitations to the interpretation of levels of albumin, prealbumin, and transferrin, as these are hepatic proteins that are influenced by non-nutritional factors, and may not be a valid reflection of a patient's nutritional status. All three proteins are negative acute-phase reactants, and their concentrations decrease in inflammatory processes. Low albumin levels can at least partially be explained by downregulation of albumin synthesis by interleukin-6, which is itself upregulated in acute stroke (123). This might be especially true in patients with more severe strokes (109). Another limitation to the use of albumin is its long half-life of about 18 days, which makes it difficult to use in the assessment of acute nutritional changes (122). Prealbumin and transferrin may be better markers than albumin because of their shorter half-lives. They should be measured in conjunction with C-reactive protein, to evaluate for the presence of a potentially confounding inflammatory response. In the FOOD trial, investigators used a combination of subjective assessment, weight/height measurements, blood tests, and anthropometry for a more complete picture of nutritional status (120). Screening for dysphagia is an integral part of the nutritional assessment in stroke patients. Often, patients are screened by a simple water swallow test at the bedside. While this is a quick, convenient, and readily accessible method, studies suggest that it could be missing up to 50% of patients who are aspirating (124). A modified barium swallow evaluation is considered the gold standard for the assessment of oropharyngeal dysphagia and should be utilized if there is any suspicion that the patient could be aspirating based on exam or the brain area infarcted. There is a novel area of neurorehabilitation research dedicated to improving swallow function recovery by the stimulation of the nervous system. In pharyngeal electrical stimulation, electrodes are placed transnasally or transorally to assist in swallowing recovery (125). In transcutaneous electrical stimulation, electrical stimulation is applied to the neck to promote the elevation of the hyolaryngeal complex (126). Undernutrition also has financial implications: hypoalbuminemia, among other factors including fever, hypokalemia, and hyponatremia, has been found to be a significant predictor for higher overall medical cost in ischemic stroke patients (17).

GLUTAMATE EXCITOTOXICITY

Glutamate is the principal excitatory neurotransmitter in the adult brain, and plays an important role in many integral neuronal processes—including neuronal growth, axon guidance, brain development and maturation, and synaptic plasticity in both health and disease (127). Glutamate is also crucial in neuronal degeneration following a stroke: excess of the neurotransmitter leads to a type of neurotoxicity referred to as excitotoxicity (127). Glutamate is released into the synapse at the axon terminal where it stimulates glutamate receptors on the postsynaptic neuron and induces depolarization via influx of calcium and sodium ions (55). Under normal conditions, the neurotransmitter is then sequestered from the synapse via active transport mechanisms, which conclude its excitatory action. During ischemia, however, inadequate adenosine triphosphate (ATP) synthesis leads to a reduction in glutamate clearance and thus results in a continual stimulation of glutamate receptors. Consequently, there is continual calcium influx into N-methyl-D-aspartate (NMDA) glutamate receptors, stimulating calcium-dependent apoptotic pathways (127,128). In animal models of ischemic stroke, there is a demonstrable upregulation of NMDA receptors in the ischemic core and surrounding cortical regions (129). Additionally, within minutes of an infarct, there is local production of proinflammatory molecules occurring at the site of occlusion (130). Upon the resolution of the vascular blockage, there is further neuronal, glial, and blood vessel injury as reoxygenation promotes the production of reactive oxygen species (131). In a mammalian cell culture study of reactive oxygen species following ischemia, an NMDA glutamate receptor antagonist significantly suppressed the reactive oxygen species generation during reoxygenation (131). There are some studies which suggest that glutamate pathways may even have a significant effect on chronic stroke, and that drugs that modulate glutamatergic activity, such as memantine, may augment synaptic plasticity and long-term potentiation (132). Memantine is an uncompetitive NMDA receptor antagonist, which preferentially blocks pathological NMDA receptor activity, and is thought to exert its neuroprotective effects through suppressing the activation of the calcium-induced calpain–caspase-3 pathway in the ischemic penumbra (133). It is currently used in human patients for the treatment of dementia. In murine models of stroke, memantine has been shown to reduce infarct size, ischemic brain injury and to enhance recovery when administered in both the acute and chronic stroke phase (133,134). In a study where mice were exposed to a middle cerebral artery occlusion and then treated with memantine

72 hours later, memantine improved motor coordination and spatial memory and was associated with reduced astrogliosis and increased capillary formation surrounding the area of the infarct (135). In a mouse study of chronic treatment with oral memantine after an experimentally induced stroke, mice were given the drug for 28 days and had improved stroke outcomes with better sensory map recovery, decreased astrogliosis, increased brain-derived neurotrophic factor, and increased vascular density (136). In a study of aphasic poststroke patients, memantine alone and the combination of memantine and intensive and prolonged speech therapy led to superior language performance. Memantine was thought to strengthen compensatory rewiring in both cerebral hemispheres and promote bilateral reorganization of language networks, making the brain better prepared for intensive poststroke therapy (137). So far, human studies of memantine in stroke patients have been largely unsuccessful in neuroprotection or the prevention of cell death beyond the infarcted core (136). The failure of the trials has been attributed to various limitations, including narrow therapeutic time windows, cognitive side effects, underdosing in order to prevent cognitive side effects, lack of studies whose observation periods exceed the acute stroke phase, and lack of studies where drug therapy is paired with speech therapy (132,135). This is a novel and promising area of research, and clinical trials of memantine for the treatment of ischemic stroke are currently under way (133).

CONCLUSION

The management of acute ischemic stroke patients goes beyond the initial thrombolytic therapy and involves the prevention and treatment of metabolic derangements that develop in the subsequent days. As we have reviewed, these may include electrolyte disturbances, changes in fluid balance, acute kidney injury, disturbance in glucose homeostasis, anemia, and complications of nutritional deficits. It is crucial to anticipate and treat these conditions accordingly in order to minimize secondary damage to ischemic areas and optimize clinical outcomes.

REFERENCES

1. Arampatzis S, Exadaktylos A, Buhl D, et al. Dysnatraemias in the emergency room: undetected, untreated, unknown? *Wien Klin Wochenschr.* 2012;124(5–6):181–183. doi:10.1007/s00508-011-0108-7
2. Funk GC, Lindner G, Druml W, et al. Incidence and prognosis of dysnatremias present on ICU admission. *Intensive Care Med.* 2010;36(2):304–311. doi:10.1007/s00134-009-1692-0

3. Robertson GL. Abnormalities of thirst regulation. *Kidney Int.* 1984;25(2): 460–469. doi:10.1038/ki.1984.39
4. Stelfox HT, Ahmed SB, Khandwala F, et al. The epidemiology of intensive care unit-acquired hyponatraemia and hypernatraemia in medical-surgical intensive care units. *Crit Care.* 2008;12(6):R162. doi:10.1186/cc7162
5. Brimioulle S, Orellana-Jimenez C, Aminian A, et al. Hyponatremia in neurological patients: cerebral salt wasting versus inappropriate antidiuretic hormone secretion. *Intensive Care Med.* 2008;34(1):125–131. doi:10.1007/s00134-007-0905-7
6. Cerda-Esteve M, Cuadrado-Godia E, Chillaron JJ, et al. Cerebral salt wasting syndrome: review. *Eur J Intern Med.* 2008;19(4):249–254. doi:10.1016/j.ejim.2007.06.019
7. Maesaka JK, Imbriano LJ, Ali NM, et al. Is it cerebral or renal salt wasting? *Kidney Int.* 2009;76(9):934–938. doi:10.1038/ki.2009.263
8. Wijdicks EF, Vermeulen M, Hijdra A, et al. Hyponatremia and cerebral infarction in patients with ruptured intracranial aneurysms: is fluid restriction harmful? *Ann Neurol.* 1985;17(2):137–140. doi:10.1002/ana.410170206
9. Chung HM, Kluge R, Schrier RW, et al. Clinical assessment of extracellular fluid volume in hyponatremia. *Am J Med.* 1987;83(5):905–908. doi:10.1016/0002-9343(87)90649-8
10. Kalita J, Singh RK, Misra UK. Cerebral salt wasting is the most common cause of hyponatremia in stroke. *J Stroke Cerebrovasc Dis.* 2017;26(5):1026–1032. doi:10.1016/j.jstrokecerebrovasdis.2016.12.011
11. Saleem S, Yousuf I, Gul A, et al. Hyponatremia in stroke. *Ann Indian Acad Neurol.* 2014;17(1):55–57. doi:10.4103/0972-2327.128554
12. Miyasaka Y, Tokiwa K, Nakayama K, et al. SIADH with hypertensive cerebral hemorrhage or cerebral infarction. *Neurol Med Chir (Tokyo).* 26(4):284–290. doi:10.2176/nmc.26.284
13. Soiza RL, Cumming K, Clark AB, et al. Hyponatremia predicts mortality after stroke. *Int J Stroke.* 2015;10(Suppl A100):50–55. doi:10.1111/ijs.12564
14. Kusuda K, Saku Y, Sadoshima S, et al. Disturbances of fluid and electrolyte balance in patients with acute stroke. *Nihon Ronen Igakkai Zasshi.* 1989;26(3):223–227. doi:10.3143/geriatrics.40.223
15. Rodrigues B, Staff I, Fortunato G, et al. Hyponatremia in the prognosis of acute ischemic stroke. *J Stroke Cerebrovasc Dis.* 2014;23(5):850–854. doi:10.1016/j.jstrokecerebrovasdis.2013.07.011
16. Huang WY, Weng WC, Peng TI, et al. Association of hyponatremia in acute stroke stage with three-year mortality in patients with first-ever ischemic stroke. *Cerebrovasc Dis.* 2012;34(1):55–62. doi:10.1159/000338906
17. Chen CM, Chang CH, Hsu HC, et al. Factors predicting the total medical costs associated with first-ever ischeamic stroke patients transferred to the rehabilitation ward. *J Rehabil Med.* 2015;47(2):120–125. doi:10.2340/16501977-1894

18. Ramthun M, Mocelin AJ, Alvares Delfino VD. Hypernatremia secondary to post-stroke hypodipsia: just add water! *NDT Plus*. 2011;4(4):236–237. doi:10.1093/ndtplus/sfr057
19. Qureshi AI, Suarez JI, Bhardwaj A, et al. Use of hypertonic (3%) saline/acetate infusion in the treatment of cerebral edema: effect on intracranial pressure and lateral displacement of the brain. *Crit Care Med*. 1998;26(3):440–446. doi:10.1097/00003246-199803000-00011
20. Zornow MH. Hypertonic saline as a safe and efficacious treatment of intracranial hypertension. *J Neurosurg Anesthesiol*. 1996;8(2):175–177. doi:10.1097/00008506-199604000-00021
21. Froelich M, Ni Q, Wess C, et al. Continuous hypertonic saline therapy and the occurrence of complications in neurocritically ill patients. *Crit Care Med*. 2009;37(4):1433–1441. doi:10.1097/CCM.0b013e31819c1933
22. Todd MM, Tommasino C, Moore S. Cerebral effects of isovolemic hemodilution with a hypertonic saline solution. *J Neurosurg*. 1985;63(6):944–948. doi:10.3171/jns.1985.63.6.0944
23. Fofi L, Dall'armi V, Durastanti L, et al. An observational study on electrolyte disorders in the acute phase of ischemic stroke and their prognostic value. *J Clin Neurosci*. 2012;19(4):513–516. doi:10.1016/j.jocn.2011.07.041
24. Bhardwaj A, Harukuni I, Murphy SJ, et al. Hypertonic saline worsens infarct volume after transient focal ischemia in rats. *Stroke*. 2000;31(7):1694–1701. doi:10.1161/01.str.31.7.1694
25. Fisher LA, Ko N, Miss J, et al. Hypernatremia predicts adverse cardiovascular and neurological outcomes after SAH. *Neurocrit Care*. 2006;5(3):180–185. doi:10.1385/NCC:5:3:180
26. Berend K, van Hulsteijn LH, Gans RO. Chloride: the queen of electrolytes? *Eur J Intern Med*. 2012;23(3):203–211. doi:10.1016/j.ejim.2011.11.013
27. Kimura S, Matsumoto S, Muto N, et al. Association of serum chloride concentration with outcomes in postoperative critically ill patients: a retrospective observational study. *J Intensive Care*. 2014;2(1):39. doi:10.1186/2052-0492-2-39
28. Mandai S, Kanda E, Iimori S, et al. Association of serum chloride level with mortality and cardiovascular events in chronic kidney disease: the CKD-ROUTE study. *Clin Exp Nephrol*. 2017;21(1):104–111. doi:10.1007/s10157-016-1261-0
29. McCallum L, Jeemon P, Hastie CE, et al. Serum chloride is an independent predictor of mortality in hypertensive patients. *Hypertension*. 2013;62(5):836–843. doi:10.1161/HYPERTENSIONAHA.113.01793
30. Testani JM, Hanberg JS, Arroyo JP, et al. Hypochloraemia is strongly and independently associated with mortality in patients with chronic heart failure. *Eur J Heart Fail*. 2016;18(6):660–668. doi:10.1002/ejhf.477
31. Bei HZ, You SJ, Zheng D, et al. Prognostic role of hypochloremia in acute ischemic stroke patients. *Acta Neurol Scand*. 2017;136(6):672–679. doi:10.1111/ane.12785

32. Cherian L, Conners J, Cutting S, et al. Periprocedural risk of stroke is elevated in patients with end-stage renal disease on hemodialysis. *Cerebrovasc Dis Extra*. 2015;5(3):91–94. doi:10.1159/000440732
33. Sluijs I, Czernichow S, Beulens JW, et al. Intakes of potassium, magnesium, and calcium and risk of stroke. *Stroke*. 2014;45(4):1148–1150. doi:10.1161/STROKEAHA.113.004032
34. Bayir A, Ak A, Kara H, Sahin TK. Serum and cerebrospinal fluid magnesium levels, Glasgow Coma Scores, and in-hospital mortality in patients with acute stroke. *Biol Trace Elem Res*. 2009;130(1):7–12. doi:10.1007/s12011-009-8318-9
35. Feng P, Niu X, Hu J, et al. Relationship of serum magnesium concentration to risk of short-term outcome of acute ischemic stroke. *Blood Press*. 2013;22(5):297–301. doi:10.3109/08037051.2012.759696
36. Siegler JE, Boehme AK, Albright KC, et al. Acute decrease in serum magnesium level after ischemic stroke may not predict decrease in neurologic function. *J Stroke Cerebrovasc Dis*. 2013;22(8):e516–e521. doi:10.1016/j.jstrokecerebrovasdis.2013.05.030
37. You S, Zhong C, Du H, et al. Admission low magnesium level is associated with in-hospital mortality in acute ischemic stroke patients. *Cerebrovasc Dis*. 2017;44(1–2):35–42. doi:10.1159/000471858
38. Liotta EM, Prabhakaran S, Sangha RS, et al. Magnesium, hemostasis, and outcomes in patients with intracerebral hemorrhage. *Neurology*. 2017;89(8):813–819. doi:10.1212/WNL.0000000000004249
39. Gariballa SE, Robinson TG, Fotherby MD. Hypokalemia and potassium excretion in stroke patients. *J Am Geriatr Soc*. 1997;45(12):1454–1458. doi:10.1111/j.1532-5415.1997.tb03195.x
40. Dorner B, Posthauer ME, Thomas D, National Pressure Ulcer Advisory Panel. The role of nutrition in pressure ulcer prevention and treatment: National Pressure Ulcer Advisory Panel white paper. *Adv Skin Wound Care*. 2009;22(5):212–221. doi:10.1097/01.ASW.0000350838.11854.0a
41. Liu CH, Lin SC, Lin JR, et al. Dehydration is an independent predictor of discharge outcome and admission cost in acute ischaemic stroke. *Eur J Neurol*. 2014;21(9):1184–1191. doi:10.1111/ene.12452
42. Schrock JW, Glasenapp M, Drogell K. Elevated blood urea nitrogen/creatinine ratio is associated with poor outcome in patients with ischemic stroke. *Clin Neurol Neurosurg*. 2012;114(7):881–884. doi:10.1016/j.clineuro.2012.01.031
43. El-Sharkawy AM, Watson P, Neal KR, et al. Hydration and outcome in older patients admitted to hospital (The HOOP prospective cohort study). *Age Ageing*. 2015;44(6):943–947. doi:10.1093/ageing/afv119
44. Bahouth MN, Bahrainwala Z, Hillis AE, et al. Dehydration status is associated with more severe hemispatial neglect after stroke. *Neurologist*. 2016;21(6):101–105. doi:10.1097/NRL.0000000000000101
45. Meyer JS, Shimazu K, Fukuuchi Y, et al. Impaired neurogenic cerebrovascular control and dysautoregulation after stroke. *Stroke*. 1973;4(2):169–186. doi:10.1161/01.str.4.2.169

46. Jauch EC, Saver JL, Adams HP Jr. Guidelines for the early management of patients with acute ischemic stroke: a guideline for healthcare professionals from the American Heart Association/American Stroke Association. *Stroke.* 2013;44(3):870–947. doi:10.1161/STR.0b013e318284056a
47. Campbell BC, Christensen S, Tress BM, et al. Failure of collateral blood flow is associated with infarct growth in ischemic stroke. *J Cereb Blood Flow Metab.* 2013;33(8):1168–1172. doi:10.1038/jcbfm.2013.77
48. Castillo J, Leira R, Garcia MM, et al. Blood pressure decrease during the acute phase of ischemic stroke is associated with brain injury and poor stroke outcome. *Stroke.* 2004;35(2):520–526. doi:10.1161/01.STR.0000109769.22917.B0
49. Lucas SJ, Tzeng YC, Galvin SD, et al. Influence of changes in blood pressure on cerebral perfusion and oxygenation. *Hypertension.* 2010;55(3):698–705. doi:10.1161/HYPERTENSIONAHA.109.146290
50. Wohlfahrt P, Krajcoviechova A, Jozifova M, et al. Low blood pressure during the acute period of ischemic stroke is associated with decreased survival. *J Hypertens.* 2015;33(2):339–345. doi:10.1097/HJH.0000000000000414
51. Gonzalez-Alonso J, Mora-Rodriguez R, Below PR, et al. Dehydration reduces cardiac output and increases systemic and cutaneous vascular resistance during exercise. *J Appl Physiol.* 1995;79(5):1487–1496. doi:10.1152/jappl.1995.79.5.1487
52. Engquist H, Rostami E, Ronne-Engstrom E, et al. Effect of HHH-therapy on regional CBF after severe subarachnoid hemorrhage studied by bedside xenon-enhanced CT. *Neurocrit Care.* 2017;28(2):143–151. doi:10.1007/s12028-017-0439-y
53. Grandjean AC, Grandjean NR. Dehydration and cognitive performance. *J Am Coll Nutr.* 2007;26(5 Suppl):549S–554S. doi:10.1152/jappl.1995.79.5.1487
54. Kelly J, Hunt BJ, Lewis RR, et al. Dehydration and venous thromboembolism after acute stroke. *QJM.* 2004;97(5):293–296. doi:10.1093/qjmed/hch050
55. Shim R, Wong CH. Ischemia, immunosuppression and infection–tackling the predicaments of post-stroke complications. *Int J Mol Sci.* 2016;17(1). doi:10.3390/ijms17010064
56. Manz F. Hydration and disease. *J Am Coll Nutr.* 2007;26(5 Suppl):535S–541S. doi:10.1080/07315724.2007.10719655
57. Salat D, Campos M, Montaner J. Advances in the pathophysiology and management of infections in the acute phase of stroke. *Med Clin (Barc).* 2012:139(15):681–687. doi:10.1016/j.medcli.2012.03.014
58. Dharmasaroja PA. Fluid intake related to brain edema in acute middle cerebral artery infarction. *Transl Stroke Res.* 2016;7(1):49–53. doi:10.1007/s12975-015-0439-1

59. Sakr Y, Dunisch P, Santos C, et al. Poor outcome is associated with less negative fluid balance in patients with aneurysmal subarachnoid hemorrhage treated with prophylactic vasopressor-induced hypertension. *Ann Intensive Care.* 2016;6(1):25. doi:10.1186/s13613-016-0128-6
60. Gentile NT, Seftchick MW, Huynh T, et al. Decreased mortality by normalizing blood glucose after acute ischemic stroke. *Acad Emerg Med.* 2006;13(2):174–180. doi:10.1197/j.aem.2005.08.009
61. Baird TA, Parsons MW, Barber PA, et al. The influence of diabetes mellitus and hyperglycaemia on stroke incidence and outcome. *J Clin Neurosci.* 2002;9(6):618–626. doi:10.1054/jocn.2002.1081
62. Jenkins JS, Buckell M, Carter AB, et al. Hypothalamic-pituitary-adrenal function after subarachnoid haemorrhage. *Br Med J.* 1969;4(5685):707–709. doi:10.1136/bmj.4.5685.707
63. Kruyt ND, Biessels GJ, Devries JH, et al. Hyperglycemia in acute ischemic stroke: pathophysiology and clinical management. *Nat Rev Neurol.* 2010;6(3):145–155. doi:10.1038/nrneurol.2009.231
64. Capes SE, Hunt D, Malmberg K, et al. Stress hyperglycemia and prognosis of stroke in nondiabetic and diabetic patients: a systematic overview. *Stroke.* 2001;32(10):2426–2432. doi:10.1161/hs1001.096194
65. Baird TA, Parsons MW, Phan T, et al. Persistent poststroke hyperglycemia is independently associated with infarct expansion and worse clinical outcome. *Stroke.* 2003;34(9):2208–2214. doi:10.1161/01.STR.0000085087.41330.FF
66. Lee SH, Lim JS, Kim N, et al. Effects of admission glucose level on mortality after subarachnoid hemorrhage: a comparison between short-term and long-term mortality. *J Neurol Sci.* 2008;275(1–2):18–21. doi:10.1016/j.jns.2008.05.024
67. Bian L, Liu L, Wang C, et al. Hyperglycemia within day 14 of aneurysmal subarachnoid hemorrhage predicts 1-year mortality. *Clin Neurol Neurosurg.* 2013;115(7):959–964. doi:10.1016/j.clineuro.2012.09.026
68. Berger L, Hakim AM. The association of hyperglycemia with cerebral edema in stroke. *Stroke.* 1986;17(5):865–871. doi:10.1161/01.str.17.5.865
69. Bruno A, Levine SR, Frankel MR, et al. Admission glucose level and clinical outcomes in the NINDS rt-PA Stroke Trial. *Neurology.* 2002;59(5):669–674. doi:10.1212/wnl.59.5.669
70. Cucchiara B, Tanne D, Levine SR, et al. A risk score to predict intracranial hemorrhage after recombinant tissue plasminogen activator for acute ischemic stroke. *J Stroke Cerebrovasc Dis.* 2008;17(6):331–333. doi:10.1016/j.jstrokecerebrovasdis.2008.03.012
71. Demchuk AM, Morgenstern LB, Krieger DW, et al. Serum glucose level and diabetes predict tissue plasminogen activator-related intracerebral hemorrhage in acute ischemic stroke. *Stroke.* 1999;30(1):34–39. doi:10.1161/01.str.30.1.34

72. Demchuk AM, Tanne D, Hill MD, et al. Predictors of good outcome after intravenous tPA for acute ischemic stroke. *Neurology*. 2001;57(3):474–480. doi:10.1212/wnl.57.3.474
73. de Rooij NK, Rinkel GJ, Dankbaar JW, et al. Delayed cerebral ischemia after subarachnoid hemorrhage: a systematic review of clinical, laboratory, and radiological predictors. *Stroke*. 2013;44(1):43–54. doi:10.1161/STROKEAHA.112.674291
74. Huang YH, Chung CL, Tsai HP, et al. Hyperglycemia aggravates cerebral vasospasm after subarachnoid hemorrhage in a rat model. *Neurosurgery*. 2017;80(5):809–815. doi:10.1093/neuros/nyx016
75. Rao AK, Chouhan V, Chen X, et al. Activation of the tissue factor pathway of blood coagulation during prolonged hyperglycemia in young healthy men. *Diabetes*. 1999;48(5):1156–1161. doi:10.2337/diabetes.48.5.1156
76. Zonneveld TP, Nederkoorn PJ, Westendorp WF, et al. Hyperglycemia predicts poststroke infections in acute ischemic stroke. *Neurology*. 2017;88(15):1415–1421. doi:10.1212/WNL.0000000000003811
77. Winklewski PJ, Radkowski M, Demkow U. Cross-talk between the inflammatory response, sympathetic activation and pulmonary infection in the ischemic stroke. *J Neuroinflammation*. 2014;11:213. doi:10.1186/s12974-014-0213-4
78. Anderson RE, Tan WK, Martin HS, et al. Effects of glucose and PaO2 modulation on cortical intracellular acidosis, NADH redox state, and infarction in the ischemic penumbra. *Stroke*. 1999;30(1):160–170. doi:10.1161/01.str.30.1.160
79. Kawai N, Keep RF, Betz AL, et al. Hyperglycemia induces progressive changes in the cerebral microvasculature and blood-brain barrier transport during focal cerebral ischemia. *Acta Neurochir Suppl*. 1998;71:219–221. doi:10.1007/978-3-7091-6475-4_63
80. Gray CS, Hildreth AJ, Sandercock PA, et al. Glucose-potassium-insulin infusions in the management of post-stroke hyperglycaemia: the UK Glucose Insulin in Stroke Trial (GIST-UK). *Lancet Neurol*. 2007;6(5):397–406. doi:10.1016/S1474-4422(07)70080-7
81. Hao Z, Wu B, Wang D, et al. A cohort study of patients with anemia on admission and fatality after acute ischemic stroke. *J Clin Neurosci*. 2013;20(1):37–42. doi:10.1016/j.jocn.2012.05.020
82. Dhar R, Zazulia AR, Videen TO, et al. Red blood cell transfusion increases cerebral oxygen delivery in anemic patients with subarachnoid hemorrhage. *Stroke*. 2009;40(9):3039–3044. doi:10.1161/STROKEAHA.109.556159
83. Barlas RS, Honney K, Loke YK, et al. Impact of hemoglobin levels and anemia on mortality in acute stroke: analysis of UK regional registry data, systematic review, and meta-analysis. *J Am Heart Assoc*. 2016;5(8). doi:10.1161/JAHA.115.003019
84. Tanne D, Molshatzki N, Merzeliak O, et al. Anemia status, hemoglobin concentration and outcome after acute stroke: a cohort study. *BMC Neurol*. 2010;10:22. doi:10.1186/1471-2377-10-22

85. Allport LE, Parsons MW, Butcher KS, et al. Elevated hematocrit is associated with reduced reperfusion and tissue survival in acute stroke. *Neurology*. 2005;65(9), 1382–1387. doi:10.1212/01.wnl.0000183057.96792.a8
86. Kumar MA, BolandTA, Baiou M, et al. Red blood cell transfusion increases the risk of thrombotic events in patients with subarachnoid hemorrhage. *Neurocrit Care*. 2014;20(1):84–90. doi:10.1007/s12028-013-9819-0
87. Kellert L, Schrader F, Ringleb P, et al. The impact of low hemoglobin levels and transfusion on critical care patients with severe ischemic stroke: STroke RelevAnt Impact of HemoGlobin, Hematocrit and Transfusion (STRAIGHT)—an observational study. *J Crit Care*. 2014;29(2):236–240. doi:10.1016/j.jcrc.2013.11.008
88. English SW, Fergusson D, Chasse M, et al. Aneurysmal SubArachnoid Hemorrhage-Red Blood CellTransfusion and Outcome (SAHaRA): a pilot randomised controlled trial protocol. *BMJ Open*. 2016;6(12):e012623. doi:10.1136/bmjopen-2016-012623
89. Sheth KN, Gilson AJ, Chang Y, et al. Packed red blood cell transfusion and decreased mortality in intracerebral hemorrhage. *Neurosurgery*. 2011;68(5):1286–1292. doi:10.1227/NEU.0b013e31820cccb2
90. Rosenberg NF, Koht A, Naidech AM. Anemia and transfusion after aneurysmal subarachnoid hemorrhage. *J Neurosurg Anesthesiol*. 2013;25(1):66–74. doi:10.1097/ANA.0b013e31826cfc1d
91. Stein M, Brokmeier L, Herrmann J, et al. Mean hemoglobin concentration after acute subarachnoid hemorrhage and the relation to outcome, mortality, vasospasm, and brain infarction. *J Clin Neurosci*. 2015;22(3):530–534. doi:10.1016/j.jocn.2014.08.026
92. Bell DL, Kimberly WT, Yoo AJ, et al. Low neurologic intensive care unit hemoglobin as a predictor for intra-arterial vasospasm therapy and poor discharge modified Rankin Scale in aneurysmal subarachnoid haemorrhage-induced cerebral vasospasm. *J Neurointerv Surg*. 2015;7(6):438–442. doi:10.1136/neurintsurg-2014-011164
93. Sun J, Tan G, Xing W, et al. Optimal hemoglobin concentration in patients with aneurysmal subarachnoid hemorrhage after surgical treatment to prevent symptomatic cerebral vasospasm. *Neuroreport*. 2015;26(5):263–266. doi:10.1097/WNR.0000000000000340
94. Ingall T, Asplund K, Mahonen M, et al. A multinational comparison of subarachnoid hemorrhage epidemiology in the WHO MONICA stroke study. *Stroke*. 2000;31(5):1054–1061. doi:10.1161/01.str.31.5.1054
95. Kim E, Kim HC, Park SY, et al. Effect of red blood cell transfusion on unfavorable neurologic outcome and symptomatic vasospasm in patients with cerebral aneurysmal rupture: old versus fresh blood. *World Neurosurg*. 2015;84(6):1877–1886. doi:10.1016/j.wneu.2015.08.024
96. Smith MJ, Le Roux PD, Elliott JP, et al. Blood transfusion and increased risk for vasospasm and poor outcome after subarachnoid hemorrhage. *J Neurosurg*. 2004;101(1):1–7. doi:10.3171/jns.2004.101.1.0001

97. Connolly ES Jr, Rabinstein AA, Carhuapoma JR, et al. Guidelines for the management of aneurysmal subarachnoid hemorrhage: a guideline for healthcare professionals from the American Heart Association/American Stroke Association. *Stroke*. 2012;43(6):1711–1737. doi:10.1161/STR.0b013e3182587839
98. Hsiao KY, Hsiao CT, Lin LJ, et al. Severe anemia associated with transient ischemic attacks involving vertebrobasilar circulation. *Am J Emerg Med*. 2008;26(3):382 e3–382 e4. doi:10.1016/j.ajem.2007.05.028
99. Shahar A, Sadeh M. Severe anemia associated with transient neurological deficits. *Stroke*. 1991;22(9):1201–1202. doi:10.1161/01.str.22.9.1201
100. Luvizutto GJ, Monteiro TA, Braga GP, et al. Low haemoglobin levels increase unilateral spatial neglect in acute phase of stroke. *Arq Neuropsiquiatr*. 2014;72(10):757–761. doi:10.1590/0004-282x20140112
101. Tomiyama Y, Jansen K, Brian JE Jr, et al. Hemodilution, cerebral O2 delivery, and cerebral blood flow: a study using hyperbaric oxygenation. *Am J Physiol*. 1999;276(4 Pt 2):H1190–H1196. doi:10.1152/ajpheart.1999.276.4.h1190
102. van Bommel J, Trouwborst A, Schwarte L, et al. Intestinal and cerebral oxygenation during severe isovolemic hemodilution and subsequent hyperoxic ventilation in a pig model. *Anesthesiology*. 2002;97(3):660–670. doi:10.1097/00000542-200209000-00021
103. Morigi M, Zoja C, Figliuzzi M, et al. Fluid shear stress modulates surface expression of adhesion molecules by endothelial cells. *Blood*. 1995;85(7):1696–1703.
104. Nagel T, Resnick N, Atkinson WJ, et al. Shear stress selectively upregulates intercellular adhesion molecule-1 expression in cultured human vascular endothelial cells. *J Clin Invest*. 1994;94(2):885–891. doi:10.1172/JCI117410
105. McLaren AT, Marsden PA, Mazer CD, et al. Increased expression of HIF-1alpha, nNOS, and VEGF in the cerebral cortex of anemic rats. *Am J Physiol Regul Integr Comp Physiol*. 2007;292(1):R403–R414. doi:10.1152/ajpregu.00403.2006
106. Felszeghy K, Banisadr G, Rostene W, et al. Dexamethasone downregulates chemokine receptor CXCR4 and exerts neuroprotection against hypoxia/ischemia-induced brain injury in neonatal rats. *Neuroimmunomodulation*. 2004;11(6):404–413. doi:10.1159/000080151
107. Moro MA, Cardenas A, Hurtado O, et al. Role of nitric oxide after brain ischaemia. *Cell Calcium*. 2004;36(3–4):265–275. doi:10.1016/j.ceca.2004.02.011
108. Kumar MA, Rost NS, Snider RW, et al. Anemia and hematoma volume in acute intracerebral hemorrhage. *Crit Care Med*. 2009;37(4):1442–1447. doi:10.1097/CCM.0b013e31819ced3a
109. Foley NC, Martin RE, Salter KL, et al. A review of the relationship between dysphagia and malnutrition following stroke. *J Rehabil Med*. 2009;41(9):707–713. doi:10.2340/16501977-0415

110. Davis JP, Wong AA, Schluter PJ, et al. Impact of premorbid undernutrition on outcome in stroke patients. *Stroke*. 2004;35(8):1930–1934. doi:10.1161/01.STR.0000135227.10451.c9

111. Mosselman MJ, Kruitwagen CL, Schuurmans MJ, et al. Malnutrition and risk of malnutrition in patients with stroke: prevalence during hospital stay. *J Neurosci Nurs*. 2013;45(4):194–204. doi:10.1097/JNN.0b013e31829863cb

112. Corrigan ML, Escuro AA, Celestin J, et al. Nutrition in the stroke patient. *Nutr Clin Pract*. 2011;26(3):242–252. doi:10.1177/0884533611405795

113. Finestone HM, Greene-Finestone LS, Wilson ES, et al. Malnutrition in stroke patients on the rehabilitation service and at follow-up: prevalence and predictors. *Arch Phys Med Rehabil*. 1995;76(4):310–316. doi:10.1016/s0003-9993(95)80655-5

114. Westergren A, Karlsson S, Andersson P, et al. Eating difficulties, need for assisted eating, nutritional status and pressure ulcers in patients admitted for stroke rehabilitation. *J Clin Nurs*. 2001;10(2):257–269. doi:10.1046/j.1365-2702.2001.00479.x

115. Finestone HM, Greene-Finestone LS, Foley NC, et al. Measuring longitudinally the metabolic demands of stroke patients: resting energy expenditure is not elevated. *Stroke*. 2003;34(2):502–507. doi:10.1161/01.str.0000053031.12332.fb

116. Zheng T, Zhu X, Liang H, et al. Impact of early enteral nutrition on short term prognosis after acute stroke. *J Clin Neurosci*. 2015;22(9):1473–1476. doi:10.1016/j.jocn.2015.03.028

117. Gomes F, Emery PW, Weekes CE. Risk of malnutrition is an independent predictor of mortality, length of hospital stay, and hospitalization costs in stroke patients. *J Stroke Cerebrovasc Dis*. 2016;25(4):799–806. doi:10.1016/j.jstrokecerebrovasdis.2015.12.017

118. Davalos A, Ricart W, Gonzalez-Huix F, et al. Effect of malnutrition after acute stroke on clinical outcome. *Stroke*. 1996;27(6):1028–1032. doi:10.1161/01.str.27.6.1028

119. Gariballa SE, Parker SG, Taub N, et al. Influence of nutritional status on clinical outcome after acute stroke. *Am J Clin Nutr*. 1998;68(2):275–281. doi:10.1093/ajcn/68.2.275

120. Collaboration, FoodTrial. Poor nutritional status on admission predicts poor outcomes after stroke: observational data from the FOOD trial. *Stroke*. 2003;34(6):1450–1456. doi:10.1161/01.STR.0000074037.49197.8C

121. Zhang J, Zhao X, Wang A, et al. Emerging malnutrition during hospitalisation independently predicts poor 3-month outcomes after acute stroke: data from a Chinese cohort. *Asia Pac J Clin Nutr*. 2015;24(3):379–386. doi:10.6133/apjcn.2015.24.3.13

122. Yoo SH, Kim JS, Kwon SU, et al. Undernutrition as a predictor of poor clinical outcomes in acute ischemic stroke patients. *Arch Neurol*. 2008;65(1):39–43. doi:10.1001/archneurol.2007.12

123. Famakin B, Weiss P, Hertzberg V, et al. Hypoalbuminemia predicts acute stroke mortality: Paul Coverdell Georgia Stroke Registry. *J Stroke Cerebrovasc Dis*. 2010;19(1):17–22. doi:10.1016/j.jstrokecerebrovasdis.2009.01.015
124. Sellars C, Campbell AM, Stott DJ, et al. Swallowing abnormalities after acute stroke: a case control study. *Dysphagia*. 1999;14(4):212–218. doi:10.1007/PL00009608
125. Jayasekeran V, Singh S, Tyrrell P, et al. Adjunctive functional pharyngeal electrical stimulation reverses swallowing disability after brain lesions. *Gastroenterology*. 2010;138(5):1737–1746. doi:10.1053/j.gastro.2010.01.052
126. Ludlow CL. Electrical neuromuscular stimulation in dysphagia: current status. *Curr Opin Otolaryngol Head Neck Surg*. 2010;18(3):159–164. doi:10.1097/MOO.0b013e3283395dec
127. Lai TW, Zhang S, Wang YT. Excitotoxicity and stroke: identifying novel targets for neuroprotection. *Prog Neurobiol*. 2014;115:157–188. doi:10.1016/j.pneurobio.2013.11.006
128. Sims NR, Muyderman H. Mitochondria, oxidative metabolism and cell death in stroke. *Biochim Biophys Acta*. 2010;1802(1):80–91. doi:10.1016/j.bbadis.2009.09.003
129. Qu M, Mittmann T, Luhmann HJ, et al. Long-term changes of ionotropic glutamate and GABA receptors after unilateral permanent focal cerebral ischemia in the mouse brain. *Neuroscience*. 1998;85(1):29–43. doi:10.1016/s0306-4522(97)00656-8
130. Yilmaz G, Granger DN. Leukocyte recruitment and ischemic brain injury. *Neuromolecular Med*. 2010;12(2):193–204. doi:10.1007/s12017-009-8074-1
131. Abramov AY, Scorziello A, Duchen MR. Three distinct mechanisms generate oxygen free radicals in neurons and contribute to cell death during anoxia and reoxygenation. *J Neurosci*. 2007;27(5):1129–1138. doi:10.1523/JNEUROSCI.4468-06.2007
132. Berthier ML, Pulvermuller F, Davila G, et al. Drug therapy of post-stroke aphasia: a review of current evidence. *Neuropsychol Rev*. 2011;21(3):302–317. doi:10.1007/s11065-011-9177-7
133. Chen B, Wang G, Li W, et al. Memantine attenuates cell apoptosis by suppressing the calpain-caspase-3 pathway in an experimental model of ischemic stroke. *Exp Cell Res*. 2017;351(2):163–172. doi:10.1016/j.yexcr.2016.12.028
134. Shih AY, Blinder P, Tsai PS, et al. The smallest stroke: occlusion of one penetrating vessel leads to infarction and a cognitive deficit. *Nat Neurosci*. 2013;16(1):55–63. doi:10.1038/nn.3278
135. Wang YC, Sanchez-Mendoza EH, Doeppner TR, et al. Post-acute delivery of memantine promotes post-ischemic neurological recovery, peri-infarct tissue remodeling, and contralesional brain plasticity. *J Cereb Blood Flow Metab*. 2017;37(3):980–993. doi:10.1177/0271678X16648971.

136. Lopez-Valdes HE, Clarkson AN, Ao Y, et al. Memantine enhances recovery from stroke. *Stroke*. 2014;45(7):2093–2100. doi:10.1161/STROKEAHA.113.004476

137. Barbancho MA, Berthier ML, Navas-Sanchez P, et al. Bilateral brain reorganization with memantine and constraint-induced aphasia therapy in chronic post-stroke aphasia: an ERP study. *Brain Lang*. 2015;145–146:1–10. doi:10.1016/j.bandl.2015.04.003

138. Khatri M, Himmelfarb J, Adams D, et al. Acute kidney injury is associated with increased hospital mortality after stroke. *J Stroke Cerebrovasc Dis*. 2014;23(1):25–30. doi:10.1016/j.jstrokecerebrovasdis.2012.06.005

139. Khwaja A. KDIGO Clinical practice guidelines for acute kidney injury. *Nephron Clin Pract*. 2012;120(4):C179–C184. doi:10.1159/000339789

140. Covic A, Schiller A, Mardare NG, et al. The impact of acute kidney injury on short-term survival in an Eastern European population with stroke. *Nephrol Dial Transplant*. 2008;23(7):2228–2234. doi:10.1093/ndt/gfm591

141. Saeed F, Adil MM, Piracha BH, et al. Acute renal failure worsens in-hospital outcomes in patients with intracerebral hemorrhage. *J Stroke Cerebrovasc Dis*. 2015;24(4):789–794. doi:10.1016/j.jstrokecerebrovasdis.2014.11.012

142. Liu M, Liang Y, Chigurupati S, et al. Acute kidney injury leads to inflammation and functional changes in the brain. *J Am Soc Nephrol*. 2008:19(7):1360–1370 doi:10.1681/ASN.2007080901.

143. Simmons EM, Himmelfarb J, Sezer MT, et al. Plasma cytokine levels predict mortality in patients with acute renal failure. *Kidney Int*. 2004;65(4):1357–1365. doi:10.1111/j.1523-1755.2004.00512.x

144. Saeed F, Adil MM, Khursheed F, et al. Acute renal failure is associated with higher death and disability in patients with acute ischemic stroke: analysis of nationwide inpatient sample. *Stroke*. 2014;45(5):1478–1480. doi:10.1161/STROKEAHA.114.004672

145. Kribben A, Witzke O, Hillen U, et al. Nephrogenic systemic fibrosis: pathogenesis, diagnosis, and therapy. *J Am Coll Cardiol*. 2009;53(18):1621–1628. doi:10.1016/j.jacc.2008.12.061

146. Balasubramanian G, Al-Aly Z, Moiz A, et al. Early nephrologist involvement in hospital-acquired acute kidney injury: a pilot study. *Am J Kidney Dis*. 2011;57(2):228–234. doi:10.1053/j.ajkd.2010.08.026

15 Poststroke Infections

Réza Behrouz

KEY POINTS

- The overall frequency of poststroke infections has been reported to be between 21% and 65%.
- Infections are responsible for 30% of all stroke-related deaths.
- Respiratory and urinary tracts are the most common sites for poststroke infections.
- Poststroke infections substantially impact stroke-related morbidity and mortality.
- Age and stroke severity are associated with increased risk of poststroke infections.
- Stroke-related immunodeficiency has been postulated as a potential underlying mechanism for infection susceptibility.
- The use of prophylactic antibiotics has not been shown to have a significant impact on stroke-related outcomes.
- Prevention of infection is a key paradigm in stroke patients.

INTRODUCTION

Infection can complicate the hospitalization course of any condition, and acute stroke is not an exception. Many patients develop infections soon after acute stroke regardless of optimal management (1). Mortality is higher in these patients and the stroke severity and age are the strongest determinants of the infectious risk (1,2). In specialized stroke units, the overall frequency of poststroke infections has been reported to be between 21% and 65% (3). Infections are responsible for 30% of all stroke-related deaths (2). With respective rates of 11% to 57% and 11% to 27%, respiratory and urinary tracts are the most common sites for poststroke infections, with the former having greater impact on clinical outcome (2). Other forms of infection after acute stroke include sinusitis

 DOI: 10.1891/9780826124791.0015

from indwelling nasogastric tubes, catheter-related bloodstream infections, and hospital-acquired enteritis (2). Because of its substantial impact on stroke-related morbidity and mortality, infection is considered a major source of complication after acute stroke.

PATHOPHYSIOLOGY

The increased risk of infection after stroke is attributable to physical disability and endogenous immunodeficiency (2). The latter explains why acute stroke patients are particularly susceptible to developing early infections, irrespective of merely stroke-related disability.

Immobility, mechanical ventilation, and indwelling tubes and intravenous/intra-arterial lines all can increase the risk for infection. Decreased level of alertness, dysphagia, and impaired cough can lead to aspiration, a common cause of pneumonia in stroke patients. The plurality of evidence suggests that poststroke pneumonia is often due to aspiration (4). Aspiration pneumonia is the most important acute complication of poststroke dysphagia (found in nearly 50% of acute stroke patients), affecting up to one-third of dysphagic patients (5). Aspiration pneumonia often occurs after aspiration of colonized oropharyngeal material. In addition, similar to nonstroke hospitalized patients, acute stroke patients are at risk for nosocomial pneumonia. Increasing age, chronic lung disease, depressed consciousness, presence of intracranial pressure monitors, and mechanical ventilation are some of the risk factors associated with hospital-acquired pneumonia (HAP) (6). In acute stroke patients who require mechanical ventilation, ventilator-associated pneumonia (VAP) is a frequent problem (7). Chronic lung disease history, severity of stroke on admission, and hemorrhagic transformation of cerebral infarctions increase the risk for VAP (7). VAP increases the duration of both mechanical ventilation and ICU (7). Risk factors for VAP include immunosuppression, chronic obstructive lung disease, and acute respiratory distress syndrome, in addition to body positioning, level of consciousness, number of intubations, and medications including sedative agents and antibiotics (8).

Urinary tract infections (UTIs) occur often after stroke and are associated with an increased risk of neurological decline during hospitalization and worse outcomes (9). Stroke patients are twice more likely to develop UTIs in the hospital, compared with the general medical and surgical population, irrespective of bladder catheterization (10). Urinary incontinence and retention are common after stroke, occurring in 29% to 58% of patients (9). Urodynamic studies reveal high rates of bladder hyperreflexia after stroke

(9). In acute stroke patients, bladder dysfunction, disability, and depressed mental status necessitate bladder catheterization, which is a well-known risk factor for UTI. Indwelling catheters are placed prior to administration of intravenous thrombolytics, or purely because of the patients' inability to properly use the commode.

Other potential causes of infection in acute stroke patients are central venous catheters and arterial lines. The frequency of line infections in acute stroke patients is similar to any other hospitalized patient who undergoes these procedures. External ventriculostomy drains (EVDs) are placed in patients who develop or are at high risk of developing hydrocephalus or for draining intraventricular blood. The frequency of EVD placement in stroke patients is highly variable across institutions and geographic locations and depends on the type and severity of stroke. The incidence rate of EVD-related ventriculitis ranges from 2% to 27% (11). It is primarily placed in patients with intraventricular hemorrhage at risk for developing hydrocephalus, or in those with cerebellar infarcts or hematomas obliterating the fourth ventricle. Predisposing factors for EVD-related infection are nonadherence to proper maintenance protocols, leakage of cerebrospinal fluid (CSF), catheter irrigation, and the frequency of EVD manipulations (11).

The theory behind "poststroke immunodepression" is complex and involves several proposed mechanisms, including poststroke systemic inflammation, giving rise to a "protective" immunosuppressive state (2). Experimental and clinical evidence suggests peripheral lymphocytopenia, decreased monocyte count and function, and interferon-gamma deficiency, which begins a few hours after ischemia and lasts for several weeks (12). There is immunological switch from proinflammatory T_{H2} response to anti-inflammatory T_{H2} response as a result of sympathetic activation after acute stroke (13). Neuroendocrine pathways involving acetylcholine and norepinephrine immediately activated after acute stroke may alter the production and function of inflammatory and anti-inflammatory cytokines, creating a state of immunologic disarray (1). This state, in turn, creates a suitable environment for pathogens causing hospital-acquired infections. As the infectious process progresses, upregulation of the systemic inflammatory response from infection leads to excessive inflammation of the brain, causing edema, elevated intracranial pressure, and possibly stroke expansion (2).

PREVENTION

Prevention of infections in acute stroke patients can be difficult, as it is often not possible to predict which patients are at risk for infection.

As mentioned earlier, patient age and the degree of stroke-related disability correlate with the risk of infection. Specifically, those with moderate-to-severe dysphagia or severe oropharyngeal dysfunction as a result of stroke may be at an increased risk of developing aspiration pneumonia.

Aspiration pneumonia can be prevented by early involvement of the dysphagia team or the speech pathologist. Objective measures of voluntary cough can identify stroke patients who are at risk for aspiration (14). The head of the bed should be placed in a position allowing adequate draining of oropharyngeal secretions. Elevating the head of the bed to an angle of 30° to 45° is recommended for patients at high risk for aspiration pneumonia (15). Frequent patient repositioning, maintaining adequate oral hygiene, diet modifications and postural compensation, prescription of appropriate fluid and solid food consistency, and expiratory muscle strengthening are some of the strategies for prevention of aspiration in acute stroke patients. In patients with feeding tubes, the position of the tube and gastric residual volume should be monitored and assessed regularly. Last, sedation should be minimized (unless the patient requires mechanical ventilation).

VAP can be prevented by oral decontamination using chlorhexidine oral rinse, saline lavage and suction of the endotracheal tube, routine frequent turning, subglottic suctioning, and monitoring of endotracheal cuff pressure. The frequency of ventilator circuit changes should be minimized (16). The use of gastrointestinal stress ulcer prophylaxis should be balanced against the potential for elevation of stomach pH, which promotes colonization with potentially pathogenic organisms (16).

For prevention of UTIs in acute stroke patients, special attention must be placed on the utility of Foley catheters. Catheters are responsible for most cases of UTIs in hospitalized patients (9). Inappropriate use of indwelling bladder catheters, for example in stroke patients who are mobile or are able to void on volition, should be avoided. If a Foley catheter is instituted in a patient, an objective plan should be formulated to promptly discontinue the device. The use of antiseptic-coated or antibiotic-impregnated bladder catheters is a promising strategy, but they have not shown to significantly reduce the incidence of UTIs (9). In men without urinary retention, condom catheters represent a noninvasive alternative.

Other measures to prevent infection in acute stroke patients include avoiding unnecessary invasive procedures and lines, and early mobilization. Venous and arterial catheters, as well as EVDs should be placed under strict sterile conditions and maintained according to institutional policies for infection control. Duration of EVD placement and frequency of CSF sampling should be minimized. The concept of antibiotic prophylaxis in stroke patients has been studied in several clinical trials. These studies showed that although antibiotic prophylaxis in acute stroke patients was associated with lower infection rates, this strategy did not have an impact on functional outcomes (17–19).

IDENTIFICATION

Identification of infection is based upon clinical findings in conjunction with diagnostic testing, which may include blood count, microbiology, and radiography. The most important marker for acute infection is fever. Between 40% and 61% of patients who experience stroke develop fever, and those patients with fever are far more likely to die within the first 10 days after a stroke than those with lower temperatures (20,21). An infectious etiology is responsible for 40% to 80% of fever in poststroke patients (22). Other clinical signs and symptoms of infection are cough, hypoxia, dyspnea, tachypnea, dysuria, altered mental status, abdominal pain, and diarrhea. Acute onset of any of these features should prompt investigation for an infectious process.

A chest x-ray should be obtained in patients with fever, clinical signs and symptoms of pneumonia, or aspiration. CT of the chest may be more sensitive for the diagnosis of community-acquired pneumonia than plain chest radiography. It should be considered in patients with a high clinical index of suspicion for pneumonia without clear infiltrates on chest x-ray. A bronchopneumonia pattern is most commonly observed, with a distribution that is characteristically gravity dependent. Chest x-ray frequently shows an infiltrate in the dependent lung segments (the superior or posterior basal segments of a lower lobe or the posterior segment of an upper lobe). Sputum Gram stain and culture are more useful in the diagnosis of nosocomial and therefore, it is rarely done for evaluation of aspiration pneumonia. In aspiration pneumonia, Gram stain and microscopy may reveal a multitude of bacteria types, which are characteristically anaerobic. However, anaerobic bacteria are difficult to culture and identification of these pathogens is time-consuming, expensive, and tedious.

The first step in the diagnosis of UTI is examination of a urine sample. Urine specimens are obtained from adult patients via the clean-catch midstream technique or via the aseptic method to remove urine from the catheter tubing with a needleless syringe. Urine Gram stain allows an estimate of the level of bacteriuria. A colony count $\geq 10^3$ colony-forming units (cfu)/mL of a bacterium is diagnostic of acute uncomplicated UTI (23). This test has a sensitivity and specificity of 97% (24). Asymptomatic bacteriuria is defined as the presence of bacteria in the urine in quantities of 10^5 cfu/mL or more in two consecutive urine specimens in women, or one urine specimen in men, in the absence of clinical signs or symptoms suggestive of a UTI. Distinguishing UTI from asymptomatic bacteriuria specifically in older adults can be challenging. A catheter-related UTI is diagnosed in a patient with UTI and an indwelling catheter, or who has had a catheter removed within the past 48 hours. Positive tests for nitrite or leukocyte esterase are helpful in supporting the diagnosis of UTI, but their accuracy is a matter of debate, especially in isolation. A positive leukocyte esterase merely depicts inflammation and not necessarily infection. Although it is associated with low specificity and positive predictive value, its absence virtually eliminates infection as a cause. A positive nitrite test is highly specific for the presence of a nitrite-reducing organism, most commonly *Escherichia coli.* However, not all uropathogens reduce nitrite. Therefore, the utility of this test is restricted to *Enterobacteriaceae.* With a positive urinalysis, cultures can be performed to identify the culprit organism and determine its antimicrobial sensitivities.

Infections associated with vascular access devices can be diagnosed via blood cultures. The diagnostic workup for EVD-associated ventriculitis typically consists of CSF analysis (cell counts, Gram staining, cultures, biochemical tests for glucose and protein). CSF typically shows a meningitis picture, with pleocytosis, elevated protein, decreased glucose, and positive Gram stain. Daily calculation of the cell index allows the timely diagnosis and initiation of antimicrobial therapy for EVD-related ventriculitis (25). The formula for cell index is

$$\text{Cell index} = \frac{\text{WBC(CSF)} \div \text{RBC(CSF)}}{\text{WBC(blood)} \div \text{RBC(blood)}}$$

where WBC depicts white blood cells and RBC indicates red blood cells. Cell index is subject to fluctuations. Therefore, an absolute cutoff for the diagnosis of infection cannot be established. Observation trends and comparison of values over time is the appropriate way of utilizing this index.

MANAGEMENT

Empirical antibiotics should be initiated on clinical suspicion. Thereafter, isolation of pathogens from relevant species should be at the center of diagnostic efforts. The choice of antibiotics has to be guided by local pathogen epidemiology and clinical features. Differentiation between aspiration pneumonia and pneumonitis is not always easy. Treatment strategies are different for the two conditions and consist of supportive management itself for aspiration pneumonitis and antimicrobial therapy for aspiration pneumonia (26). However, it is common practice to use antibiotics with the potential for aspiration pneumonia in mind. Common pathogens in aspiration pneumonia are bacteria that normally reside in the upper airways or stomach, primarily oral anaerobes and streptococci (27). Broad-spectrum antibiotics are usually initiated with a plan to de-escalate the regimen based on definitive and quantitative culture in the following 72 hours. Examples of empirical treatment for hospital-acquired aspiration pneumonia are intravenous piperacillin–tazobactam or ampicillin–sulbactam (Table 15.1).

Early HAP in acute stroke patients is typically caused by gram-negative bacteria, such as *Haemophilus influenzae*, and gram-positive bacteria such as *Staphylococcus aureus* or *Streptococcus pneumonia* (28). Late-onset HAP is usually attributed to higher level antibiotic-resistant gram-negative bacteria such as *Pseudomonas aeruginosa, Acinetobacter* spp. and gram-positive bacteria such as methicillin-resistant *Staphylococcus aureus* (28). Empiric therapy for HAP and VAP should include antimicrobials against *Staphylococcus aureus, Pseudomonas aeruginosa,* and

Table 15.1 Options for Antimicrobial Therapy in the Treatment of Aspiration Pneumonia

Piperacillin–tazobactam		3.375 g IV every 6 hours		
Ampicillin–sulbactam		1.5–3.0 g IV every 6 hours		
Cefoxitin		2 g IV every 6–8 hours		
Cefotetan		1–2 g IV every 12 hours		
Cefotaxime	2 g IV every 8 hours	*Plus*	Clindamycin	600 mg IV every 6–8 hours
Ceftriaxone	2 g IV every 24 hours	*Plus*	Clindamycin	600 mg IV every 6–8 hours
Ciprofloxacin	400 mg IV every 12 hours	*Plus*	Clindamycin	600 mg IV every 6–8 hours
Levofloxacin	500–750 mg IV daily	*Plus*	Clindamycin	600 mg IV every 6–8 hours

IV, intravenous.

other gram-negative bacilli. Third-generation cephalosporins (e.g., cefotaxime, ceftriaxone, and ceftazidime), broad-spectrum penicillins (e.g., piperacillin/tazobactam), fluoroquinolones (e.g., ciprofloxacin and levofloxacin), aminoglycosides (e.g., gentamicin), and carbapenems (e.g., imipenem and meropenem) have broad-spectrum activity against the common aerobic pathogens causing HAP or VAP (29).

Typical organisms implicated in hospital-acquired UTI (which are largely catheter related) are *Escherichia coli, Candida* spp., *Enterococcus* spp., *Klebsiella* spp., and *Pseudomonas aeruginosa.* Antimicrobial treatment of asymptomatic bacteriuria does not influence patient outcomes or increase the risk of complications and subsequent development of UTI symptoms (30). Nitrofurantoin monohydrate, trimethoprim–sulfamethoxazole, and fosfomycin trometamol are used as first-line, and fluoroquinolones are used as second-tier antibiotics for uncomplicated UTI (31). Treatment duration should not exceed 7 days.

For the treatment of EVD-associated infections, intravenous vancomycin plus an antipseudomonal beta-lactam (cefepime, ceftazidime, or meropenem) is typically used as empiric therapy; the choice of empiric beta-lactam agent should be based on local in vitro susceptibility patterns (Table 15.2). For patients allergic to beta-lactam, intravenous aztreonam or ciprofloxacin is used. CSF cultures are important for establishing the diagnosis of EVD

Table 15.2 Empirical Therapy for Ventriculostomy-Related Infections

Vancomycin	15–20 mg/kg IV	Every 8–12 hours*
	Plus	
Ceftazidime	2 g IV	Every 8 hours
	Or	
Cefepime	2 g IV	Every 8 hours
	Or	
Meropenem	2 g IV	Every 8 hours
	For Patients With Beta-Lactam Allergy	
Aztreonam	2 g IV	Every 6–8 hours
	Or	
Ciprofloxacin	400 mg IV	Every 8–12 hours

*Adjusted to a trough level of 15–20 mcg/mL; not to exceed 2 g per dose.
IV, intravenous.

infections and should be obtained before starting antibiotics. This is for organism identification and performing antibiotic susceptibility testing that steers antibiotic therapy. No randomized controlled trial of the efficacy of intraventricular (intrathecal) antibiotics in EVD-related infections has been performed. Intrathecal vancomycin or gentamicin is sometimes used in situations in which conventional intravenous therapy has failed. The colonized EVD catheter should be removed and replaced with a new catheter, preferentially at a new site (32).

CONCLUSION

Infections in acute stroke patients are common, and increase the length of hospital stay and prevent early participation in rehabilitation. Prevention of infection is paramount, but can be difficult. Predicting infection in acute stroke patients is not always possible. Patient characteristics and disability scores are useful in identifying patients who are at high risk for poststroke infections. Once infection is suspected, appropriate antimicrobial agents should be initiated with a solid plan to de-escalate the regimen based on microbiology.

REFERENCES

1. Chamorro A, Urra X, Planas AM. Infection after acute ischemic stroke: a manifestation of brain-induced immunodepression. *Stroke*. 2007;38:1097–1103. doi:10.1161/01.STR.0000258346.68966.9d
2. Miller CM, Behrouz R. Impact of infection on stroke morbidity and outcomes. *Curr Neurol Neurosci Rep*. 2016;16:83. doi:10.1007/s11910-016-0679-9
3. Meisel C, Schwab JM, Prass K, et al. Central nervous system injury-induced immune deficiency syndrome. *Nat Rev Neurosci*. 2005;6:775–786. doi:10.1038/nrn1765
4. Armstrong JR, Mosher BD. Aspiration pneumonia after stroke: intervention and prevention. *Neurohospitalist*. 2011;1:85–93. doi:10.1177/1941875210395775
5. Dziewas R, Schilling M, Konrad C, et al. Placing nasogastric tubes in stroke patients with dysphagia: efficiency and tolerability of the reflex placement. *J Neurol Neurosurg Psychiatry*. 2003;74:1429–1431. doi:10.1136/jnnp.74.10.1429
6. Celis R, Torres A, Gatell JM, et al. Nosocomial pneumonia. A multivariate analysis of risk and prognosis. *Chest*. 1988;93:318–324. doi:10.1378/chest.93.2.318
7. Kasuya Y, Hargett JL, Lenhardt R, et al. Ventilator-associated pneumonia in critically ill stroke patients: frequency, risk factors, and outcomes. *J Crit Care*. 2011;26:273–279. doi:10.1016/j.jcrc.2010.09.006

8. Augustyn B. Ventilator-associated pneumonia: risk factors and prevention. *Crit Care Nurse.* 2007;27:32–36.
9. Poisson SN, Johnston SC, Josephson SA. Urinary tract infections complicating stroke: mechanisms, consequences, and possible solutions. *Stroke.* 2010;41:e180–e184. doi:10.1161/STROKEAHA.109.576413
10. Ersoz M, Ulusoy H, Oktar MA, et al. Urinary tract infection and bacteriurua in stroke patients: frequencies, pathogen microorganisms, and risk factors. *Am J Phys Med Rehabil.* 2007;86:734–741. doi:10.1097/PHM.0b013e31813e5f96
11. Beer R, Lackner P, Pfausler B, et al. Nosocomial ventriculitis and meningitis in neurocritical care patients. *J Neurol.* 2008;255:1617–1624. doi:10.1007/s00415-008-0059-8
12. Wartenberg KE, Stoll A, Funk A, et al. Infection after acute ischemic stroke: risk factors, biomarkers, and outcome. *Stroke Res Treat.* 2011;2011:830614. doi:10.4061/2011/830614
13. Hannawi Y, Hannawi B, Rao CP, et al. Stroke-associated pneumonia: major advances and obstacles. *Cerebrovasc Dis.* 2013;35:430–443. doi:10.1159/000350199
14. Smith Hammond CA, Goldstein LB, Horner RD, et al. Predicting aspiration in patients with ischemic stroke: comparison of clinical signs and aerodynamic measures of voluntary cough. *Chest. 2009*;135:769–777. doi:10.1378/chest.08-1122
15. Tablan OC, Anderson LJ, Besser R, et al. Guidelines for preventing health-care—associated pneumonia, 2003: recommendations of CDC and the Healthcare Infection Control Practices Advisory Committee. *MMWR Recomm Rep.* 2004;53:1–36.
16. Hellyer TP, Ewan V, Wilson P, et al. The Intensive Care Society recommended bundle of interventions for the prevention of ventilator-associated pneumonia. *J Intensive Care Soc.* 2016;17:238–243. doi:10.1177/1751143716644461
17. Harms H, Prass K, Meisel C, et al. Preventive antibacterial therapy in acute ischemic stroke: a randomized controlled trial. *PLoS One.* 2008;3:e2158. doi:10.1371/journal.pone.0002158
18. Westendorp WF, Vermeij J, Zock E, et al. The Preventive Antibiotics in Stroke Study (PASS): a pragmatic randomized open-label masked endpoint clinical trial. *Lancet.* 2015;385:1519–1526. doi:10.1016/S0140-6736(14)62456-9
19. Laban KG, Rinkel GJ, Vergouwen MDI. Nosocomial infections after aneurysmal subarachnoid hemorrhage: time course and causative pathogens. *Int J Stroke.* 2015;10:763–766. doi:10.1111/ijs.12494
20. Azzimondi G, Bassein L, Nonino F, et al. Fever in acute stroke worsens prognosis. A prospective study. *Stroke.* 1995;26:2040–2043. doi:10.1161/01.STR.26.11.2040

21. Castillo J, Dávalos A, Marrugat J, et al. Timing for fever-related brain damage in acute ischemic stroke. *Stroke*. 1998;29:2455–2460. doi:10.1161/01.STR.29.12.2455
22. Phipps MS, Desai RA, Wira C, et al. Epidemiology and outcomes of fever burden among patients with acute ischemic stroke. *Stroke*. 2011;42:3357–3362. doi:10.1161/STROKEAHA.111.621425
23. Stamm WE. Criteria for the diagnosis of urinary tract infection and for the assessment of therapeutic effectiveness. *Infection*. 1992;20 Suppl 3:S151–S154. doi:10.1007/BF01704358
24. Lipsky BA, Ireton RC, Fihn SD, et al. Diagnosis of bacteriuria in men: specimen collection and culture interpretation. *J Infect Dis*. 1987;155:847–854. doi:10.1093/infdis/155.5.847
25. Pfausler B, Beer R, Engelhardt K, et al. Cell index—-a new parameter for the early diagnosis of ventriculostomy (external ventricular drainage)-related ventriculitis in patients with intraventricular hemorrhage? *Acta Neurochir (Wien)*. 2004;146:477–481. doi:10.1007/s00701-004-0258-8
26. Raghavendran K, Nemzek J, Napolitano LM, Knight PR. Aspiration-induced lung injury. *Crit Care Med*. 2011;39:818–826. doi:10.1097/CCM.0b013e31820a856b
27. Bartlett JG. How important are anaerobic bacteria in aspiration pneumonia: when should they be treated and what is optimal therapy. *Infect Dis Clin North Am*. 2013;27:149–155. doi:10.1016/j.idc.2012.11.016
28. Harms H, Hoffmann S, Malzahn U, et al. Decision-making in the diagnosis and treatment of stroke-associated pneumonia. *J Neurol Neurosurg Psychiatry*. 2012;83:1225–1230. doi:10.1136/jnnp-2012-302194
29. Rotstein C, Evans G, Born A, et al. Clinical practice guidelines for hospital-acquired pneumonia and ventilator-associated pneumonia in adults. *Can J Infect Dis Med Microbiol*. 2008;19:19–53. doi:10.1155/2008/593289
30. Hooton TM, Bradley SF, Cardenas DD, et al. Diagnosis, prevention, and treatment of catheter-associated urinary tract infection in adults: 2009 International Clinical Practice Guidelines from the Infectious Diseases Society of America. *Clin Infect Dis*. 2010;50:625–663. doi:10.1086/650482
31. Gupta K, Hooton TM, Miller L; Uncomplicated UTI IDSA Guideline Committee. Managing uncomplicated urinary tract infection—making sense out of resistance data. *Clin Infect Dis*. 2011;53(10):1041–1042. doi:10.1093/cid/cir637
32. Dey M, Jaffe J, Stadnik A, et al. External ventricular drainage for intraventricular hemorrhage. *Curr Neurol Neurosci Rep*. 2012;12:24–33. doi:10.1007/s11910-011-0231-x

Index